Language

Issues in the Biology of Language and Cognition
John C. Marshall, editor

Language

Structure, Processing, and Disorders

David Caplan

A Bradford Book
The MIT Press
Cambridge, Massachusetts
London, England

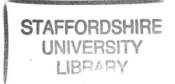

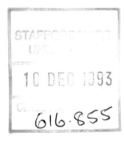
Second printing, 1993

This book was set in Trump by Asco Trade Typesetting Ltd., Hong Kong
and was printed and bound in the United States of America.

Library of Congress Cataloging-in- Publication Data

Caplan, David, 1947–
  Language: structure, processing, and disorders / David Caplan.
    p. cm.
  "A Bradford book."
  Includes bibliographical references and index.
  ISBN 0-262-03189-2
  1. Language disorders. 2. Psycholinguistics. 3. Linguistics.
I. Title.
    [DNLM: 1. Cognition. 2. Language Disorders.
3. Psycholinguistics. 4. Speech Disorders. WL 340 C244l]
RC423.C26   1992
616.85'5—dc20
DNLM/DLC
for Library of Congress   91- 31225
                                                               CIP

Contents

Series Foreword

The MIT Press series on Issues in the Biology of Language and Cognition brings new approaches, concepts, techniques, and results to bear on our understanding of the biological foundations of human cognitive capacities. The series includes theoretical, experimental, and clinical work that ranges from the basic neurosciences, clinical neuropsychology, and neurolinguistics to formal modeling of biological systems. Studies in which the architecture of the mind is illuminated by both the fractionation of cognition after brain damage and formal theories of normal performance are specifically encouraged.

John C. Marshall

Preface

This book presents a synopsis of recent linguistic and psycholinguistic research on language disorders in adults with neurological disease. It deals with language structures and psycholinguistic experiments that explore how these structures are processed, and then discusses language disorders in relation to these linguistic and psycholinguistic models of language. I have attempted to present an accurate summary of the major concepts and results in the fields of linguistics and psycholinguistics, in order to provide the reader with the basis for understanding both the studies of language disorders that are discussed here and those that are likely to be discussed in the psycholinguistic literature in the foreseeable future. The primary readership to which the book is directed are clinicians who work with language-impaired adults—speech-language pathologists, neuropsychologists, neurologists, other medical professionals, and students in these disciplines—and researchers and students in experimental psychology, linguistics, and related fields.

The book reflects my view of what is important to understand about normal language in order to approach contemporary studies of language disorders. Accordingly, I have gone into detail regarding some aspects of linguistics, psycholinguistics, and aphasiology, and not others. For instance, I place considerable emphasis on what are known as "on-line" studies of language processing—studies that measure what representations a subject is computing while he or she is in the middle of accomplishing a language-related task. I believe these studies provide the best guides to the nature of many psycholinguistic processes. Even though few studies of language disorders presently incorporate on-line observational methods, studies using these methods are likely to become important to understanding language impairments in the very near future. Similarly, I have discussed the evidence in favor of many psycholinguistic models of aspects of language processing. I have done so because many papers in psycholinguistic aphasiology make reference to specific models, and I believe the reader should be in a position to judge the strength of the evidence supporting the assumptions about normal processing that underlie these papers. On the other hand, for the most part, I have not attempted to present different theories of linguistic representation or the justifications for these different theories, because the differences between these theories figure very little in contemporary studies of language disturbances.

I want to emphasize that, even in the areas where I present the most detail, this book is intended to be introductory in nature. My goal in presenting these studies is to help the reader become informed about the work of linguistically and psycholinguistically oriented researchers who study normal and disordered language; I have not attempted to deal exhaustively with every controversy in the field. I hope to have presented a responsible overview of contemporary ideas about language and its processing and of how these ideas are related to language disorders. I hope to convince clinicians that it is worthwhile to keep abreast of the literature on language and language processing in order to understand language disorders and to indicate to cognitive scientists that the study of language impairments can provide data relevant to models of normal language processing.

Two comments on subjects that are not included in this book are in order.

First, though this book is intended to be useful for clinicians and students in clinical disciplines, it is not a guide to clinical practice. I have included a final chapter that touches on aspects of diagnosis (and even more briefly on therapeutics), but this book does not tell the clinician what tests to use to diagnose a particular type of language disorder, or how to choose, create, or apply therapeutic materials once a diagnosis has been made. This book describes the disorders that affect language processing, as they have been viewed by psycholinguistically oriented researchers in the past few years. My hope is that this volume will provide enough knowledge of what language is, how it is processed, and how it breaks down, to allow the clinician to use diagnostic and therapeutic materials within a psycholinguistic perspective.

Second, this book is not directly about what is sometimes called "functional communication." It does not deal with the goals and intentions that lead people to use language or, for the most part, with whether their use of language is successful in satisfying these intentions and achieving these goals. It is mainly about the largely unconscious processes that underlie the activation of the elements of the language code by speakers, listeners, readers, and writers. My focus on disorders of the language code and its associated processors should not be taken to imply that there is nothing to be said about the nature of disorders that primarily affect the ability of patients to accomplish their goals through the use of the language code. There is an extensive literature on the nature of functional communication and its disorders. I mention these issues briefly in chapter 9, but have not attempted go into them in detail. In part, this is because to cover these types of disorders would add considerably to the material covered in this book. Also, these disorders involve analyses of motivational states, intentions, social considerations, and many other topics that begin to get farther and farther removed from the processing of the language code itself. There is more than enough to cover regarding the narrower topic itself.

Aspects of this book were prepared while I received support from the National Institutes of Health (Grants No. DC00776-01 and DC00942-01), and the Medical Research Council of Canada (Grant 9761). Research of my own that is reported here was also partially supported by these grants. This support is gratefully acknowledged.

I am grateful to many people for their help with aspects of this book. In particular, I wish like to thank Hiram Brownell, Alfonso Caramazza, Verne Caviness, Barbara Grosz, Merrill Garrett, Nancy Hildebrandt, Susan Kohn, Steven Kosslyn, Pim Levelt, Maryellen MacDonald, Mark Seidenberg, Stephanie Shattuck-Hufnagel, Janet Sherman, Ken Stevens, and Gloria Waters for discussions that have greatly clarified my understanding of aspects of the material presented here, and Mary Andreonopolis, Joan Arsenault, Jennifer Aydelotte, William Badecker, Cynthia Bogatka, Hiram Brownell, Alfonso Caramazza, Nancy Hildebrandt, Susan Kohn, Nancy Lefkowitz, Pim Levelt, Carol Leonard, Elizabeth Rochon, Janet Sherman, Nina Silverberg, Ken Stevens, and Gloria Waters for reading parts of the manuscript and providing helpful comments and criticisms. John Hennen and Eileen Centofanti provided indispensible help with the preparation of the manuscript. Joy Hanna prepared the subject index, and Amy Biel the author and patient indices. By far my greatest debt is to Daniel Bub. While we were colleagues at the Montreal Neurological Institute, Dan and I were close collaborators in efforts to apply research in psycholinguistic aphasiology to clinical practice. This book was conceived of and begun as a result of this work. Dan's work on disorders of reading, writing, and lexical semantics contributed heavily to my understanding of these areas. He wrote extensive drafts of chapters 3 and 5. This book is very much the better for the help of these colleagues and friends.

1 Introduction

Human language is a unique mental entity. It is a system of symbols that greatly enhances the ability of humans to represent aspects of the world, to think, and to communicate with each other. Linguists, philosophers, psychologists, and other researchers have all contributed to our understanding of what language is, and how it is acquired and used. These studies show that language has a complex structure and that its use involves many diverse, interacting psychological operations. In recent years, researchers have made considerable progress in understanding language disorders by approaching them in terms of the models of language structure and language processing developed by linguists and psycholinguists. In turn, some of these studies of language disorders shed light on the nature of normal language structure and language processing. This book is designed to provide an introduction to this recent work.

The structure of this book follows the structure of the language code and its processing. The topics move from simple words, through word formation processes, sentences, and discourse. Chapters 2 through 9 deal with disorders of recognition, comprehension, or production of these elements of the language code, in both the auditory-oral and written modalities of language use. I begin each chapter with a discussion of features of the language code and their processing, and follow this presentation with a description of disorders affecting these representations and processes. In this introductory chapter, I prepare the ground for what follows by outlining the language code, its processing, and their disorders.

LANGUAGE PROCESSING AND ITS ROLE IN COMMUNICATION

In this book, language is viewed as a code that connects certain forms (the sounds of words, sentence structures, and so on) to meanings. There is evidence that the different forms of the language code are computed by a set of processors, or "components" of a language processing system, each dedicated to activating particular elements of the code. The inputs into these processors are other representations of the language code as well as nonlinguistic representations. For instance, a particular language processor activates the phonological forms of words from their meanings; another activates aspects of sentence form from syntactic information derived from spoken words. These processors can be thought of as being "dedicated" to these tasks, in the sense that they cannot be used to accomplish other mental operations. For instance, the two processors mentioned above—the one that activates the phonological forms of words from their meanings, and the one that activates aspects of sentence form from syntactic information derived from spoken words—are not interchangeable, and neither is used in nonlinguistic tasks such as recognizing visually presented objects. The language processors each make use of cognitive "processing resources." It is an open question whether they all make use of one and the same set of resources or whether each has its own processing resource "pool", and whether the resource pool available for language processing is also used for any nonlinguistic tasks.

These language processors can be used in different combinations to accomplish language-related tasks such as auditory comprehension, reading, repeating what has been heard, taking written notes on a lecture, etc. The use of these processors in these tasks is under the control of other cognitive systems, such as those that deploy and shift attention, search knowledge stored in memory, match motivations to actions, etc. These control mechanisms apply to affect the use of all levels of the language code. We exercise control over the entire language processing system when we decide whether to use language to convey our thoughts and intentions, and when we decide to pay attention to a particular linguistic input. We exercise control over the choice of vocabulary elements in our speech on the basis of our estimation of our listener's ability to understand different sets of words. We control the rate of our speech, the formality of the vocabulary and syntax we choose, etc. We enunciate differently for different listeners. We can place emphatic stress on any part of the sound of a word, if we think we need to (as in: I said, "*bat* the ball, not *pat* the ball!"). Some of this control is exercised consciously, but a great deal is exercised unconsciously. Unfortunately, though they are of great importance to language processing, the control mechanisms involved in language use—especially those that are activated unconsciously—are not well understood. I therefore have little to say about their disturbances in this book, and can only hope that the study of these mechanisms and their disorders develops significantly in the near future.

The normal use of language also requires nonlinguistic processing. When we speak, we continuously engage in searches through our semantic memory for information about the world; we continuously reason about what we are saying and hearing; we take note of our immediate environment and incorporate information about it into our language productions. Language processing does not take place in a cognitive vacuum. However, processing the language code itself is separable from undertaking these other cognitive tasks, and its disorders must be separated from those affecting these related tasks.

Functional communication involving the language code occurs when people undertake language-related tasks to accomplish specific goals—to inform others, to ask for information, to get things done. The use of language is thus a special instance of intentional action. The ability to use the language code to accomplish one's goals confers enormous advantages upon an individual, and upon the human species as a whole. It allows us to make reference to items and events not in our immediate physical environment, to reason, to update our knowledge of the world on the basis of what we are told, to think privately, to share our thoughts with others, and so on. These functions would be very much more limited were it not for the availability of the language code and the ability of humans to use it. Imagine, for instance, that a chimpanzee discovered the Newtonian laws of motion (assuming, even, that such a discovery is possible in a member of a species that does not have a natural language). This discovery would almost certainly die with that individual chimpanzee for lack of a means to convey it to other members of the species. On the other hand, the language code is not adequate for every activity that falls under the heading of human intentional action. Using language might be helpful in explaining to someone how to change a flat tire, for instance, but it would not be sufficient to actually change a real flat tire. For that, physical action itself is needed.

DISORDERS OF LANGUAGE PROCESSING AND THEIR FUNCTIONAL CONSEQUENCES

This book is about psycholinguistic disorders of language; that is, disorders that affect the language processors themselves. When neurological disease affects the forms and meanings that make up the language code, or disrupts the processors devoted to their activation, the ability to perform language-related tasks and to use language to accomplish goals is compromised. Therefore, an understanding of these disorders is important in the diagnosis and rehabilitation of patients with language impairments.

To make these points more concrete, consider what goes on when a speaker utters the sentence "I'm hot" as an answer to a question put to him by his physician, and as a statement directed toward the driver of the car that he is riding in. In the first case, the speaker's intention is presumably to answer the physician's question; presumably, this intention is related to the speaker's goal in seeing the physician in the first place—to deal with some medical problem. In the second case, the speaker's intention is presumably to add to the driver's knowledge about the present situation; presumably, this intention is also related to a goal the speaker has—to have the driver act to reduce the speaker's discomfort by opening a window, putting on the air conditioning, stopping as soon as possible, etc. At the level of motivations and intentions, these are very different speech acts, and it is possible for a patient to have trouble saying "I'm hot" in one of these settings and not the other because of a difficulty he or she has in dealing with the motivations or communicative requirements found in one of these settings and not the other. The two speech acts also require different control mechanisms—e.g., they involve different deployments of attention—and different ancillary cognitive operations—e.g., they require quite different searches through memory—and a patient may fail to produce the correct utterance on one occasion because something has gone wrong with these aspects of cognitive processing. However, at the level of using the language code—accessing words, forming a sentence, pronouncing words, etc.—the two speech acts involve many identical linguistic forms and psycholinguistic processors. A patient who could not use those aspects of the language code that are found in the sentence "I'm hot" would probably have trouble with both of these speech-act uses of this sentence. He might compensate for his impairment—and these compensations are likely to be quite different in these different cases—but some degree of ease of communication, at the least, would be affected.

As the intentions and motivations of the language user become more complex, functional communication is more and more affected by disturbances of the language code and its processors. Thus, though "high-level" language-impaired patients may be able to function well in many settings, their language impairments can cause significant functional limitations. Imagine an investment counselor trying to explain the pros and cons of investing in growth stocks as opposed to municipal bonds without being able to use language efficiently. I have seen several elementary school teachers with very mild disturbances in accessing the forms of spoken words, who felt they could not function in the classroom setting because of the demands it makes on them to retrieve specific words under considerable time pressure. The language code is a remarkably powerful code with respect to the semantic meanings it can encode and convey, and psycholinguistic processors are astonishingly fast and accurate. Without this code and the ability to use it quickly and accurately, our functional communicative powers are extremely limited, no matter how elaborate our intentions and motives. This is the situation many patients who have disorders affecting the language code and the processors dedicated to its use find themselves in.

There is no simple, one-to-one relationship between impairments of elements of the language code or of psycholinguistic processors, on the one hand, and abnormalities in performing language-related tasks and accomplishing the goals of language use, on the other. Patients adapt to their language impairments in many ways, and some of these adaptations are remarkably effective at maintaining at least some aspects of functional communication. Conversely, patients with neurological disease who have intact language processing mechanisms may fail to communicate effectively (as is true of some normal persons!). Nevertheless, most patients who have disturbances of elements of the language code or psycholinguistic processors experience limitations in their functional communicative abilities.

With this as background, let us turn to an overview of the central topics to be discussed in this book.

THE LANGUAGE CODE

Human language can be viewed as a code that links a set of linguistic forms to a number of aspects of meaning. The basic levels of the language code include the *lexical level*, the *morphological level*, the *sentential level*, and the *discourse level*. Linguistics is the study of the nature of the representations that make up each of these levels of the language code.

The lexical level of language makes contact with concepts and categories in the nonlinguistic world. Lexical items (simple words) designate concrete objects, abstract concepts, actions, properties, and logical connectives. The basic form of a simple lexical item consists of a phonological representation that specifies the segmental elements (phonemes) of the word and their organization into metrical structures (e.g., syllables). The form of a word can also be represented orthographically. Simple words are assigned to different syntactic categories, such as nouns, verbs, and adjectives. Chapters 2 though 5 are devoted to different aspects of processing at the lexical level.

The morphological level of language allows words to be formed from other words (e.g., the word *destruction* is derived from the word *destroy*). This allows the meaning associated with a simple lexical item to be used as a different syntactic category without coining a huge number of new lexical forms that would have to be learned. Other word formation processes (inflection) play roles in encoding syntactic relationships. Chapter 6 deals with processing morphologically complex words.

The sentential level of language expresses propositions that convey aspects of the structure of events in the world (e.g., thematic roles convey who did what to whom; attribution of modification conveys which adjectives go with which nouns; the reference of pronouns and other referentially dependent categories determine which words in a set of sentences refer to the same items or actions). The propositional content of a sentence is determined by the way the meanings of simple and derived words combine in syntactic structures—hierarchical sets of syntactic categories (e.g., noun phrase, verb phrase, sentence). Sentences expressing propositions are a crucial level of the language code because they make assertions about the world. These assertions can be entered into logical systems, and can be used to add to a person's knowledge of the world. Comprehension of sentences is discussed in chapter 7 and sentence production in chapter 8.

The propositional meanings conveyed by sentences are entered into higher-order structures that constitute the discourse level of linguistic structure. Discourse includes information about the general topic under discussion, the focus of a speaker's attention, the novelty of the information in a given sentence, the relationship of events and actions to each other (e.g., the temporal order of events, causation), and so on. Information conveyed by the discourse level of language also serves as a basis for updating a person's knowledge of the world and for reasoning and planning action. Discourse processing is the subject of chapter 9.

Many of the representations that make up the language code appear to be unique to this code. To the best of our knowledge, the representations that are needed to describe the structures of objects, of concepts, of logical inferences, etc., are different from those needed to describe elements and structures in the language code. This raises the question of whether the language code is a special and separate component of mental life. Many theoretical linguists believe that it is, and argue for its uniqueness in part on the grounds that its structure is different from that needed to describe elements and operations in other cognitive domains (Chomsky, 1985). Other researchers disagree (Bates and MacWhinney, 1989). They maintain that the forms of language result from the interaction of the different factors that constrain the use of the language code. These factors include the semantic values that the language code expresses (derived from human cognitive abilities), the nature of the input and output channels in which language use usually takes place (derived from the human auditory and articulatory systems), and the nature of the computations the human mind can perform (derived from physiological operations in the brain). The language code is thought to be an "emergent property" derived from these other functional systems.

Whatever the final outcome of this debate, it is fair to say that, at least at present, many of the properties of the language code are not derivable from properties of other cognitive systems. The student of language disorders who wishes to characterize the linguistic structures that are impaired and intact in a patient must therefore rely upon characterizations of these elements and structures that are

[margin handwritten notes: "each combining to form a whole :: producing coherent speech lang."]

provided by linguistic theory. I provide descriptions of key aspects of this code in chapters 2 through 9.

MODELS OF LANGUAGE PROCESSING

As conceived of here, psycholinguistics is the study of the processors dedicated to the activation of linguistic representations. As indicated above, current models of language processing subdivide functions such as reading, speaking, auditory comprehension, etc., into many different, semi-independent components or "modules." Each component is thought to perform a particular function in the overall system. The components of the language processing system perform highly specialized operations. For instance, the operations involved in processing an auditory stimulus appear to be different if that stimulus is being treated as a linguistic entity or as a nonlinguistic item (see chapter 2).

Information-processing models of language are now widely expressed as flow diagrams (or *functional architectures*) that capture the sequence of operations of the different components performing a language-related task. We identify the *major components of the language processing system* as those processes that activate the lexical, morphological, sentential, and discourse levels of the language code in the usual tasks of language use—speech, auditory comprehension, reading, and writing. This approach to defining language processing components groups together different operations that all activate a similar type of linguistic representation into a single processor. The major components of the language processing system for simple words are listed in table 1.1, and of language processing for morphologically complex words and sentences in table 1.2. Figure 1.1 presents a model indicating the sequence of activation of components of the lexical processing system. Figure 1.2 presents a similar model of the processing system for morphologically complex words and sentences. Models of this general type will be developed in greater detail in chapters 2–9.

First, the way in which the linguistic structures are activated by each processor needs to be specified. For instance, the forms of words may be listed and searched for as separate entries in a mental dictionary, or they may be recognized as levels of activation of units in a set of nodes in which individual words are not represented (Seidenberg and McClelland, 1989). Many models maintain that some linguistic representations, such as syntactic structures, are stored as rules that are applied when we recognize and generate particular structures, while other models of language processing never develop rules relating linguistic elements to each other. These details of processing within individual modules are discussed throughout this book.

Second, there are important interactions between different components that are not indicated in these elementary models. These interactions greatly affect the way information is translated between different levels in the system. Figures 1.1 and 1.2 suggest that processing primarily occurs sequentially through the system, each component executing its function after termination of the previous stage. This greatly underestimates the extent to which these components of the system operate in parallel. In addition, these components are subject to feedback from later processes (Samuel, 1981; Dell, 1986). These factors must be incorporated into processing models, as we shall see in many places in our discussion.

Leaving these questions about the detailed nature of the representations activated by these processors, their internal operations, and their organization aside for the moment, let us consider several important operating characteristics of the components of the language-processing system.

One characteristic is that each processor accepts only particular types of representations as input and produces only specific types of representations as output. The processor that activates syntactic structures from auditory input may use as input many features derived from the speech signal—the syntactic categories of the words presented to it, the meanings of these words, intonational contours, etc.—but it does not make use of those acoustic properties that indicate that the speaker is a man or a woman. Fodor (1983) uses the term *encapsulation* to refer to this property of components of the language processing system. Similarly, the output of this processor is a syntactic structure; it is not a representation of the logical entailments of a sentence. Fodor (1983) uses the term *domain specificity* to refer to this property. A major research area is to determine what the input and output representations that are paired by the operation of a given language processor are.

Second, most processors are obligatorily activated when their inputs are presented to them. For instance, if the control and supervisory components of cognition lead us to attend to a sound that

Table 1.1
Summary of Components of the Language-Processing System for Simple Words

Component	Input	Operation	Output
Auditory-Oral Modality			
Acoustic-phonetic processing	Acoustic waveform	Matches acoustic properties to phonetic features	Phonological features and segments (phonemes, allophones, syllables)
Input-side lexical access	Phonological units	Activates lexical items in long-term memory on basis of sound	Phonological forms of words
Input-side semantic access	Words (represented as phonological forms)	Activates semantic features of words	Word meanings
Output-side lexical access	Word meanings ("lemmas")	Activates the phonological forms of words	Phonological forms of words
Phonological output planning	Phonological forms of words (and nonwords)	Activates detailed phonetic features of words (and nonwords)	Speech

Written Modality

Written lexical access	Abstract letter Identities	Activates orthographic forms of words	Orthographic forms of words
Lexical semantic access	Orthographic forms of words	Activates semantic features of words	Word meanings
Accessing orthography from semantics	Word meanings	Activates orthographic forms of words	Orthographic forms of words
Accessing lexical orthography from lexical phonology	Phonological representations of words	Activates orthographic forms of words from their phonological froms	Orthographic forms of words
Accessing sublexical orthography from sublexical phonology	Phonological units (phonemes, other units)	Activates orthographic units corresponding to phonological units	Orthographic units in words and nonwords
Accessing lexical phonology from whole-word orthography	Orthographic forms of words	Activates phonological forms of words from their orthographic forms	Phonological forms of words
Accessing sublexical phonology from orthography	Orthographic units (graphemes, other units)	Activates phonological units corresponding to orthographic units	Phonological units in words and nonwords

Table 1.2
Summary of Components of the Language-Processing System for Derived Words and Sentences (Collapsed Over Auditory-Oral and Written Modalities)

Component	Input	Operation	Output
Processing Affixed Words			
Accessing morphological form	Word forms	Segments words into structural (morphological) units; activates syntactic features of words	Morphological structure; syntactic features
Morphological comprehension	Word meanings; morphological structure	Combines word roots and affixes	Meanings of morphologically complex words
Accessing affixed words from semantics	Word meanings; syntactic features	Activates forms of affixes and function words	Forms of affixes and function words
Sentence Level Processing			
Lexico-inferential processing	Meanings of simple and complex words; world knowledge	Infers aspects of sentence meaning on basis of pragmatic plausibility	Aspects of propositional meaning (thematic roles; attribution of modifiers)
Syntactic comprehension	Word meanings; syntactic features	Constructs syntactic representation and combines it with word meanings	Propositional meaning
Construction of sentence form	Word forms; propositional meaning	Constructs syntactic structures; inserts word forms into structures	Sentence form (including positions of lexical items)

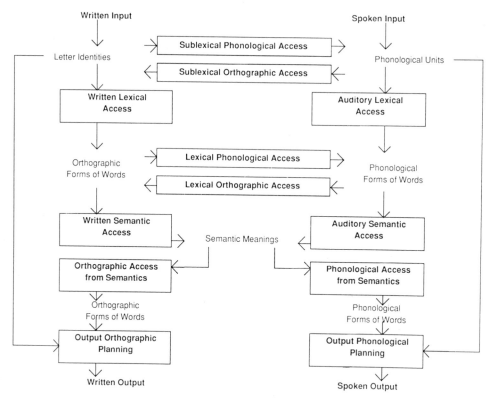

Figure 1.1
Diagrammatic representation of the sequence of activation of components of the processing system for single words. Processing components are presented in boxes in **boldface**; representations are presented in lightface. *Arrows* represent the flow of information (representations) from one processing component to another.

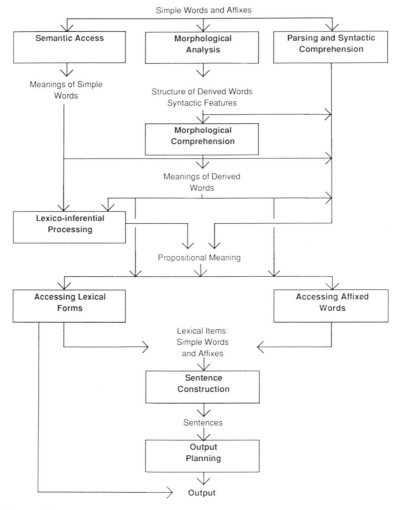

Figure 1.2
Diagrammatic representation of the sequence of operation of components of the language-processing system for morphologically complex words and sentences. Processing components are presented in boxes in **boldface**; representations are presented in lightface. *Arrows* represent the flow of information (representations) from one processing component to another.

happens to be the word *elephant*, we must hear and understand that word; we cannot hear this sound as just a noise (Marslen-Wilson, 1987).

Third, language processors generally operate unconsciously. The unconscious nature of most language processing can be appreciated by considering that when we listen to a lecture, converse with an interlocutor, read a novel, or engage in some other language-processing task, we usually have the subjective impression that we are extracting another person's meaning and producing linguistic forms appropriate to our intentions without paying attention to the details of the sounds of words, sentence structure, etc.

Finally, components of the system operate remarkably quickly and accurately. For instance, it has been estimated on the basis of many different psycholinguistic experimental techniques that spoken words are usually recognized less than 125 milliseconds after their onset (i.e., while they are still being uttered (Marslen-Wilson and Welsh, 1978; Tyler and Wessels, 1983; Marslen-Wilson, 1987). Similarly, normal word production in speech requires searching through a mental word production "dictionary" of over 20,000 items, but still goes on at the rate of about three words per second with an error rate of about one word misselected per million and another one word mispronounced per million (Levelt, 1989). The speed of the language-processing system as a whole occurs because of the speed of each of its components, but also is achieved because of the massively parallel functional architecture of the system, which leads to many components of the system being simultaneously active.

In general, cognitive processes that are limited to a specified domain, obligatory, unconscious, and fast, are thought to be "automatic" and to require relatively little allocation of mental resources (Shiffrin and Schneider, 1977). However, whether the concept of automaticity, as it has been developed in some parts of the contemporary experimental and theoretical psychological literature, can be applied to language processing without undergoing some modification, is unclear. Many experimental results indicate that language-processing requires the allocation of processing resources (Wanner and Maratsos, 1978). It has been suggested that there is a maximum level of resource utilization of which each language-processing component is capable, and that a reduction in the resources available to a component diminishes that component's ability to perform its normal operations (Shallice, 1988).

In summary, the language-processing system consists of a set of semi-independent components that act together to accomplish language-related tasks. We will be dealing with disorders of this complex and highly efficient processing system.

PSYCHOLINGUISTIC ANALYSES OF LANGUAGE DISORDERS

These linguistic representations and psycholinguistic models provide the basis for an analysis of a patient's language disorders. The term *aphasia* refers to language impairments. It is very often restricted in use to refer to certain types of language impairments, or to certain types of language disorders in patients with certain types of neurological diseases (mostly stroke). I use the term *aphasia* here to refer to any language processing deficit. The disorders I will be presenting here are *primary* aphasic impairments—those due to disturbances of language-processing mechanisms themselves. *Secondary* aphasic disturbances can result from disorders of memory, attention, perception, motor functions, etc. Secondary aphasias may affect language functions selectively. A disturbance that has become known as "neglect dyslexia," for instance, is secondary to a visual attention disturbance, and only affects written, not spoken, language processing (Shallice, 1988).

The psycholinguistic approach to aphasia consists of trying to identify the disturbances in the components of the language processing system that are present in each patient and to describe the nature of a disturbance that affects a component of the system. This is accomplished by detailed analyses of the linguistic elements, structures, and rules that are affected in a given task (or set of tasks), and of the patterns of responses that a patient produces. In practice, the types of tasks that are set for a patient, and the type of linguistic representation that is tested in a task—or that is postulated to be deficient in a patient as a result of the performance on a task—are heavily influenced by a researcher's ideas about what linguistic representations are and how they are processed. That is, tasks and analyses of tasks and of performances on tasks are always "theory-dependent." A researcher may be more or less explicit about the theory he or she is testing, or even be unaware that the test is based on a theory at all. But there is no escaping reliance on some theory (perhaps a very simple theory that a researcher may not even think of as a theory) if we set tasks for a patient and use performance on those tasks as a guide to the patient's deficits.

Let us consider a very simple example of this sort of approach. In 1976, Caramazza and Zurif described a set of patients who could match sentences like (1) to pictures, but not sentences like (2):

(1)   The apple the boy is eating is red.

(2)   The woman the boy is chasing is tall.

These researchers claimed that the difference between (1) and (2) is that a patient needs to assign syntactic structure to understand (2), but not to understand (1). This is because a patient can understand (1) simply by knowing that apples are inanimate and can be eaten and that boys are animate and can eat, but no such knowledge about the meanings of the words in (2) will indicate who is doing the chasing and who is tall. There are a number of technical questions about whether this is the only way to interpret these results. I deal with several of these questions in chapter 7. Here I simply want to point out that this experiment and its analysis depends on a theory that maintains that: (1) sentences have syntactic structures that determine aspects of their meaning; (2) sentences can be understood in two ways—by constructing a syntactic structure and using it to determine aspects of meaning or by inferring aspects of meaning from understanding individual words and putting together the meanings of words to make a sensible sentence. This is a fairly simple theory. It does not specify what types of syntactic structures there are, how they are constructed, or how breakdown of the mechanism involved in assigning syntactic structures happens. Much work since this seminal paper has been directed to these questions. This work, which is reviewed in chapter 7, has relied on more detailed theories of syntax and syntactic processing and on many other types of experiments in aphasic patients to describe and explain more specific patterns of comprehension disturbances.

I shall examine many analyses of aphasic performances in many language tasks. The conclusions that are drawn about what is wrong with a patient are based upon four features of these performances. The first is the documentation of a patient's ability to accomplish one language-related task and his inability to perform another language-related task normally. Under some circumstances, this pattern provides evidence for a selective deficit in one language-processing operation and not another. The second part of a database is poor performance on the part of a patient on two tasks. Under some circumstances, this pattern suggests that a single processing impairment underlies both abnormal performances. Third, comparison of performances of groups of patients on different types of linguistic stimuli within a given task, or on different language tasks, provides evidence regarding the relative difficulty of processing those representations or accomplishing those tasks, and an individual patient's level of performance can be compared with that of the group to obtain an estimate of the degree to which there is a reduction in processing resources available to that patient on a given task. Finally, analyses of error types provide evidence regarding the nature of a patient's disorder. We shall come across the use of all these lines of reasoning in this book.

The reader should keep in mind that none of these approaches to finding out what is wrong with a patient are foolproof. For instance, when we find what is known as a double dissociation between performance on two language-related tasks (patient A does well on task 1 but poorly on task 2 and patient B performs in the opposite fashion), we may draw the conclusion that, in at least one of the patients, one or more specializations within the cognitive system are affected by disease while others remain intact (Caplan, 1987; Shallice, 1988). We do not necessarily know, however, what the affected functions are. Similarly, observing poor performance on two tasks in a single patient does not necessarily imply that a single functional disturbance underlies both abnormal performances, and the qualitative nature of errors made on a task may reflect the nature of the compensations a patient makes to his deficit, not the deficit itself. We shall find examples of these problems in interpreting data from patients in this book. The moral is that only a detailed analysis of a patient's performance, based on a variety of tasks that the patient has undertaken that are themselves chosen on the basis of what is known about normal language, its processing, and its breakdown, is likely to arrive at a plausible and defensible analysis of the patient's deficit. Psycholinguistic aphasiology requires some hard intellectual work. We now turn to a survey of this work.

2   Recognition of Spoken Words

Many aphasic patients fail to understand spoken words normally. Bedside clinical assessment frequently shows that patients are unable to point to objects in a hospital room in response to the names of these objects, or to carry out simple commands. More formal language testing frequently reveals that a patient is not able to select a picture from a set of foils upon presentation of a single spoken word, or answer questions about the meanings of words. These disturbances are signs that a patient does not understand spoken words.

Failure to understand a word can have two broad sources: a patient may fail to recognize the word or he or she may fail to extract the meaning from a word that is recognized. In this chapter, we deal with disturbances affecting patients' abilities to recognize auditorily presented words, leaving to chapter 3 the discussion of failures to appreciate the meanings of individual words because of problems of "semantic access" or "semantic activation."

Researchers and clinicians have recognized several different reasons for the failure of a patient to recognize a single spoken word. First, the patient may have a disturbance of early auditory processing. Second, patients may have disturbances of more linguistically specific aspects of sound processing, leading to difficulties in discriminating or identifying the sounds of their language. Several theorists, beginning with Wernicke (1874), have also thought that patients may have disturbances of the permanent representations of the sound patterns of words in their language, preventing them from recognizing spoken input as a lexical item despite intact auditory and acoustic-phonetic processing mechanisms.

I begin this chapter with a description of the sound structure of words and normal lexical access mechanisms, and then review the literature on disturbances of auditory and acoustic-phonetic processing and the relationship of these disturbances to auditory single word recognition.

Table 2.1
The Distinctive Feature Content of English Phonemes

	ɪ	ī	ū	ē	ō	æ	ā	ǣ	ɔ̃	i	u	e	ʌ	o	æ	ɔ	y	w	ε	r
Vocalic	+	+	+	+	+	+	+	+	+	+	+	+	+	+	+	+	−	−	−	+
Consonantal	−	−	−	−	−	−	−	−	−	−	−	−	−	−	−	−	−	−	−	+
High	+	+	+	−	−	−	−	−	−	+	+	−	−	−	−	−	+	+	−	−
Back	+	−	+	−	+	−	+	−	+	−	+	−	+	+	−	+	−	+	−	−
Low	−	−	−	−	−	+	+	+	+	−	−	−	−	−	−	+	+	−	−	−
Anterior	−	−	−	−	−	−	−	−	−	−	−	−	−	−	−	−	−	−	−	−
Coronal	−	−	−	−	−	−	−	−	−	−	−	−	−	−	−	−	−	−	−	+
Round	−	−	+	−	+	−	−	+	+	−	+	−	−	+	−	+	−	+	−	
Tense	+	+	+	+	+	+	+	+	+	−	−	−	−	−	−	−	−	−	−	
Voice																			+	
Continuant																			+	
Nasal																			−	
Strident																			−	

Reproduced with permission from Chomsky and Halle, 1968, pp. 176–177.

THE SOUND STRUCTURE OF WORDS

Phonemes and Distinctive Features

phonemes = basic sound units!

Simple words are primarily defined and distinguished from each other by their constituent phonemes. A phoneme is a sound that contrasts with another to determine the existence of a word in a language. For instance, in English, /p/ and /b/ are different phonemes, because they determine the separate existence of word pairs such as *pat-bat*, *pale-bale*, *pull-bull*, *lap-lab*, etc. The phonemes /p/ and /b/ are minimally different from each other, varying only in whether voicing occurs during the production of the segment (/b/) or not (/p/). Other contrasts involve larger articulatory and acoustic contrasts (e.g., the contrast between /p/ and /g/—*pot/got*—involves both voicing and place of articulation).

The phonemes of each language are selected from a fairly small set of sounds that can be produced by the human vocal tract. Since the pioneering work of Jakobson (1941), Troubetskoy, (1939), Jakob-

l	p	b	f	v	m	t	d	θ	ə	n	s	z	c	č	j	š	ž	k	g	x	ŋ	h	kʷ	gʷ	xʷ
+	−	−	−	−	−	−	−	−	−	−	−	−	−	−	−	−	−	−	−	−	−	−	−	−	−
+	+	+	+	+	+	+	+	+	+	+	+	+	+	+	+	+	+	+	+	+	−	+	+	+	+
−	−	−	−	−	−	−	−	−	−	−	−	−	+	+	+	+	+	+	+	+	−	+	+	+	+
−	−	−	−	−	−	−	−	−	−	−	−	−	−	−	−	−	+	+	+	+	−	+	+	+	+
−	−	−	−	−	−	−	−	−	−	−	−	−	−	−	−	−	−	−	−	−	−	+	−	−	−
+	+	+	+	+	+	+	+	+	+	+	+	+	+	−	−	−	−	−	−	−	−	−	−	−	−
+	−	−	−	−	−	+	+	+	+	+	+	+	+	+	+	+	+	−	−	−	−	−	−	−	−
																		−	−	−			+	+	+
+	−	+	−	+	+	−	+	−	+	+	−	+	−	−	+	−	+	−	+	−	+	−	−	+	−
+	−	−	+	+	−	−	−	+	+	−	+	+	−	−	−	+	+	−	−	+	−	+	−	−	+
−	−	−	−	−	+	−	−	−	−	−	+	−	−	−	−	−	−	−	−	−	−	+	−	−	−
−	−	−	+	+	−	−	−	−	−	−	+	+	+	+	+	+	+	−	−	−	−	−	−	−	−

son, Fant, and Halle (1963), and others, most phonologists have argued that all phonemes consist of sets of "distinctive features"— features of sound production such as voicing, aspiration, roundedness, the location and degree of maximal constriction of the vocal tract, the nature of the constriction of the vocal tract, etc. A list of the phonemes of English and their distinctive features is found in table 2.1.

In table 2.1, we have represented each distinctive feature along a binary axis. A phoneme either has the positive or negative value of this feature. For instance, /b/ is marked as [+voiced] and /p/ is marked as [−voiced]. This aspect of the distinctive feature framework we have adopted forces us to code certain aspects of the structure of phonemes in particular ways. For instance, although the stop consonants /p/, /t/, and /k/ represent stopped, voiceless consonants whose point of closure of the vocal tract is progressively more posterior (/p/ represents closure at the lips, /t/ at the alveolar ridge behind the teeth, and /k/ at the velum), we cannot represent this difference between these phonemes as three different values of a single distinctive feature representing "point of articulation" in a and /k/ are represented in terms of binary values of two distinctive features, [± anterior] and [± coronal].

The fact that we use a binary system for representing distinctive features indicates that distinctive features are abstractions— idealizations of the articulatory and acoustic content of the phonemes of languages. Though phrased in terms of positions and manners of articulation of the vocal tract, distinctive features are not easily mapped onto articulatory or acoustic phenomena. This is basically because, though distinctive features are related to articulatory gestures, specific theories of what distinctive features there are have been postulated in an effort to account for regularities in the sound systems of languages, not articulation itself.

There is another reason why distinctive features are abstract representations of articulatory gestures. The vocal tract does not move instantaneously from one position to another, and speech continues to be produced while the vocal tract is between target positions. This has the effect of "spreading" the speech output associated with a particular feature in a particular phoneme over time. This phenomenon is known as "co-articulation." Consider, for example, the sound /p/ in the words *pit* and *pool*. The /p/ is quite different in these two words. In *pool*, there is rounding of the lips at the onset of the /p/, and there is no rounding at this point in the word *pit*. This is because the vowel following the /p/ is rounded in the case of *pool* and unrounded in the case of *pit*; rounding "spreads" from the /u/ to the preceding /p/ in the first case but not in the second. When one looks at the details of the articulatory gestures involved in producing phonemes and of the resulting acoustic waveforms, every phoneme is affected in some way by every different context in which it occurs. Thus, not only is the /p/ different with respect to rounding in *pit* and *pool*, it also varies in terms of its associated articulatory gestures and acoustic features across the entire set of rounded consonants in words such as *pool, pole, pull,* etc.[1]

Each language uses a restricted number of phonemes—its "phonemic inventory"—to construct words. The phonemes of a given language are partially selected on the basis of language-universal factors and in part by language-specific processes. The language-universal factor dictates that some phonemes are more likely to occur in a language than others, for two reasons: they are easier to produce and they represent more extreme contrasts of articulatory gestures. All languages have at least a vowel-consonant

(VC) distinction, reflecting the extreme contrast between an open vocal tract (the vowel) and a closed tract (the consonant). If a language has only three vowels, it likely to have the high front unrounded vowel /i/ (as in *beet*), the high back rounded vowel /u/ (as in *pool*), and the low back partially rounded vowel /ɑ/ (as in *father*)—vowels that are maximally distinguished with respect to their articulatory gestures. If a language has a single consonant, it is likely to be /t/—a consonant that differs maximally from the vowels in having a total occlusion of the vocal tract and being voiceless. If a language has a large phonemic inventory, it is likely to have both the more common, basic phonemes and a number of phonemes not found in all languages. For instance, English has phonemes not found in French (e.g., the /th/ sounds in words such as *this* and *thimble*), and vice versa (e.g., the high rounded front vowel found in the French word *queue* (*tail*) is not found in English). These are language-specific "choices" that form part of the basis for the differences and similarities between languages.

Word-Level Phonology

Phonemes and their distinctive features are the elementary segments out of which words are built. Simple, underived words consist of sequences of phonemes structured into higher-order units (Goldsmith, 1976; McCarthy, 1979; Halle and Vergnaud, 1980; Clements and Keyser, 1983; Selkirk, 1984). The higher-order phonological structure of the phonemes in the words *cat* and *reconciliation* is represented in figure 2.1. As can be seen, *cat* is a monosyllabic word, made up of an onset (/k/), and a rime (/at/). The rime is itself made up of a nucleus (/a/) and a coda (/t/). In the multisyllabic word *reconciliation*, the syllables are further organized into "feet."

The sequence of phonemes in a word is partially determined by the laws regulating syllable structure in a language. Both universal and language-specific features of the organization of sounds are involved in syllable-structure rules. Universal factors dictate that syllables tend to become more "sonorant" from onset to nucleus, and less sonorant from nucleus to coda. Sonorance reflects the degree of unimpeded flow of air through the vocal tract. Thus sonorance is directly related to the articulation of the phonemes of a word. Distinctive features such as [high], [back], [low], [continuant] characterize the degree of closure of the vocal tract during the production of

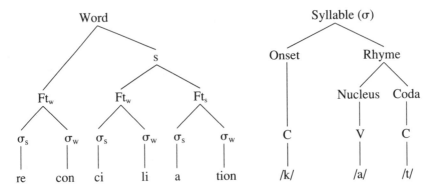

Figure 2.1
The phonological structure of words and syllables. (Adapted from Selkirk, 1984.)

a particular phoneme; features such as [tense] and to a lesser extent [voiced] characterize the force with which air is expelled through the vocal cavity. These distinctive features thereby determine the sonorance of each phoneme of the language, and place each phoneme on a "sonorance hierarchy." In each syllable, there is a strong tendency for less sonorant items to occur in onset and coda positions relative to the nucleus of the syllable.

Language-specific rules further constrain the internal organization of syllables and thus the order of phonemes in the words of a language. For instance, Italian has a language-specific rule that indicates that, with a few exceptions, morpheme-final syllables end in a vowel; English has a variety of language-specific rules that regulate the possible phonemes in syllabic onsets (such as the rule that indicates that the liquid following syllable-initial /st/ must be /r/ and not /l/). For the most part, these language- specific rules are in keeping with language-universal tendencies such as the sonorance hierarchy, although there are some cases in which they produce exceptions to language-universal factors (as in English tolerating the unusual sequence of consonants which terminates the word *sixths*). Other phonological features of words include stress and tone. In English and many other languages, word stress contours are determined by the phonemes in a word and their organization into syllables (Halle and Vergnaud, 1980). English has a complex set of rules determining stress assignment that are derived from the stress-assignment rules of Romance and Anglo-Saxon languages. The for-

Table 2.2
Patterns of Assignment of Stress in English Words with Different Types

I	II	III
astónish	maintaín	collápse
édit	eráse	tormént
consíder	caróuse	exháust
imágine	appéar	eléct
intérpret	cajóle	convínce
prómise	surmíse	usúrp
embárrass	decíde	obsérve
elícit	devóte	cavórt
detérmine	achíeve	lamént
cáncel	careén	adápt

Reproduced with permission from Chomsky and Halle, 1968, p 69.

mer, derived from Latin, place stress toward the end of a word, as in French, Italian, and Spanish, while the latter place stress toward the beginning of words, as in German. These stress-assignment rules apply to syllables (Liberman and Prince, 1977; Halle and Vergnaud, 1980), and the phonemic nature of the syllables of a word determines the application of these rules. For instance, in English, "heavy" syllables are distinguished from "weak" syllables and have different consequences for stress assignment. Heavy syllables are those with a tense vowel or more than one consonant in coda position; weak syllables are those with a lax vowel followed by a coda consisting of not more than one consonant. Heavy syllables in word-final position attract stress by the Latinate (Romance) stress rule; weak syllables in word-final position do not attract this stress. Thus, we have patterns such as those shown in table 2.2.

In table 2.2, the words in columns II and III have heavy syllables in word-final position, and stress appears in the final syllable in these words, while the words in column I, with weak final syllables, have stress placed on the second-to-last (penultimate) syllable. If a word is sufficiently long, such as *hurricane, anecdote, pedigree,* or *matador,* the final determination of the stress contour of the word is affected by the Anglo-Saxon stress-assignment process, which "retracts" stress from its position at the end of a word to a more dominant position at the beginning of a word. Stress assignment also affects phonemic distinctive feature content. In English, all vowels which have not been assigned any stress whatsoever during the process of stress assignment in a word are reduced to a neutral vowel known as "schwa" (/ə/). Thus, the vowel sounds almost the same in the second syllables of *anecdote, matador,* and *Canada.* However, quite clearly, these vowels are not all the same at *some* level of phonemic representation. For instance, the second vowel in the word *Canada* takes on its "true" phonemic value in the word *Canadian.*

In general, the phonemes that we actually produce and hear are not necessarily the "underlying" distinctive feature values that phonologists assign to phonemes. Aside from unstressed vowel reduction and the allophonic variation discussed above, other instances of changes in underlying distinctive features include the diphthongization of tense vowels in English (i.e., tense vowels are followed by glides: *cry, bay, bow, blue*), and a process known as "vowel shift" that affects the features [high] and [low] in tense diphthongized vowels. Indeed, most theories of phonology assume that the abstract representation of the phonemes of a word consists of just enough distinctive feature information to allow each phoneme to be uniquely determined by the application of the general phonological rules of the language (Pesetsky, 1979; Halle and Monahan, 1985; Pulleyblank, 1986). Thus, most phonological theories maintain that the surface phonological form of a word is not an accurate description of the sound structure of a word. On the one hand, the surface form contains too much information (as in allophonic detail that is not relevant to the identity of phonemes in a word) and, on the other hand, the surface form does not contain either enough or the correct information (as when different underlying vowels are reduced to schwa or changed by vowel shift).[2]

With this background regarding the sound structure of words, we can now turn to the way words are recognized.

PROCESSING THE ACOUSTIC SIGNAL FOR PHONETIC FEATURES AND PHONOLOGICAL SEGMENTS

Most studies of word recognition assume that words consist of phonemes defined in terms of distinctive features, and that these features are somehow extracted from the acoustic waveform and matched to those of stored lexical forms. Acoustic-phonetic studies have been directed toward the question of how the acoustic signal is processed to identify distinctive features and phonemes. However, despite great progress in this field, the goal of specifying the acoustic correlates of distinctive features has remained elusive. Researchers have therefore explored other analyses of the acoustic waveform that might be relevant to word recognition. Some work explores the possibility that the recognition of syllable structure and stress play important roles in identifying phonemes. Studies of lexical access investigate how the phonological information derived from the waveform interacts with stored representations of the sound patterns of words and with information in the previous discourse context to allow a listener to identify a word (and ultimately extract its meaning). We briefly review this literature before discussing disturbances of word recognition in aphasia.

The human auditory system can detect and process a wide range of sounds, in the range of approximately 50 to 18,000 cycles-per-second (cps), or Hertz (Hz). Different parts of the system from the cochlea through the auditory cortex are sensitive to different aspects of sound. The complex nature of auditory processing is beyond the scope of this chapter. We shall focus on those aspects of processing that are relevant to speech.

Speech produces vibrations in the ambient air as a function of the pattern of airflow escaping from the vocal tract. Unimpeded airflow, as in sighing, is minimally audible; resonance set up by the vibration of air within the vocal tract is needed for normally audible speech. Vibration of the air column is caused by rapid movements of the vocal cords as air is forced through them from the lungs, creating the fundamental frequency (F_0) of each utterance by a speaker. Fundamental frequencies normally vary from approximately 100 to 200 cps in adult males; F_0 is higher in females and children. In its passage though the vocal tract, the waveform that is produced in this way activates the natural resonances of the various cavities of the tract—the mouth, pharynx, nasal cavities, etc. These resonances are determined both by several (relatively) fixed features of the vocal tract (e.g., the length of the cavity from the vocal cords to the teeth and lips) and by features of the cavity that are modifiable (e.g., the position of the tongue). The resonances produce the formant frequencies of the acoustic waveform associated with speech.

Our understanding of the acoustic properties of speech advanced significantly with the use of the sound spectrograph, a device that enabled researchers to display acoustic energy as a function of time (along the horizontal axis of a graph) and frequency (along the vertical axis). Spectrographic recordings allowed the formants of the speech waveform to be seen and correlated with phonemes and features. More advanced computer analyses are based upon digitized waveforms. Spectrographic and other analyses of the acoustic correlates of distinctive features in various contexts have been extensively studied. The following brief discussion presents some basic results in this field of research (it is beyond the scope of this chapter to provide a detailed description of all that is known about acoustic phonetics).

The first three formants play critical roles in determining the speech sounds that are identifiable in the waveform. Since vowels are produced with little change in the configuration of the vocal tract, they are associated with regions of the waveform in which the formants are relatively stable. Conversely, since consonants are produced by active movements of the articulators, they are associated with areas of change in formant frequencies. Stevens (1986) has suggested that the process of identification of distinctive features in the acoustic waveform begins by noting where these major changes in the character of the formants occur. This process demarcates more sonorant stretches of the waveform, which are likely to be relevant to the nature of vowels and other syllabic peaks, from less sonorant stretches of the waveform, which are likely to be relevant to the nature of consonants.

Within any portion of the waveform, various properties of the formants (and other acoustic features such as aspects of bursts, etc.) define individual speech sounds. For vowels, the relationship between the formant frequencies gives a vowel its characteristic sound. For instance, a high front vowel (/i/, as is *see*) is associated with a low first formant and a high second formant. For consonants, different features have different acoustic correlates. For instance, the feature [± voiced] in syllable-initial stop consonants correlates with the time of onset of periodic voicing relative to the release of the energy burst associated with vocal tract closure (so-called voice onset time, VOT; see later discussion); the point of closure in stop consonants correlates with the direction and duration of the transi-

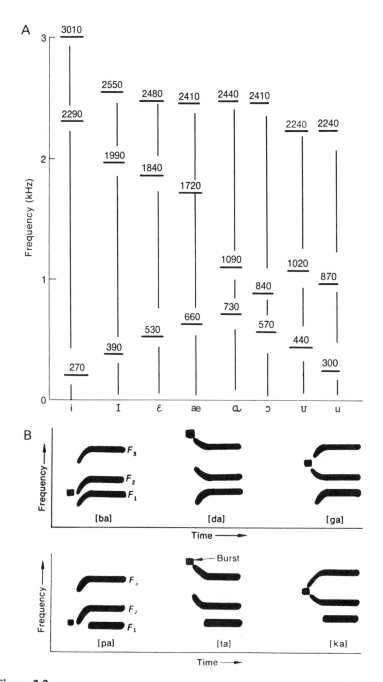

Figure 2.2
A: Mean values of formant frequencies for adult males of vowels of American English. B: Formant transitions and bursts for stop consonants in English. (Reproduced with permission from Lieberman and Blumstein, 1990, p. 224.)

tions in the acoustic formants, the shape of the burst of energy that accompanies the release of air after the closure is ended, the frequency of the maximum portion of the waveform at the burst, and the bandwidth of the burst (Pisoni and Luce, 1987). Some of these features of vowels and consonants are shown in figure 2.2.

Acoustic correlates of distinctive features are specific to particular sets of phonemes and particular phonemic contexts. For instance, VOT differences are much less marked in syllable-final and intervocalic stops than in syllable-initial stops, and other acoustic features (such as the duration of the preceding vowel) correlate with voicing of stops in these contexts. Voicing also has different acoustic correlates for different consonants. The duration of voicing at the boundary between sonorant and nonsonorant portions of the waveform is important in determining voicing in intervocalic fricatives, rather than VOT or vocalic lengthening (Stevens, Fant, and Hawkins, 1987). The existence of these different cues to distinctive features in part reflects the fact, mentioned above, that the articulatory gestures associated with any particular phoneme are not all restricted to one temporal interval, but rather carry over into the production of neighboring sounds (co-articulation).

One fundamental question in the study of acoustic phonetics is whether identification of phonetic features and phonemes is totally based upon these contextually variant cues or whether there are any invariant acoustic features that are used in the identification of individual sound units. Early research documented listeners' abilities to discriminate and identify sounds on the basis of context-variant acoustic cues (Liberman et al., 1967). More recently, research has suggested that there may be some invariant properties of the acoustic waveform that correspond to distinctive features. Stevens and Blumstein (1981) and Mack and Blumstein (1983) have provided evidence for invariant properties of the acoustic waveform. For instance, for the feature [± continuant], the size of the increase in the amount of acoustic energy at the moment of consonant release relative to acoustic energy in the surrounding waveform distinguishes the [−continuant] stop consonant /b/ from the [+continuant] glide /w/. In forced-choice and free identification tasks for segments in five vowel environments, subjects identified stops and glides on the basis of these differences in amplitude envelope in synthetic CV sequences with high degrees of reliability. These and other results are the basis of claims by Blumstein and her colleagues that there are important invariant aspects of the acoustic waveform which serve as the basis for the identification of the distinctive features that make up phonemes.

The relative importance of invariant and context-sensitive cues to the identification of the sound segments that make up words is not entirely clear at present. For one thing, the accuracy rates for identification of stop consonants and liquids in the studies of Blumstein et al. sometimes run as low as 75%, and it is not clear that the invariant features of the waveform that have been described so far are sufficient to ensure identification of particular distinctive features reliably enough for the purpose of word identification. Second, though Blumstein and her colleagues have provided evidence in favor of acoustic invariance for some distinctive features of potential relevance to perception, there are very few distinctive features that have been explored in this respect, and it is not clear that the invariance noted by Blumstein and her colleagues will continue to hold up for a wide range of distinctive features across different positions of phonemes and syllables.

In addition to variation in the acoustic correlates of phonemes due to different co-articulatory effects in different phonemic contexts, word pronunciation also varies as a function of sentence- and discourse-level factors. Church (1987) has suggested that it may be worthwhile to distinguish between phonemic and phonetic variation. The former, discussed above, is related to variation due to the position of phonemes in lexical phonological structures, and it is possible that the acoustic correlates of distinctive phonemic features are at least partially invariant. The latter reflects changes in phonemes related to resyllabification due to discourse and other factors. For instance, the utterance "Did you hit it to Tom?" can come out as: / dɪdjəhɪʕɪ?tʰɪtʰam /. A speech recognition system can make use of the facts that /h/ and /tʰ/ are always syllable initial and /ʕ/ and /?/ always syllable final. This leads to a syllabification of the utterance as / dɪdjə#hɪʕ#ɪ?#tʰɪ#tʰam /, which can help in identifying the phonemes in the words of the utterance. Church argues that variable acoustic cues to phonetic features (such as aspiration, flapping, etc., see note 1) can help establish syllable boundaries and that these boundaries then serve to help identify other segments.

Intonational contours beyond the level of the single word also provide important cues for recognizing derived and compound words, the syntactic structure of sentences, and other linguistic structures (see chapters 7 and 8). Intonational contours strongly affect the acoustic values of phonemes and distinctive features, and identifying them may also interact with the processes involved in identifying phonemes themselves. These interactions are just beginning to be studied.

One of the most important aspects of auditory processing for speech is that the auditory system rapidly distinguishes speech from nonspeech sounds, and appears to process speech sounds differently than nonspeech sounds. Where this separation first occurs in the anatomical structures that make up the auditory system is unknown, but the evidence that it occurs comes from several sources.

The discovery of the phenomenon known as "categorical perception" was one of the first indications of the special nature of speech perception (Cooper et al., 1952; Liberman et al., 1967). Categorical perception refers to the fact that humans do not seem to be able to discriminate sounds that vary along acoustic dimensions within an individual phonemic category, but can do so when these same variations in acoustic features cross over phonemic boundaries. The classic examples of categorical perception arise in studies of the role of VOT in discriminating and identifying voiced and voiceless stop consonants. Studies using synthetic speech sounds have varied the onset of periodic voicing relative to the release of the burst of high-frequency energy that signals consonantal onset, as illustrated in figure 2.3. Variations in voice onset time of 20 ms produce different identification functions when they occur at a critical point after consonantal onset (between points at 20 and 40 ms in figure 2.3). Subjects identify stimuli with VOTs of 20 ms or less as voiced consonants, and those with voice onset times of 40 ms or more as voiceless stop consonants. Subjects are also excellent at discriminating synthetic stimuli with VOTs of 20 and 40 ms. On the other hand, 20-ms differences in voice onset time that fall *within* each of these consonantal areas (the difference between points at 0 and 20 ms in figure 2.3, both of which lie within the /b/ consonantal area, and between points at 40 and 60 ms figure 2.3, both of which lie within the /p/ consonantal area) cannot be discriminated, even though the physical difference between these two synthetic stimuli is the same as the physical difference between the stimuli with VOTs of 20 and 40 ms. Several investigators have argued that this

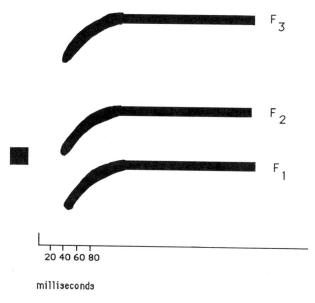

Figure 2.3
Illustration of formant patterns in synthetic consonants in which voice onset time can be varied to produced stimuli perceived as unvoiced or voiced stop consonants.

phenomenon of categorical perception—the ability of humans to discriminate acoustic values that are relevant to distinctive feature identity only at the points at which they create differences in phoneme identification—is an important aspect of the mechanisms involved in speech perception (Liberman, 1970; Eimas et al., 1971).

Contrary to initial speculation, it does not appear that categorical perception is confined to speech perception; a similar mechanism can be found in the perception and discrimination of tones (Cutting, 1972) and is present in some infrahuman species (Kuhl and Miller, 1974, 1975). Nonetheless, this mechanism is not known to be important in recognizing natural nonspeech stimuli, and does seem to be an important characteristic of speech perception processes. Together with other phenomena, it provides evidence for the existence of a special mode of processing for speech.

In one of these related phenomena, "duplex perception," listeners simultaneously hear a dichotically presented auditory stimulus (i.e., a stimulus that is partly presented to one ear and partly to the

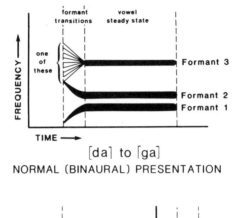

[da] to [ga]
NORMAL (BINAURAL) PRESENTATION

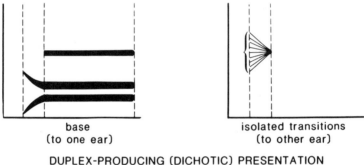

base
(to one ear)

isolated transitions
(to other ear)

DUPLEX-PRODUCING (DICHOTIC) PRESENTATION

Figure 2.4
Schematic representation of the stimulus pattern used to study duplex perception. (From Studdert-Kennedy, 1982, p. 12.)

other) as both a speech sound and a nonspeech sound. A typical stimulus that produces this effect would be one in which the transitions and steady-states of the first and second formants and the steady-state portion of the third formant for the sound /da/ are presented to one ear, and the transition of the third formant is presented to the other (Liberman, Isenberg, and Rakerd, 1981; figure 2.4). In isolation, the first stimulus is heard as /da/ and the second as a chirp. Together, they are heard as both /da/ and a chirp— so-called duplex perception. Varying the direction and rate of change of the third formant transition changes the perception of the phoneme in the duplex condition from /da/ to /ga/, exactly as would be the case if the stimulus were presented as a whole. In addition, discrimination of differences in the direction and rate of change of the third

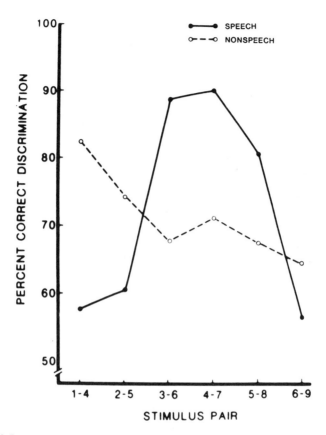

Figure 2.5
Discriminability of formant transitions when perceived as stop consonants and as chirps. (From-Studdert-Kennedy, 1982, p. 12.)

formant transition shows categorical perception and follows that found for the entire stimulus when the subject is asked to attend to the phonemic percept, but shows a totally different pattern when the subject is asked to attend to the perceived chirp (figure 2.5). These results have been taken as a strong indication that there is both a linguistic (phonetic) and a nonlinguistic mode of processing auditory stimuli (Liberman et al., 1967; Liberman and Studdert-Kennedy, 1978).

In summary, one vital task of the auditory system, as far as linguistic processing is concerned, is converting the acoustic waveform into a form that allows the listener to activate stored representations of words. Though phonemes are organized into higher-order structures, we have emphasized studies that deal with the acoustic correlates of phonemes and acoustic-phonetic processing mechanisms, because most models of auditory word recognition make use of phonemes and distinctive features. We now turn to research on the way words are activated from the phonological features that are extracted from the acoustic signal.

AUDITORY WORD RECOGNITION

A framework for viewing the process of word recognition has been suggested by Frauenfelder and Tyler (1987). They identify four stages in lexical processing. The first is lexical *contact*, the stage at which some representation derived from analysis of the incoming waveform makes initial contact with the lexicon. The second process is the *activation* of lexical entries and deals with how lexical entries are activated. The third phase consists of the *selection* of the appropriate lexical entry from the set of activated candidates. The fourth stage is the *accessing* of the entirety of the information listed in the lexical entry—semantic, syntactic, etc. We will deal with the first three processes here, leaving the matter of accessing meaning to chapter 3. The reader is encouraged to consult an excellent review of work on models of speech perception and lexical access by Klatt (1989) for additional discussion.

The Contact Representation

As noted above, most researchers work within a model of lexical access that assumes that the contact representation is, or at least includes, a sequence of phonemes specified as to their distinctive features. According to these models, aspects of the waveform such as those outlined above are recognized as distinctive phonemic features or combined into phonemes. Entries in the auditory input lexicon are represented in terms of their phonemes and the constituent distinctive features of each phoneme. The results of the bottom-up analysis of the waveform are matched to lexical entries. A problem for the view that the contact representation is a series of phonemes is the limitations of bottom-up analyses in unambiguously identifying phonemes in the waveform. As noted above, the difficult task of specifying how mapping of acoustic values onto phonetic and phonemic units occurs has yet to be accomplished in its entirety. Partly because of these and other limitations of feature-based models of lexical access, other models have been proposed that specify quite different contact representations.

The oldest of these models is the "motor theory of speech perception," which has recently been revised (Liberman et al, 1967; Liberman and Mattingly, 1985). According to this theory, the acoustic waveform is analyzed into units that correspond to either observed or underlying articulatory gestures. This theory emphasizes the link between perception and production, and solves the problem of acoustic-phonetic conversion by eliminating the process from the model. However, this solution creates the new problems of defining what acoustic-articulatory conversion is and how it takes place. Klatt (1989) discusses some of the difficulties in establishing a direct mapping between acoustic properties of the waveform and articulatory gestures. In the absence of models of the direct link between aspects of the acoustic waveform and articulatory gestures, this theory remains primarily a theoretical possibility.

A quite different response to the "front-end" problem—the problem of analyzing the acoustic waveform into linguistically relevant units—has come from Klatt (1979, 1986). He proposed that the acoustic waveform is not analyzed into distinctive features and phonemes, but only as far as acoustic spectra, representing the energy of different bandwidths in the waveform over time. He suggested that the entire lexicon is "precompiled" into a set of spectral properties, and that the match between input and stored representations occurs at the spectral level as shown in figure 2.6. This proposal requires enormous storage space for lexical representations, but it eliminates the acoustic-phonetic stage of processing. Klatt (1989) argues that it enhances the accuracy of the system, and considers it to be the optimum engineering solution to the problem of speech recognition. However, it has not yet been investigated for its psychological plausibility.

A somewhat hybrid model that lies between the standard acoustic-phonetic conversion model and Klatt's lexical-access-from-spectra (LAFS) model is Stevens's (1986) lexical-access-from-features (LAFF) model. This model is similar to the acoustic-phonetic conversion model in that features are extracted from the waveform. As we saw above, Stevens has a model of how this is done

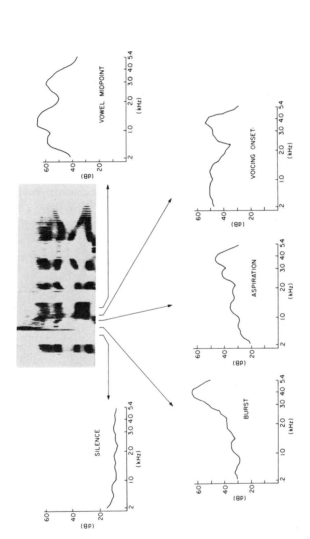

Figure 2.6
Illustration of how the transition from the middle of [t] to the middle of [a] in the spectrogram can be approximated by a sequence of five static critical-band spectra. (Reproduced with permission from Klatt, 1989, p. 193.)

that includes identifying areas of change from sonorance to non-sonorance and inspecting the areas of each type for acoustic features that correlate with distinctive features. Stevens's model differs from the more usual models in that these features are located at different points in time within these regions. The lexicon in Stevens's model contains a description of the features associated with each phoneme of each word, but these features are also distributed along a temporal axis, as in figure 2.7. Thus, Stevens's model retains the advantages of binary features for phonological theory and incorporates the results of acoustic-phonetic studies. It requires that the lexicon be precompiled into a form more directly isomorphic to the temporal location of the acoustic correlates of distinctive features.

At this point in time, it seems most likely that some form of acoustic-phonetic conversion does occur in speech recognition (though even this point remains uncertain). The most pressing questions are how this is accomplished bottom-up and whether lexical phonological entries are modified in some way that makes the task of matching bottom-up analyses of the waveform to lexical entries easier. More work is needed to answer these questions.

Whatever the units of analysis of the acoustic waveform that are involved in speech recognition (we shall henceforth assume these units include distinctive features organized into phonemes), another basic question is how much of the incoming waveform must be analyzed to begin the process of lexical access. Marslen-Wilson and Tyler (Marslen Wilson and Tyler, 1980; Marslen Wilson, 1987), Elman and McClelland (1984, 1986), and others have suggested that activation of the lexicon begins as soon as the first features or phonemes are identified. The contact representation is a sequence of sets of distinctive features. In Marslen-Wilson's model, all the lexical entries that begin with the phonemes defined by these distinctive feature sets—a so-called word initial cohort of lexical entries—are activated. For instance, if a listener hears the sound /ba/, he will activate the words *bat, bad, battle, ballot*, etc. As more acoustic information arrives, some of these words will become more activated (because the phonemes and features that are extracted from the acoustic signal match those in these words), while others will see their activation levels decline (because the phonemes and features that are extracted from the acoustic signal do not match those

Conventional lexical representation

	p	ɔ	n
high	−	−	−
low	−	+	−
back	−	+	−
nasal	−	−	+
spread glottis	+	−	−
sonorant	−	+	+
voiced	−	+	+
strident	−	−	+
consonantal	+	−	+
coronal	−	−	+
anterior	+	−	+
continuant	−	+	−

Modified lexical representation

	p	ɔ	n
high		−	
low		+	
back		+	
nasal			+
spread glottis		+	
sonorant	−		
voiced	−		
strident			
consonantal	+		+
coronal	−		+
anterior	+		+
continuant	−		−

Figure 2.7
A conventional lexical representation of the word "pawn" (top panel) modified to reflect expectations of the temporal locations of the acoustic information important in feature detection. (Reproduced with permission from Klatt, 1989, p. 190.)

in these words). Eventually, a single word will be left from the initial cohort of activated words.

Marslen-Wilson's and Elman and McClelland's models contrast with others in which the contact representation is not the word-initial phonetic sequence. Grosjean and Gee (1987) have suggested that lexical contact is based upon the stressed syllable of a word in a phonological phrase. Church (1987) has argued that phonetic variation is used to achieve an initial segmentation of the acoustic waveform and that syllable parts organized hierarchically are the contact representations for lexical access (see above). These proposals require that considerably more of the waveform be analyzed before lexical contact is made than the cohort and other similar models postulate.

There is considerable evidence that words are activated very soon after their onsets (Marslen Wilson, 1987, 1989). For instance, Marslen-Wilson studied the ability to shadow speech—to repeat a tape-recorded speech stimulus as quickly and as accurately as possible while it is being presented. Fast shadowers, who repeat passages with delays of as little as 250 ms, correct both form and semantic errors in target passages, indicating that they are accessing lexical phonological and semantic codes within this time period (Marslen-Wilson, 1973). This is well before words in the utterance being shadowed are completely over. Word-monitoring experiments, in which a subject must indicate that he has heard a word in a sentence, show the same effects: words can be identified before they are over (Marslen-Wilson and Tyler, 1980). Another technique, known as "gating," involves having subjects complete word-initial fragments of various lengths. Gating studies show that lexical identification can be determined as early as 200 ms after the onset of a word (Tyler and Wessels, 1983).

Zwitserlood (1985) performed a more complicated experiment using a technique known as "priming." In a priming experiment, a subject sees or hears a stimulus (say, a word) and then must make a response to a second stimulus. If the two stimuli are related, the response to the second is usually faster than it would be if the second stimulus had been presented in isolation. Zwitserlood presented the first few gated forms of words auditorily and then displayed a series of letters on a computer screen to subjects. Their task was to say if the letters formed a word (a "lexical decision" task).

Half the letter strings were words and half were not; some of the real words were semantically related to the gated spoken word, and others were not. Zwitserlood found that the word-initial gated stimuli produced semantic priming to all members of the word-initial cohort in the cross-modal lexical decision task, but stimuli gated from the ends of words did not. This indicates that early contact with the lexicon can be based upon a left-to-right access mechnism operating over a limited temporal window.

Lexical Activation

Given that some units extracted from the waveform can be matched to stored lexical entries, how does this matching take place? We shall consider three types of models: the analysis-by-synthesis model; activation models (the logogen model, the cohort model, and the "TRACE" model); and serial search models.

An older model of lexical activation is the analysis-by-synthesis model (Halle and Stevens, 1964). A newer, modified version is proposed by Zue (1986). This model proposes that the waveform be analyzed to the point where several possible words can be associated with a particular stretch of sound. These are matched to words generated internally in the listener's mind. If the match is sufficiently close, the word is "recognized." This model shifts part of the burden of speech recognition to the task of speech synthesis, because generating the forms of words from their lexical representations is relatively easy compared to the acoustic-to-phonetic transformation problem. The challenge of the analysis-by-synthesis model is to limit the number of words that need to be synthesized to be compared with the analyzed waveform. It is not clear what triggers the synthesis of these words (see discussion in Klatt, 1989).

A whole family of models of lexical activation make use of the concept of thresholds. Morton (1969, 1970, 1979a; Morton and Patterson, 1980) was the first to propose that the basic mechanism of lexical activation was to raise the resting activation level of a word above some critical level (a "threshold"). In his "logogen" model, logogens are information-collecting units that serve to activate lexical items. These units have resting activation levels that are determined by factors such as their frequency of occurrence in the language. When information of any sort—semantic, syntactic, phonological—that is related to a lexical item is presented to the logogen, its resting activation level rises. This level decays over time but remains above its resting level for some time once any activation has occurred. When enough information related to the logogen has been presented, the activation level of the logogen passes threshold, and the logogen fires. This causes a word to be activated. This model was designed to account for the fact that high-frequency words are more easily recognized than low-frequency words (Morton, 1969), that words that have just been presented are more easily recognized than words that have not just been presented (repetition priming effects) (Morton, 1979b), that words are more easily recognized when they have just been preceded by semantically similar words (semantic priming effects, Meyer and Schvanevelt, 1971), and other phenomena.

The idea that words have resting activation levels has been incorporated into computer-based models of lexical access in a number of ways. In some models of this sort, each word is connected to a set of feature detectors. When the feature detectors fire (due to bottom-up analyses), they activate the words that contain the active features. Each feature and each word simultaneously inhibits all other features and words with a strength equal to the strength of its activation. To see how this works, suppose the word *bat* is presented to the model. Each feature in each phoneme will activate all words containing that feature. Thus, since the first phoneme is a voiced stop consonant, all words that begin with stop consonants and all words that begin with voiced consonants will become slightly activated. However, the words beginning with /b/ will be more active than any other word, and the features corresponding to /b/ eventually cause the activation of any words beginning with other consonants to dampen out. The word that most closely matches the output of the feature detectors will be the most highly activated. If its activation passes threshold, it will be "recognized." This model explains why nonwords are sometimes recognized as words (they are close to some words in phonological form) and why words can be recognized even if some sounds are misidentified (the threshold for a word can be reached even if not every sound is correctly perceived). The latest version of the cohort model (Marslen-Wilson, 1987, 1989) includes an activation mechanism. In this respect, it is similar to the logogen model. However, the present version of the cohort model differs from the logogen model in that lexical activation does not make use of semantic (contextual) information, but is entirely based upon bottom-up analyses of the incoming waveform that yield elements of word form.

Activation models tend to have in common the notion that all possible lexical candidates that have features produced by the feature detectors are activated simultaneously, and the one that best fits the incoming signals is recognized. In contrast, serial search models maintain that lexical entries are examined one by one on the basis of representations derived from the input. These models were originally proposed to account for certain effects in tasks in which subjects were asked to say whether a letter string is or is not a word (lexical decision tasks; see above). The most extreme versions of these models will not work: it is obviously implausible that each word in a person's lexicon should be searched in sequence during speech recognition. However, no one ever proposed such extreme models. Both the earliest and contemporary models of this sort assume that the lexicon is divided into a number of "bins," all of which are examined in parallel for a match to features of the input, and that a serial search goes on in the appropriate bin. The issue dividing serial search from parallel activation models is thus not whether some parallel processing occurs (both types of models have this feature), but whether any sequential search occurs within a limited set of lexical items. Forster (1989) provides a scholarly account of the differences between these models and a description of the difficulties facing experimental psychologists who would like to know which model is correct.

We present these capsule sketches of models of lexical activation because some of the notions incorporated in these models are of interest in relationship to disturbances of word recognition. Chief among these is the fact that frequency affects the speed of lexical access, and the fact that lexical access apparently begins—and can entirely depend upon—the recognition of the first few phonemes of a word. At present, there has been very little exploration of these factors has gone on in the study of aphasic disturbances, but future work will likely include consideration of these aspects of word recognition.

Lexical Selection

In any model that maintains that more than one word is activated during speech recognition (such as all the activation models), some process must operate to select the best item from the set of words that has become active. We shall focus on how this is accomplished in the cohort model, which provides an explicit and interesting account of the selection process.

The selection stage in the cohort model consists of two processes. Items in the set of candidates drop out as additional phonetic information becomes inconsistent with them and as these words cannot be accomodated by the antecedent context. For any given word, a purely linear phonemic analysis allows one to establish its "recognition point"—the point at which it differs from all other words in the language. This point correlates well with the point at which speakers converge on a single word in gating tasks and with recognition latencies for words presented in isolation. The effect of semantic context in the selection process is seen in the ability of subjects to identify words before this recognition point in context. Marslen-Wilson (1987) has argued that the roles of the accruing phonological analysis and semantic context in the selection process are quite different. Accruing phonological analyses can determine lexical access: a listener can recognize a word that he does not expect to hear. Context cannot operate in this definitive way. In the cohort model, items in the word-initial cohort that are appropriate to the context are integrated into the representation of the discourse, and are thus further activated. Those that are not appropriate to the developing context see their activation levels decline.[3] Marslen-Wilson cites as evidence for this aspect of his model the fact that subjects need *some* acoustic information to make a response in monitoring tasks; they do not appear to guess that a word is about to occur. He also points to the fact that bottom-up information overrides context when it has to: we recognize words that we do not expect to hear.

Evidence supporting the view that the form of a word and the sentential context in which it occurs play different roles in perceptual processes also comes from phoneme restoration experiments. Samuel (1981) presented subjects with word and nonword stimuli in which a phoneme was either replaced by noise or in which the same phoneme was partially masked by noise. The subjects' task was to say whether the phoneme had been replaced or was still present and masked. Subjects were much better at detecting the absence of the phoneme in nonwords than in words (the so-called phoneme restoration effect) but, in a later experiment, were not affected by whether or not the word occurred in a highly predictable context.

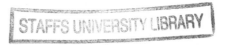

This indicates that perception of word forms affects perception of their constituent phonemes, but that sentential context does not feed back to the level of phoneme perception. (For more discussion of the role of sentential and discourse context on aspects of lexical processing, see chapters 7 and 9.)

Summary

This brief review of models of single word recognition indicates that researchers agree that the ability to analyze the acoustic waveform in terms of phonological elements—features, phonemes, allophones, syllables, and possibly other structures—is probably vital to the ability to recognize spoken words. The exact way that these phonological elements are activated from the acoustic waveform and how they contribute to word recognition are areas of active investigation. If the basic theory is correct, we can expect that disturbances of both acoustic processing—in particular those disturbances of acoustic-phonetic processing that affect a patient's ability to extract phonological information from the spoken signal—will affect word recognition. We can also expect that word recognition will be affected by disturbances of the permanent representations of the forms of words and the way these representations become activated on the basis of phonological input. We now turn to disorders of these processes.

DISTURBANCES OF AUDITORY FUNCTIONING

We begin our discussion of disorders of word recognition by considering patients who have disturbances of auditory processing that are not specific to the conversion of the auditory signal into linguistically relevant units. Many researchers and clinicians have claimed that these disturbances may affect word recognition.[4]

Several patients have had documented problems with a variety of complex auditory functions. For instance, Jerger et al. (1969) followed a patient who had had two strokes, one in each posterior temporal region. Originally, pure tone audiometry showed a bilateral severe hearing loss. Over time, the picture improved so that there was a high frequency loss in the right ear but improved hearing in the speech frequencies. Loudness discrimination and perception of temporal order were abnormal. Kanshepolsky, Kelley, and Wagner

(1973) described a patient in whom audiometry showed significant loss of acuity for pure tones and unilaterally impaired loudness discrimination; tests of perception of temporal ordering showed normal function. Albert and Bear (1974) documented a disturbance of "temporal discrimination" in a patient: their case showed abnormal fusion of two clicks separated by up to 15 ms. Chocolle et al. (1975) published a report of a patient who could not discriminate differences in rhythms, performed poorly in sound localization, and showed an increased effect of masking upon auditory performances. Auerbach et al. (1982) described a patient with abnormal click fusion and click counting, as well as deficits in phonemic processing. Divenyi and Robinson (1989) documented disturbances of frequency discrimination, gap detection, gap discrimination, frequency sweep discrimination, assessment of the magnitude of the frequency uncertainty effect in the detection of tones in noise, and assessment of frequency selectivity through simultaneous masked thresholds in stroke patients with and without aphasia. No doubt, there are many other disturbances of auditory processing that arise after brain damage.

The consequences of these types of disturbances for speech perception and word recognition are not entirely clear. Jerger's patient complained that although he could hear words, he could not understand them. Interestingly, at the bedside, this patient did not show word deafness—a feature raising the question of the relationship between these low-level acoustic processing deficits and disturbances in comprehension. In the patient of Kanshepolsky et al., speech audiometry showed severely impaired perception. Albert and Bear's patient showed severe auditory comprehension problems, which improved with slower rates of presentation of materials. The patient of Auerbach et al. had several disturbances in phoneme discrimination (see below) and an auditory comprehension disorder. Divenyi and Robinson found that three auditory capacities— frequency discrimination, frequency sweep discrimination, and the frequency uncertainty effect in the detection of tones in noise—best predicted aphasic patients' auditory verbal comprehension abilities. However, they did so relatively weakly, accounting for only 54% of the variance in a regression analysis.

One focus of recent work is the relationship between the rate at which speech is presented and patients' ability to comprehend utterances (see Blumstein, Katz, Goodglass, Shrier, and Dworetsky,

1985, for review). Tallal and Newcombe (1978) found that stretching out the formant transitions in stop consonants improved patients' abilities to identify the syllables /ba/ and /da/. Subjects who were unable to identify these syllables with normal transition durations also were negatively affected by short interstimulus intervals between two tones in another task in which they had to indicate the order of presentation of the tones. Performance on this tone-ordering task correlated well with comprehension on a sentence comprehension task (the Token Test: DeRenzi and Vignolo, 1962). The authors argued that increasing the duration of formant transitions and slowing down the speech rate might improve comprehension in some patients, whose problem, they argued, consists of an inability to process the acoustic signal at normal speeds. A similar conclusion was reached by Gardner, Albert, and Weintraub (1975). This idea, however, has been questioned by many other researchers who have failed to replicate these results (e.g., Blumstein et al, 1985; Riedel and Studdart-Kennedy, 1985). Perhaps the most specific correlation between slowing of the speech signal and improved comprehension has been documented by Blumstein and her colleagues (Blumstein et al., 1985), who showed that subjects with Wernicke's aphasia improved in a sentence comprehension task requiring comprehension of semantically reversible sentences (e.g., *The boy pushed the girl who touched the woman*; see chapter 7), when the phrases in those sentences were separated by pauses. Metz-Lutz and Dahl (1984) reported that introducing pauses between morphemes improved comprehension in a single case, but adding pauses between syllables did not. Thus, the relationship between limitations of the ability to process speech at the rate at which it is normally presented and impairments of auditory comprehension remains unclear. In addition, exactly which patients benefit from slowing down the rate of speech, and what types of slowing down of the speech signal these patients do benefit from, are subjects that will have to investigated further.

DISTURBANCES OF ACOUSTIC-PHONETIC PROCESSING

Several studies show that disturbances of acoustic-phonetic processing are common in aphasic patients. Varney (1984) found that 18% of aphasic patients had phonemic discrimination disturbances.

Though the full range of disturbances of acoustic-phonetic perceptual processing has yet to be explored in even a single patient, it is clear from studies in the literature that a variety of disturbances can exist in individual patients at this level of sound processing.[5]

For instance, Blumstein and her colleagues (Blumstein et al., 1977b) identified two basic patterns of disturbed acoustic-phonetic processing in 16 aphasic patients. The authors investigated their patients' abilities to discriminate and identify synthetic stop consonants. Stimuli consisted of three formant patterns in which voice onset time varied from −20 ms to +80 ms. For identification, the locus of the VOT boundary discriminating voiced from unvoiced stop consonants and the steepness of the identification function in the labeling task were noted. In the discrimination task, the VOT differences which led to maximal discriminatory capacity (local peaks in the discrimination function) were noted for each VOT difference, and these peaks were compared to the VOT boundaries separating voiced from voiceless consonants on the identification task.

One group of patients performed normally on both tasks, indicating both normal discrimination and labeling capacities. A second group of patients performed normally on the discrimination tasks, but were unable to label phonemes normally. In this case, the discrimination results showed a single peak in discriminatory capacity at the VOT boundary that separates voiced from voiceless stop consonants, the normal pattern for discrimination functions on this test. A third group of patients were unable to perform normally on either the discrimination or the labeling tasks. No patients could identify but not discriminate these stimuli.

These results indicate that there can be disturbances affecting the earliest linguistically relevant discriminatory perceptual capacities such as VOT discrimination, and others affecting linguistically relevant labeling of speech sounds. Blumstein and her colleagues emphasized the difference between not being able to achieve elementary aspects of discrimination and not being able to identify a phoneme. They argued that the latter ability required a subject to "assign a stable category label to a speech stimulus, i.e., to use phonological information in a linguistically relevant way" (Blumstein et al., 1977b, p. 381). Blumstein et al. suggested that these results showed that intact discrimination capacities are necessary for intact labeling, but that they do not necessarily guarantee intact labeling.

Further research has shown that there are a variety of different disturbances affecting phoneme discrimination and identification. In part, these different patterns fall out along phonological lines, such that different linguistically relevant acoustic parameters are subject to disturbances at each of these levels.

These patterns emerge from the work of several authors who studied acoustic-phonetic processing disturbances over a wider range of stimuli in individual patients than did Blumstein and her colleagues. One of the most extensive studies of a patient with an acoustic-phonetic processing disturbance is that by Saffran, Marin, and Yeni-Komshian (1976), who reported a patient with "pure word deafness." This patient had no evidence of peripheral hearing loss by audiometry and could identify musical instruments and environmental noises as well as the gender of a recorded voice and whether a spoken language was English or foreign. Clinically, he had extremely poor auditory comprehension and repetition performances but only a mild speech output disturbance consisting of dysnomia and occasional phonemic paraphasias. In contrast to his intact reading ability, he was unable to identify familiar monosyllabic words presented auditorily on a multiple choice test.

Saffran and her colleagues administered a variety of tests of acoustic phonetic abilities to their patient. They found that he was impaired in identifying stop consonants in CV sequences, with greater difficulty experienced for consonants followed by back vowels than front vowels. They interpreted this trend as possibly indicating an acoustic- rather than a phonetic-based mode of processing, since the formant structure of the acoustic signal becomes much more compressed as the vowel is produced further back in the vocal tract. There was also a strong tendency to identify voiced stops as voiceless. The authors repeated this identification process with synthetic CV sequences varying in VOT. They found the same trends as in natural speech with an even stronger bias toward voiceless responses, especially /ka/. Errors in identification were distributed over the entire VOT spectrum, indicating that errors were not occurring because of a resetting of the normal phoneme category boundary. The authors took this as evidence that a phonetic mode of processing was operating "extremely noisily or perhaps not at all" (Saffran et al., 1976, p. 219).

Discrimination of stop consonants was also grossly impaired, using the materials from the experiment on synthetic CV identification. Closely related pairs (/pa/-/ba/, /ga/-/ka/, /ta/-/da/) were particularly confused. Discrimination of pairs differing in voicing was worse than those differing in place of articulation, though both were much poorer than normals. An interesting feature of the patient's performance was that discrimination depended upon the order of presentation of these synthetic stop consonants, with sequences beginning with /ka/ being better than sequences that began with /ta/. The authors suggest that /k/ was particularly salient for this patient. The patient's performance was not entirely due to random effects in discrimination or identification, but appeared to reflect some systematic misanalysis of a variety of consonants as the consonant /k/. The authors report several preliminary studies with fricatives and sibilants indicating that voiceless consonants were identified as voiced in this group (the opposite of the pattern for stops), and that vowels seemed to be easier to identify than the consonants. However, these studies were not pursued in detail.

Context affected the patient's performance favorably, with improved performance once a topic had been firmly established in a conversation and poor performance as topics shifted. Similarly, repetition and multiple choice recognition tests were performed better when the patient had been previously exposed to the auditorily presented stimuli. Repetitions improved for items presented in lists blocked by superordinate categories, and identification of words was better for words in sentences than for isolated words. The authors argued that this indicated that the patient's problem was not simply one involving the temporal resolution of auditory stimuli.

Caramazza et al. (1983) reported a patient, J.S., who could not discriminate synthetic auditory sounds, but who had several disturbances in acoustic-phonetic processing. J.S. could discriminate natural non-speech sounds. However, he could not discriminate synthetic CV stimuli or identify either natural or synthetic consonants or vowels. The question of what acoustic features were present in the natural sounds that were absent in the synthetic stimuli that allowed J.S. to identify the former but not the latter was not explored.

Friedrich, Glenn, and Marin (1984) described a patient, E.A., who did not show the normal sharp identification function for synthetic acoustic continua varying in VOT. She also had a mild disturbance in discrimination of natural speech vowels and consonants. She was not tested for her ability to discriminate synthetic stimuli. E.A.

showed extremely poor ability to maintain phonemes in memory, being unable to report the phoneme in a specified position of a three-phoneme word or indicate the order of three phonemes by arranging colored blocks in order. Friedrich et al. analyzed E.A.'s deficit as one of phonological analysis, and concluded that she was operating with a "pre-categorical" code—i.e., an acoustic, rather than a phonemic, code.

The patient of Auerbach et al. (1982), whose click fusion and click counting disturbances were mentioned above, also had acoustic-phonetic impairments. He performed poorly in discrimination of synthetic CV stimuli that differed in place of articulation and in VOT. Surprisingly, however, he was able to identify VOT continua, and to discriminate natural speech vowels, digits, and words.

In summary, these studies show that individual patients differ with respect to their acoustic-phonetic disturbances; i.e., acoustic-phonetic processing disturbances can be partial. Our own research results are in agreement with this claim. Table 2.3, showing the results of discrimination tests using different phoneme pairs in seven patients, illustrates multiple double dissocations—instances where one patient can make one discrimination and another patient cannot, and in which the patients' performances are reversed on another pair.

In addition to these specific disturbances in phoneme discrimination, there are central tendencies in the group and case data regarding both the ease of discrimination of different segments and the relationship of discrimination to identification. Some of these are seen in the data in table 2.3. Discrimination of vowels is easier than consonants (see also Shankweiler and Studdert-Kennedy, 1967). There is strong evidence that discrimination of phonemes that differ in only one distinctive feature is more difficult than discrimination of phonemes that differ in more than one feature in both normal subjects (Miller and Nicely, 1955) and aphasic patients (Blumstein Baker, and Goodglass, 1977a). However, there are contradictory reports regarding the difficulty of particular feature contrasts. Blumstein et al. (1977a, b), Miceli et al. (1980), and Perecman and Kellar (1981) found that performance was worse on discriminations that differed in place of articulation than on those that differed in voicing, but Carpenter and Rutherford (1973) reported the opposite result. Discrimination of stops appears to be easier than dis-

Table 2.3
Discrimination of Various Phonemic Contrasts by Aphasic Patients (A'
Values)

	Patient						
Phoneme	G.Z.	L.D.	F.C.	J.L.	E.M.	M.D.	P.M.
i-u	.91	1.00	1.00	1.00	.99	.70	1.00
u-o	1.00	1.00	1.00	1.00	.99	.81	.98
b-p	.93	.98	.99	1.00	.99	.96	.93
b-d	.83	.99	1.00	1.00	.98	.94	.94
s-sh	.91	1.00	.92	1.00	0	.83	.94
s-z	.72	.97	.86	.86	.79	.78	.55
f-v	.68	.89	.85	.86	.82	.89	.67
m-n	.36	.95	.76	1.00	.60	.92	.90

crimination of fricatives (see table 2.3). More needs to be learned
about which phonemes are harder to recognize.

Neither the traditional clinical classes of aphasic patients nor
lesion sites are related in any clearly systematic way to disturbances
of acoustic-phonetic processing. For instance, Blumstein et al.
(1977b) point out that the ability to discriminate VOT differences
but not to label voiced and voiceless synthetic stops normally was
more characteristic of patients with Wernicke's aphasia than any
other group (three out of four Wernicke's aphasia patients showed
this pattern), but one of five patients with Broca's aphasia showed
the same pattern, and one of the four in the Wernicke's aphasia
group performed normally on both the discrimination and labeling
tasks. A study by Basso, Casati, and Vignolo (1977) reported the
somewhat surprising finding that patients with Broca's aphasia
performed worse than those with Wernicke's aphasia in phoneme
discrimination. Acoustic-phonetic perceptual processing deficits
apparently occur in all the traditional categories of aphasia.

The data regarding the effect of lesion site are more complex.
Some authors have suggested there may be some systematic differences in phonemic processing as a function of a lesion location. The
12 patients with anterior lesions in the study of Blumstein et al.
(1977a) showed abnormalities with both place of articulation contrasts and voicing contrasts, while the 13 patients with posterior

lesions had greater difficulty discriminating place than voicing contrasts. However, these correlations between patterns of performance and lesion sites are also very tenuous, based as they are upon very small numbers of patients in whom lesion sites were determined by imaging techniques now considered inadequate. To the extent that fluency reflects the locus of lesion (nonfluency being associated with anterior lesions and fluency with posterior lesions), the patterns of performance that arise in each of the syndromes reported by Blumstein et al. (1977b) and Basso et al. (1977) indicate that a wide variety of acoustic-phonetic perceptual processing disturbances can occur with either anterior or posterior lesions.

ACOUSTIC-PHONETIC PROCESSING AND DISTURBANCES OF LEXICAL ACCESS AND COMPREHENSION

If the ability to extract distinctive features and phonemes from the speech waveform is required for words to be accessed, we would expect that patients with disturbances of acoustic-phonetic processing would have impairments in lexical access. In turn, these disturbances should lead to comprehension impairments. If single words are not accessed at all, they should not be understood. If acoustic-phonetic disturbances only lead to words being accessed inefficiently, however, the consequences of acoustic-phonetic processing disturbances will be more subtle. Patients may be slowed in understanding a word, but be able to identify and understand a word in context (see the discussion of the role of context in word recognition above and in note 3). Patients may also have trouble with complex aspects of sentence comprehension. If word recognition is slowed and all the syntactic and semantic information associated with a word is not delivered to the language-processing systems devoted to constructing sentence structure, these latter processes may lag behind the incoming speech signal and operate poorly.

Several studies appear to bear this out. In the studies we described above, Saffran and her colleagues (Saffran et al., 1976) interpreted their results as indicating that disturbances of acoustic-phonetic processing led to impairments in auditory word comprehension. Similar conclusions were reached by Caramazza et al. (1983), Auerbach et al. (1982), and Albert and Bear (1974).

However, not all authors have reached the same conclusion.

Blumstein and her colleagues (Blumstein et al., 1977a) examined 16 aphasic patients for their abilities to perform phoneme discrimination, syllable discrimination, and phoneme order discrimination tasks, and correlated performance with single word auditory comprehension. They studied auditory comprehension using the four subtests of the auditory comprehension scale of the Boston Diagnostic Aphasia Examination (BDAE) (Goodglass and Kaplan, 1972). They found that, for the group as a whole, there was a significant correlation between the phoneme discrimination results and the comprehension results, and a further significant correlation between the results on phoneme order discrimination and syllable discrimination and the auditory comprehension measures. However, when the six patients with Broca's aphasia, who showed very good performance on both the discrimination and comprehension tasks, were removed from the patient group, no significant correlation was found between comprehension capacities and discrimination capacities. In particular, the mixed anterior aphasic patients showed a random relationship between phoneme discrimination and comprehension. Similar results—a failure of the degree of impairment in acoustic-phonetic processing to correlate with the degree of impairment in comprehension—were also reported by Basso et al. (1977), Jauhiainen and Nuutila (1977), and Gandour and Dardarananda (1982) for Thai. Miceli et al. (1980) reported only a weak correlation between these two impairments in their Italian population.

Blumstein et al. (1977b) were particularly interested in the possibility that phonemic and syllable discrimination impairments were the reason for the comprehension deficit of the patients with Wernicke's aphasia, as suggested by some authors (e.g., Luria, 1947). They concluded that this could not be the sole reason for these patients' disturbances of auditory comprehension. The Wernicke's aphasia group did have the most severe comprehension deficit on the BDAE, but were not overall the most impaired in the discrimination tasks. In addition, Blumstein et al. argued that, if the comprehension deficit in Wernicke's aphasia were based solely upon a phonological perception deficit, the meaningfulness of the stimuli used in discrimination tasks should not affect a patient's performance. They observed, however, that the discrimination performances in the Wernicke's aphasia group depended upon the lexical status of the stimuli (real word vs nonword) as much as was the case in any of the other aphasic groups. They concluded that semantic disturbances played an important role in creating the comprehension problems of the Wernicke's aphasia group.

Blumstein et al. (1977a) tried to account for the fact that the meaningfulness of the stimuli used in discrimination tasks affected the phoneme discrimination performances of patients with Wernicke's aphasia. They suggested that, if phoneme discrimination capacities were partially intact, this might be adequate for lexical access to be achieved. Once lexical access was achieved, the lexical status of a stimulus might, in turn, influence performance on phoneme discrimination tasks. This type of effect has been simulated for written language in a computer-implemented model in which the lexical level of representation feeds back onto the level of processing at which letters are processed (McClelland and Rumelhart, 1981). Similar models are beginning to be developed for the auditory language system (Elman, 1989).

Blumstein et al. (1977a) contrasted their results with those of Schuell and her colleagues (Schuell, Vekins, and Jimenez-Pabon, 1964). In the Blumstein et al. research, patients with Wernicke's aphasia showed a lexical effect—they were able to discriminate phonemes in words better than in nonwords. Schuell et al. found, however, that the Wernicke's aphasia patients were impaired on a word-picture matching task when the picture foils in such a task consisted of phonemically similar items. Blumstein et al. tried to explain this difference by suggesting that phoneme identification, not merely discrimination, might be needed to allow auditory word comprehension to be achieved. This is because, as we have seen, they conceived of phoneme identification as reflecting the ability to "assign a stable category label to a speech stimulus, i.e., to use phonological information in a linguistically relevant way" (Blumstein et al., 1977b, p. 381). Blumstein et al. suggested that the word-picture matching task is a comprehension task in which the ability to maintain "a stable phonemic configuration or label" is required, and that the difficulties they had documented in the abilities of patients with Wernicke's aphasia to identify phonemes might reflect a disturbance of that ability, leading to a failure to achieve a record of word form that is sufficiently stable to allow semantic representations to be accessed and manipulated in a word-picture matching task.

This interpretation of the performance of patients with Wernicke's aphasia runs into difficulties, however, with the observation of Baker, Blumstein, and Goodglass (1981) that patients with Wernicke's aphasia were more likely to select a semantic foil than a phonological foil on a word-picture matching test. If phoneme identification problems cause their auditory word comprehension deficits, these patients should select phonologically related foils. The account of Blumstein et al. also is contradicted by the case of Freidrich et al., E.A., who showed abnormal identification of stop phonemes in synthetic continua that varied in VOT but who nonetheless performed well on the comprehension portions of several aphasia batteries and the Token Test. This should not happen if phoneme identification is required for auditory word comprehension to take place.

What, then, is the relationship between disturbances in acoustic and phonetic perceptual processing and comprehension disturbances? The literature is contradictory. There are several considerations which may ultimately provide the basis for reconciling these different results.

First, we must remember that there is a fairly wide range of disturbances of acoustic-phonetic perceptual processing that has been documented in different aphasic patients. It is conceivable, as suggested by Blumstein and her colleagues, that certain of these disturbances affect later stages of word processing more than others. However, contrary to the hypothesis of Blumstein et al., that phoneme identification abilities are the crucial correlates of word comprehension, it may be that the ability to discriminate phonetic categories is needed for comprehension. Though Blumstein et al. (1977b) found that the ability to identify phonemes in synthetic continua—not discrimination abilities—correlated most strongly with comprehension scores, these studies were undertaken in groups of patients who had complex aphasic disorders. The significance of these correlations is very hard to determine.

Second, we must keep in mind that the tests of comprehension that have been used in all the patients with acoustic-phonetic discriminatory problems reported as cases of "word deafness" are not ideally suited to examining the consequences of phonemic processing disturbances on auditory word comprehension. For instance, in the study by Blumstein et al. (1977a), comprehension was assessed using the four auditory comprehension subtests of the BDAE. However, the auditory comprehension subtests of the BDAE do not test matching of single words against phonological foils, which would be the simplest and most direct assessment of the effect of phonemic processing disturbances on word recognition. The auditory comprehension subtests of the BDAE also test comprehension of both sentences and paragraphs, and it is not clear from the report by Blumstein and her colleagues to what extent patients' performances on the sentence and paragraph level sections of the BDAE comprehension battery are responsible for the lack of correlation between acoustic-phonetic perceptual processing and comprehension.

Finally, none of the reports we have reviewed have attempted to document a relationship between acoustic-phonetic perceptual processing disturbances and word recognition; all these studies have focused on comprehension rather than word recognition. One would expect that a disturbance affecting acoustic-phonetic perceptual processing would have a direct effect upon the identification of words; that is, a disturbance of this sort should affect lexical access directly and semantic access only secondarily. None of the reports we have reviewed establish that lexical access itself is abnormal in patients with acoustic-phonetic processing disturbances. Tasks such as lexical decision, word monitoring, gating, and others used in the experimental psycholinguistic literature to examine the activation of lexical forms, could be used to explore the consequences of an acoustic-phonetic processing disturbance upon lexical access. Ideally, the consequences of acoustic-phonetic processing deficits upon word recognition and comprehension would be explored by looking systematically for the specific acoustic-phonetic processing disturbance found in an individual patient and examining its specific effect upon lexical access, using the models of lexical access described above to generate predictions and interpret results. Exploring this possibility may also clear up some of the contradictions in the literature.

DISTURBANCES OF AUDITORY WORD RECOGNITION

The earliest account of a disturbance of word comprehension, that of Wernicke (1874), postulated that a patient may lose the ability to recognize a word despite good auditory and acoustic-phonetic processing. Wernicke believed that he had described patients who had sustained damage to the permanent representations of the sound patterns of words, and that this damage led to disturbances of word recognition (and production). In principle, disturbances of *accessing* permanent phonological representations could also exist, as well as these hypothesized disturbances of *storage* of permanent phonological representations (see chapter 3 for discussion of these different types of disturbances).

To my knowledge, there is no clear case of a patient who has intact acoustic-phonetic processing and who cannot access the auditory lexicon. The patient whose deficit comes closest to this is a case (E.D.E.) described by Berndt and Mitchum (1990). E.D.E. performed well on phoneme discrimination and identification in natural speech nonwords (CV syllables) but showed a persistent tendency to accept nonwords as words in a lexical decision task, even when she had been warned that she was making false-positive errors. Looked at in a superficial way, one might say that E.D.E. showed good acoustic-phonetic processing but poor lexical activation, because of her poor performance on the lexical decision task. However, it is unlikely that this pattern of performance resulted from an inability on the part of E.D.E. to access her phonological lexicon, because she correctly identified and interpreted real words. Berndt and Mitchum (1990) concluded that E.D.E.'s "access to real words within the lexicon is achieved normally" (p. 139), and proposed that her problem in rejecting nonwords was related to her limited auditory-verbal short-term memory. In addition to being able to recognize real words, E.D.E. did quite well on word-picture matching tests, even when the target was paired with up to three phonological distractors. Thus, this case is not a good example of a failure to access the lexicon without an acoustic-phonetic processing disturbance.

It is possible that the absence of reports of patients with disturbed auditory word recognition and intact acoustic-phonetic processing reflects inadequacies of the materials used to test patients, not the non-existence of such patients. As more studies appear in which acoustic-phonetic processing and lexical activation are both tested in detail, patients with primary disturbances in the activation or permanent storage of the phonological forms of words may yet be described.

OVERVIEW

Accessing words is a crucial part of the language comprehension process. It is well established that patients can have disturbances in auditory and acoustic-phonetic processing, and that these disturbances can co-occur with disturbances in single word comprehension. However, the relationship between these two types of impairments is not clear. We expect that disturbances in auditory and acoustic-phonetic processing will lead to disturbances of word recognition, but this has never been clearly proved. Many patients with disturbances of the first sort will have disturbances of the second, but this does not prove that one disturbance causes another, or that therapy aimed at improving auditory and acoustic-phonetic processing will be enough to ensure better lexical or semantic access. More research is needed to increase our understanding of acoustic-phonetic processing, word recognition, the relationship between the two, and their disorders.

NOTES

1. We do not identify all these different sounds as phonemes, only those sounds that can substitute for each other in a given position to create different words. Variants of a phoneme whose occurrence is predictable from the position of the phoneme in the phonological structure of a word are known as *allophones*. Different languages make use of different features to create phonemes and allophones. For instance, aspiration (designated by /^{h}/) occurs on morpheme-initial voiceless stop consonants (e.g., /$p^h at$/) and not on these same consonants in morpheme-final position (e.g., /tap^o/, where /^{o}/ indicates nonaspiration), as the reader can verify by placing his hand in front of his mouth while pronouncing these words and feeling the amount of air that strikes it while producing the /p/ sound. Because /p/ and /b/ can substitute for each other in the same phonological context and thereby create different words, they are phonemes of English; because /p^h/ and /p^o/ cannot occur in the same context, they are not phonemes of English, but allophones of the phoneme /p/. Voicing is thus a phonemic feature of English, and aspiration is not. In Hindi, however, both voicing and aspiration are phonemic features, and there are both aspirated and unaspirated voiced and voiceless stops—/p^h/, /p^o/, /b^h/, and /b^o/that can occur in the same position to create different words.

2. Linguists have argued that, if words consist of these complex and abstract phonological structures, learning the words of a language is easier in certain respects. For instance, if the stress patterns of English words can be partially determined by general rules, a child does not need to learn the stress pattern of each word of English individually. Rather, he can learn the rules that determine the assignment of stress, and apply them to each new word that he acquires. He will have to learn that words consist of phonemes, defined in terms of distinctive features, that are organized into higher-order structures such as syllables, and he will have to learn the rules that apply to these

structures to yield stress contours, vowel quality, etc. Still, it might be easier to learn these structural features and general rules than to acquire all this information about each word separately.

On the other hand, if the *sole* permanent representation of the sound pattern of a word is one which consists of the most abstract description of the sounds of the word, the processes of producing the word or recognizing it will be much more complicated. A speaker would have to compute the actual value of each segment of the word from a very abstract representation of the sound of the word, and a listener would have to do the reverse computation—constructing the abstract representation of the sound of the word to match it to an entry in his or her mental dictionary (Lahiri and Marslen-Wilson, 1991). It may be that the simplest solution to the problem of learning the sound patterns of words in a language does not result in a representation of the sound pattern of words that makes for the simplest solution to the problem of recognizing and producing the sound patterns of words.

3. Words are not "identified" as such in the Marslen-Wilson model; rather they fit into the context or they do not. The goal of the entire word recognition process (and of all other processes related to computation of linguistic structures) is to arrive at a representation of the developing discourse. This model captures the subjective feeling that most words are not identified at all in running speech, in the sense of a single lexical item emerging as a conscious percept. Rather, as Marslen-Wilson puts it "the bottom-up and selection processes provide the essential basis for rapid on-line comprehension processes, but they provide no more than a partial input to an integrative system that is only peripherally concerned with identifying word-forms, and whose primary function is to uncover the meanings that the speaker is trying to communicate" (Marslen-Wilson, 1987, p. 99).

4. We exclude from this discussion the consequences of hearing loss on word recognition. The reader can find discussions of this issue in many audiology texts.

5. It should be noted that though most researchers who have observed these disturbances assume that lower-level auditory functioning is intact, the more complex aspects of auditory functioning mentioned above (e.g., click fusion) have not been tested in most of these cases.

3   The Meanings of Words

Comprehension of words requires that the visual or auditory form of a word be connected to a concept; in most speech settings, producing a word requires that a concept be mapped onto the form of a word. This chapter provides a discussion of the structure and processing of concepts related to concrete objects and the language impairments that follow breakdown of these structures and processes. We begin by examining the traditional theoretical view of object concepts that dates back to Aristotle (termed *the classical view*). I then summarize empirical work that has conflicted with this approach to the representation of concepts, and consider a number of theoretical alternatives of how concrete concepts are represented. After this review of normal function, we turn to disorders affecting concepts. I discuss the distinction that some researchers have made between impairments affecting access and those affecting storage of items in semantic memory, the view that disturbances may affect the meanings of words and visual objects separately because they are processed in different functional subsystems, and the recent evidence for category-specific disorders in semantic memory (the claim that different superordinate categories, such as animals vs. objects, can be separately affected in brain-damaged patients).[1]

This chapter concentrates on concepts related to concrete objects, avoiding the concepts associated with abstract words, verbs, function words, etc. There are several reasons for restricting our discussion of word meaning to concepts related to concrete objects. First, the bulk of the experimental literature on normal concepts deals with the representation and encoding of object concepts. The nature of an object's conceptual description in semantic memory and the procedures that gain access to this knowledge system remain as formidable questions that have received few definitive answers. Progress on the semantics of abstract words, involving even greater theoretical challenges, is unlikely to occur without a substantial grasp of the underlying representation of concrete objects. A second reason for the focus is that brain-damaged patients often have trouble with concrete concepts. Many patients exist, of course, whose comprehension deficit is greater for abstract words (see, for example, the deep dyslexic patients described in chapter 5), but it is not impossible to observe the reverse dissociation, where words referring to familiar concrete objects are poorly understood in the face of remarkably preserved comprehension for less frequent abstract words (e.g., Warrington, 1975). Thus, how concrete concepts are represented, how these representations are processed, and how these mechanisms are disturbed by brain damage, are sufficiently substantial and important issues to occupy this chapter.

THE CLASSICAL VIEW OF CONCEPTS AND CHALLENGES TO THIS VIEW

How are objects represented in semantic memory? Are they stored in terms of constituent properties (i.e., properties that refer to parts of the object), or in terms of a more holistic, unanalyzed description? If object concepts are structured according to their properties, how are these properties to be characterized? Finally, how do we identify different instances of a concept—by interrogating a fixed set of properties for all possible examples of a concept, or a variable set that depends on a given exemplar? These are some of the basic questions that have begun to be addressed in the literature on the nature of concepts.

The classical view of what concepts are can be traced back to Aristotle, and is sometimes known as the Aristotelian theory of concept structure. Three main assumptions define the classical theory of concept representation:

1. The various exemplars of a concept are described in terms of a list of properties that apply to all members. For example, the description of the category BIRDS is identical for all the different instances of the concept (robins, chickens, owls, parrots, etc.).

2. A second fundamental assumption is that the meaning of an object is represented in terms of features (e.g. "beak," "feathers," "wings," etc. for the concept BIRD). These features are present in every instance of the concept (the features are taken to be *singly necessary*), and they can be used to uniquely classify any given instance of the concept (the features are together *jointly sufficient*). This statement amounts to the claim that object concepts can never be

disjunctive in form; we *cannot* define an instance as having features A, B, C, D *or* A, B, E, F, because all instances must have exactly the same basic features in common.

3. Lastly, if concept B (e.g., OWL) is represented as a subset of concept A (e.g., BIRD), then it follows that the features of A must all emerge in the description of B. The defining features of BIRD must be carried over into the definition of OWL, because owls are a subset of the more general concept.

This classical view has been subjected to a great number of counterarguments during its long and turbulent history. Some of them can be met with a plausible rebuttal; others are not so easily dismissed (see Smith and Medin, 1981, for an excellent summary). Perhaps the most widely cited point (Wittgenstein, 1953) is that the "essence" of a particular object concept—a set of necessary and sufficient features—has eluded description in the vast majority of cases. This rather surprising fact, that it is by no means a trivial intellectual challenge to define the essence of even the simplest natural object, has implications that extend well beyond the question of semantic representations in memory.[2] However, though the failure to define a set of necessary and sufficient features for an object concept is obviously disturbing, it does not, by itself, force us to abandon the classical view. After all, the fact that the defining features of a given object have not been isolated need only imply that no one has yet been clever enough to determine them.

The most compelling reasons for the now widespread dissatisfaction with classical theories of categorization are empirical. The performance of normal subjects in a variety of experiments cannot be easily reconciled with the idea that all instances of a concept are classified by referring to a fixed set of properties. In what follows, we present a summary of the evidence on this point, borrowing heavily from the detailed review by Smith and Medin (1981). None of the individual findings provides overwhelming proof against the classical approach; however, our confidence in the Aristotelian theory diminishes to the extent that it must undergo repeated adjustment to account for each new set of results.

Typicality Effects in Categorization

Normal raters are able to assign a value to different instances of a concept on the basis of how typically each instance represents the category (Rips, Shoben, and Smith, 1973; Rosch, 1973). For example, a robin is considered to be a much better exemplar of the concept BIRD than an owl, and would be rated accordingly on a scale from 1 to 5. A great deal of evidence now indicates that typicality ratings predict the speed with which a target word is categorized as an instance of a concept. Thus, it takes less time to evaluate the sentence "A robin is a bird" than "An owl is a bird" (Collins and Loftus, 1975), because robins appear to be closer to our prototypical notion of bird.[3] The implication for the classical view is that not all members of a concept have equal status, a conclusion that does not easily fit with the premise that all positive instances of a concept are classified by referring to a single set of necessary and sufficient features.

Measures of Family Resemblance

Additional evidence by Rosch and Mervis (1975) indicates that typicality judgments are highly correlated with the number of common features that are produced by normal raters when they are asked to list the relevant semantic features of various category members (e.g., to produce the features associated with various items of furniture, such as sofa, chair, rug, vase.). Variation in these feature listings is based on the occurence of attributes that are not held in common by all members of the category (furniture), and is closely related to judgments of the typicality of items within the category. Less typical items produce less frequently cited features. This suggests that typicality differences are due to the fact that *non-necessary* features enter into the description of a concept.

We could raise the objection, of course, that asking subjects to list the semantic properties of natural objects does not provide an accurate index of the concept's true features. Responses for CHAIR might be "made of wood," "has four legs," etc., neither of which need necessarily be true of a subject's concept of all chairs. Rosch and Mervis (1975), however, repeated the experiment using artificial concepts made up of written letter combinations that exemplified different instances of a "category" (higher family resemblance strings contained letters that were more often shared by other members of the group). For alphabetic test items, the relevant features of each exemplar were unambiguous, and the results confirmed the importance of family resemblance: letter strings with a high family resemblance score were learned more easily as members of a category, could be more rapidly categorized, and were given higher ratings of typicality (but see Martin and Caramazza, 1980, for a different result and a discussion of this issue).

Nonnecessary Features in Categorization

When normal subjects are asked to set down the relevant features of a concept, they list properties that are clearly not possessed by all legitimate instances. For example, the feature "made of wood" does not apply to all tables, nor does the attribute "flies" apply to every instance of the concept BIRD. Feature listings are reliable predictors of categorization times; the more features shared by a concept and one of its members, the faster the instance can be categorized (see, e.g., Hampton, 1979). This outcome suggests that *nonnecessary* features are involved in categorization.

Further support for the role of nonnecessary features in semantic processing comes from studies that use multidimensional scaling techniques to compute the relationships between concepts (e.g., Caramazza, Hersch, and Torgerson, 1976). Subjects are asked to judge pairs of concepts (e.g., HAWK ROBIN) for their similarity of meaning. These values then undergo statistical treatment that creates a geometric space where members of the category are positioned in terms of their rated semantic proximity. From this analysis, the dimensions that vary between members of the group may be uncovered. Results of multidimensional scaling also reveal the presence of nonnecessary features (e.g., birds may cluster along dimensions of size and ferocity), without the complication inherent in the subjective listing of features (but see Tversky, 1977, for other weaknesses in the interpretation of multidimensional analyses). Taken together, the two methods point to the conclusion that the properties of an object concept (e.g., BIRD) used in classification are not limited to a set that necessarily applies to all exemplars.

Nested Concepts in Categorization

One prediction derived from the classical view is that any instance of a concept should be judged more similar to an immediate superordinate category than to a distant category. Thus, OWL should be judged more similar to BIRD than ANIMAL because the defining features of BIRD must all be carried over into the definition of OWL, making the two concepts more analogous than concepts sharing fewer defining features. Normal subjects, however, produce the same number of distant superordinates (e.g., plant) as immediate superordinates (flower) when asked to define the category of an object (e.g., daffodil), a finding that provides no support for nested concepts (Smith, Shoben, and Rips, 1974). In addition, the speed with which subjects categorize objects does not consistently vary according to the objective distance between the target item and the superordinate. Thus, while ROBIN is classified as a bird more rapidly than it is classified as an animal, the reverse holds true for CHICKEN (e.g., Roth and Shoben, 1980). The classical theory cannot provide a straightforward account of the difference, because the two instances of the concept BIRD are assumed to be equivalent with respect to the superordinate.

We have summarized four converging experimental results that cause significant problems for the idea that objects are categorized by referring to a set of features that are singly necessary and jointly sufficient for the definition of the concept. Faced with this outcome, we could abandon the classical theory as psychologically unrealistic, or we could try to defend it by making some plausible assumptions about the way normal categorization takes place that would allow us to explain the range of data we have described without completely rejecting the classical position. We shall consider both these options.

ALTERNATIVE MODELS OF CONCEPTS

If we reject the classical view of concepts and assume that the description of an object involves a set of properties that are not uniformly shared by the members of a concept, then categorization must depend on probabilistic criteria. For example, not all birds can fly (i.e., the ability to fly is not a *necessary* one for group membership), but many do and it is therefore desirable to include this attribute in the representation of the concept BIRD. A particular instance may be classified without having to meet all the relevant criteria that make up the definition of the target concept; it is sufficient that the object and the concept share a large enough percentage of them to establish group membership. Thus, an ostrich cannot fly, but it does share many other properties (e.g., wings, feathers, a beak) with the concept BIRD and the match is sufficiently good for an ostrich to be classified as a bird.

We may distinguish between two different forms of this general approach to categorization, termed the *probabilistic view*. One approach is based on the premise that the representation of a concept is made up of abstract and perceptual features like <animate>, <feathered>, <rigid>, <sharp>, etc. These are originally established by isolating the semantic features that recur most commonly among the different instances of a category. The features are then assigned weights that provide a measure of their salience (e.g., the attribute <can fly> is met by the majority of birds and is therefore highly salient), and reliability (e.g., all birds are feathered, and this attribute is given a rating that indicates maximum probability over different exemplars). Classification requires a comparison of the features listed for the category and the relevant instance; the weights are combined and evaluated against a criterion that is used to determine membership in the group.

The alternative probabilistic framework emphasizes continuous dimensions instead of features as the "conceptual units" of an object, representing the numerical average for the individual members of the class.[4] Birds may vary, for example, in their size, predatoriness, and so forth. We can capture these differences by assigning each concept from the category (e.g., robin, owl, woodpecker) to a point in an abstract mathematically defined space relative to the other members of the group. An object (e.g., ROBIN) is categorized as an instance of a concept if its position from the concept (e.g., BIRD), defined according to scaled values on the dimensions of interest, is less than a criterial number.

Both the featural and the dimensional viewpoints depart radically from the assumption that the definition of an object concept includes only necessary and sufficient properties. Thus, probabilistic models of categorization have little difficulty accounting for the central findings that create so many problems for the classical theory. The approach is not without its own weak points, however. Chief among these is the lack of constraints associated with the failure to admit either necessary or sufficient properties into the representation of an object concept. It seems likely that some features or dimensions exist that would be found in every instance of a concept and which are therefore a necessary part of a concept's definition (e.g., animacy would presumably be a characteristic of *all* instances of the concept "person"). Similarly, while other properties may not be *necessary* for concept membership, their occurrence may be *sufficient* to guarantee admission into the category. Thus, any creature that is animate, has feathers, and can fly must be a bird, even though the attribute <can fly> does not apply to every instance. Further development of the probabilistic view requires imposing limits on the degree of disjunctiveness found in natural concepts.

Let us consider one final view on the representation of object concepts. Concepts might be represented in terms of *specific exemplars* rather than a more abstract summary description involving features or dimensions. The particular instances that form the concept would presumably be those that are the most typical of the category (Rosch, 1975). For classification, all exemplars of the concept would be available for comparison with the test item.[5] Classifying an item would require matching it to at least one exemplar, and the probability of such a match is determined by the similarity between the presented item and the exemplar.

The exemplar approach is just as capable of dealing with the "nonclassical" results from experiments on categorization as the probablistic framework. Concepts are disjunctive because a number of possible exemplars, incorporating different properties, can be used to ascertain membership. Like the probabilistic models, however, the exemplar viewpoint suffers from a lack of constraint on the properties that are necessary or sufficient for the definition of a concept. In addition, there is a further lack of restriction on the kind of the exemplars that can be conceptually linked. What information is needed to prevent unrelated exemplars from being stored under the same heading? The most reasonable assumption is that knowledge common to all the instances of a concept is maintained, a proposal that implies the existence of a general description beyond the presence of discrete exemplars.

CORE CONCEPTS AND IDENTIFICATION PROCEDURES

It thus appears that both the classical view of concepts and its chief rivals run into problems. Let us therefore consider one model of the nature of concepts that includes aspects of both the classical and probabilistic views in an effort to avoid these problems. This approach draws a distinction between the "core" definition of a concept and the procedures required to actually identify exemplars. The distinction may later help us understand some of the dissociations in performance manifested by patients with semantic deficits.

The distinction arises from the idea that the underlying representations of *object concepts* are not necessarily the knowledge structures that are required for the identification of *visual instances*. It seems implausible that everything we know about an object concept (e.g., that bears have hearts) must enter into the identification of visually presented objects (so-called perceptual or visual instances). The representation of many objects is most likely to include *abstract* as well as more perceptual attributes.

On the other hand, some of these abstract properties are relevant to recognizing visual instances of a concept. Miller and Johnson-Laird (1976), for example, argue convincingly that even so elementary an object as a table cannot simply be recognized by means of perceptual features like (1) is connected and rigid, (2) has a flat and horizontal top, and (3) has vertical legs. Their reasoning proceeds as follows. Some of these features are not true of many objects we would unhesitatingly classify as tables (e.g., drafting tables do not have a horizontal top). This problem seems to exist no matter how we juggle with the kinds of perceptual attributes included in the list. Furthermore, the same object may be treated as an instance of two different concepts, depending on the circumstances, without any change in its form. A table may be used one day as a kitchen table, on another as a worktable, and on the third day as a card table; it may even be used as a bench or a raft. According to Miller and Johnson-Laird, these facts indicate that *functional* as well as perceptual attributes are part of the definition of an object. If we include features like "has a surface capable of providing support," the flexibility of a concept like TABLE when applied to different exemplars, and the changeable role of a particular instance, become more readily understandable.

However, if the representation of an object includes both physical and abstract properties, how do we actually recognize a visually presented object, where the input is exclusively perceptual in nature? The solution proposed by many theorists is that some ancillary knowledge must exist for translating between physical and abstract levels of representation. Each object concept with abstract properties forming part of its definition would then have two semantic components associated with it. One is its *core meaning*, which includes both functional and perceptual attributes, and yields a description that captures the semantic relationship between different objects (e.g., between a boy and a girl). The second is an *identification procedure*, which is responsible for categorizing visual exemplars, and therefore has access to perceptual features plus information about any abstract properties (e.g., young, human) instantiated by these features.

The relevance of the distinction between core concepts and identification procedures for the classical view of object concepts is that it provides a possible escape route from the evidence that conflicts with the main assumptions behind this theory. If we assume that the identification procedure related to a concept is more readily accessible than the core definition of that concept, we can argue that semantic categorization tasks are often not performed by looking up core features but by comparing the features in the identification procedure of the target and those associated with the probe items. This assumption then allows us to explain many of the results that have embarrassed the classical approach. For example, the properties of an object represented in an identification procedure may often not be essential to its definition, so that many features that determine semantic categorization will be nonnecessary ones. The effects of typicality can now be interpreted to reflect the degree of similarity between the identification features of a concept and the target exemplar. The fact that typical members of a category have many features in common (Rosch and Mervis, 1975) can be accounted for simply by arguing that the identification features shared by many exemplars of a concept (e.g., sparrow, robin, chickadee, pigeon) are the most likely features to be part of the identification procedure for the general concept (BIRD). Finally, there is no reason to expect that the identification features of a concept will be equally applicable to all of its instances, so that the similarity relationship between objects and superordinates derived from the classical view may not always be upheld. On the other hand, the constraints on which properties are necessary or sufficient for the definition of a concept can reflect the concept's core meaning.

Research by Armstrong and her colleagues (Armstrong, Gleitman, and Gleitman, 1983) provides evidence that this may be the right way to think about concepts. These researchers studied concepts that do, in fact, meet the Aristotelian criteria for membership of their items: for instance, the man-made categories of even and odd numbers are well-defined concepts that meet the Aristotelian criteria. Armstrong et al. found that subjects knew that this was the case: asked, for instance, if it made any sense to say that one odd number was a better example of the concept ODD NUMBER than another, the subjects said that it did not. Nonetheless, these subjects ranked certain numbers as better examples of these categories than others. This indicates that even when a category has a well-defined structure and subjects know that it has, they assign typicality ratings to instances of that category. These ratings must be assigned on the basis of some representation other than that which characterizes the core concept itself. In the case of odd and even numbers, this representation may not be part of an identification procedure that categorizes perceptual instances of these categories. However, in other, natural, categories, it may well be derived from an identification procedure, at least in part.

In summary, we began this chapter by examining a traditional view of concepts that argues for a set of properties shared by every member of a category and that, if present in an object, guarantees its membership in the group. We then described some experimental findings that conflicted with this approach, obliging us to consider a number of alternative suggestions. These involve a different view of concepts themselves. One theory is that the attributes of a given object concept are defined probabilistically, either in terms of features or continuous dimensions, or both, and that instances vary in the number of attributes they share with the target concept. A drawback to the general probabilistic model is the lack of any constraints on the disjunctiveness of a category; it seems unlikely that there are neither sufficient nor necessary conditions that are used for establishing membership of natural concepts. A second tack relies on the assumption of discrete exemplars—corresponding to specific instances or the average of a subset of instances—to represent the knowledge of an object concept. In addition to suffering from the same lack of constraint as the probabilistic framework, this viewpoint also requires some way of predefining the relationship between exemplars that coexist in a particular representation. We have considered a way out of these problems that retains the traditional notions about concepts. The solution is to hypothesize that the empirical findings that cannot be explained by the classical theory result from subjects' use of identification procedures to accomplish a variety of categorization tasks, while core concepts still remain as the basis of a concept. We shall return to this analysis in our discussion of certain patient performances.

MODALITY-SPECIFIC REPRESENTATIONS OF CONCEPTS

Up to this point, we have been assuming that the stored descriptions of object concepts are maintained in a single store, which is accessed by both words and perceptual instances of a concept. This view of an *amodal* semantic system mediating the categorization and semantic processing of words, visually presented objects, tactile modes of input, etc., is not shared by every theorist. Paivio (1971), for example, has argued against the existence of a single semantic code. Instead, he claims that components of the language processing system that recognize and produce the forms of words contain information about abstract properties of the items that the words refer to, while components of the perceptual system involved in object recognition contain information about perceptual features of a concept. Verbal semantic codes include nonsensory properties of an object, such as the fact that a carrot is edible, that is is a vegetable that can be used in salads, that it usually costs less than 50 cents, and so on. Nonverbal semantic codes contain information about properties of objects such as their shape, color, and texture. The processing of a word allows direct contact with the properties of the associated concepts that are maintained in the verbal semantic store, but further processing is required to access those properties maintained in the nonverbal semantic store. The converse is the case when a perceptual instance of a concept is recognized.

A great number of experimental tests of the dual-code theory of semantics have been carried out. Most of these tests rely on differences between reaction times in semantic judgments made to words and pictures. These experiments have produced mixed results (see Potter, 1979, and Snodgrass, 1984, for reviews of this literature). Paivio (1975), for example, demonstrated that size judgments of pictured objects, adjusted to eliminate perceptual cues to actual size, were performed more rapidly than the same task applied to written words for the same objects. This result was taken as confirmation of Paivio's model: pictures were said to produce faster reaction times because they made direct contact with physical properties such as size (even if these properties were not actually perceptually available in the presented picture), while words made primary contact with verbal semantics and required extra processing time for the extraction of these properties from nonverbal semantics.

Unfortunately for the dual-code theory, later experiments indicated that the advantage for pictures over words could be found even when the judgment required information that was entirely nonperceptual, which was ostensibly derived from the verbal semantic system. Banks and Flora (1977) showed that pictures yielded faster reaction times than words for judging which of two animals was more intelligent, and Paivio himself reported an advantage for pictures in mental comparisons involving dimensions like pleasantness and monetary value (Paivio, 1978). To maintain the dual-code theory in the face of these and similar results (see Potter and Faulconer, 1975; Friedman and Bourne, 1976), Paivio has suggested that more abstract properties like category membership, pleasantness, intelligence, and the like are more relevant to the visual object than to the word and may therefore be represented in the nonverbal semantic system. It is far from clear why this should be true. Moreover, there is another explanation of the advantages of pictures in these judgment tasks. Many other researchers have argued that the advantages of pictures over words in these tasks is due to their greater discriminability, which allows pictures to be recognized faster and gain access to an amodal semantic system sooner than words.

In general, then, the data obtained from normal subjects provide little clear support for a dual-code theory of the representation of concepts. We shall see that some performances of brain-damaged patients have been explained by invoking the notion of separate verbal and nonverbal semantic systems. We will review these data, and offer our own account of them based on a theory that contains a single semantic component (see also Caramazza et al., 1990, for a discussion of these issues).

Our brief review of the literature has barely scratched the surface of the complex issues relating to object identification and categorization. The models we have discussed should each be seen as a preliminary framework within which a more precise account can be developed. Some phenomena cannot be easily interpreted by any of these rudimentary approaches. For example, semantic features of objects become more or less salient depending on contextual influences. A sentence like "The container held the juice" implies a bottle of some kind, whereas "The container held the apples" indicates a much larger container (e.g., a box or basket). How the relevant properties of "juice" and "apples" become transferred onto the idea of container, altering the features that are activated, remains mysterious. A related problem involves combinatorial properties of concepts: a typical value for the concept GREEN APPLE is neither a typical apple (typical apples are considered to be red, not green, in the United States) nor a typical shade of green. However, although our understanding of the nature of object concepts is limited, we have enough knowledge to approach the research on the breakdown of semantic processing, which is described in the next section in relationship to work on the normal structure and processing of object concepts.

One important point that emerges from our discussion is that accessing concepts is likely to be quite different depending upon whether the input is a word on an object. Objects have properties that are themselves parts of many concepts (their physical features), and the process of accessing a concept from a perceptual instance (i.e., from the object itself) is likely to involve an identification procedure that makes use of these features. In contrast, words do not usually themselves contain features that are part of the concepts they stand for. Therefore, accessing concepts from words is likely to involve a look-up process of some kind that is more arbitrary than that involved in recognizing an object. We shall see whether these differences affect patients' abilities to access meanings from words and to recognize objects.

SEMANTIC DEFICITS

Disturbances affecting object concepts show up as impairments in numerous language-related tasks, but are usually apparent in single word comprehension and naming tasks.[6] A very large number of brain-damaged patients are impaired on one or the other of these tasks. However, not all patients with disturbances of single word comprehension or naming have semantic deficits.

Failure to correctly extract the meaning of an object or a word can be due to impairment at a number of possible stages of processing. Damage to components outside the semantic mechanism may prevent the extraction of a visual or auditory word form, or the synthesis of a three-dimensional description for a visual object from sensory input. The kinds of deficits that are seen when the phonological or orthographic structure of a word is not reliably activated for recognition are described in chapters 2 and 5. Other disorders exist that specifically involve the perceptual analysis of objects, resulting in a range of visual agnosias. We cannot review this literature here, but we direct the reader to a number of valuable publications on the topic (Marr, 1982; Warrington, 1982; Humphreys and Riddoch, 1984; Humphreys, Riddoch, and Quinlan, 1985, 1988; Kosslyn, et al., 1990; Farah, 1990). The main point about these deficits is that they all concern the processing of physical structure *before* actual contact is made with the semantic mechanism. As such, the deficit is perceptual in nature and confined to a single modality of input (visual or auditory).

Similarly, though brain-damaged patients frequently have difficulty assigning the correct names to objects, naming deficits in aphasic patients often result from a disturbance affecting the retrieval or production of the form of a word rather than a failure to determine the precise semantic decription of the target (Wiegel-Crump and Koenigsknecht, 1973; Goodglass and Geschwind, 1976). Several lines of evidence support this interpretation: erroneous responses frequently include parts of the form of the target word; repeated attempts to produce the target result in closer and closer approximations to the target; cuing with the first sound of the target helps the patient produce the word. We discuss these disturbances of accessing and producing phonological forms in chapter 4.

The simplest indication that a patient may have a disturbance affecting semantic representations or their processing is the co-occurrence of an anomia and a single word comprehension deficit. However, though suggestive of a disturbance affecting semantics, even this combination of deficits may be due to separate input- and output-side processing disturbances that affect word recognition and production. For instance, a case reported by Howard and Orchard-Lisle (1984) was a patient with global aphasia with very poor comprehension of spoken and written words, who also made many semantic errors when naming objects. The patient, however, was found to be quite normal on a relatively high-level conceptual task involving the matching of depicted objects that were functionally related (e.g., THIMBLE matched to NEEDLE rather than COTTON REEL).[7] Nor is the association of anomia and impaired performance on some nonverbal test of semantic categorization adequate evidence for the claim that the naming errors are directly linked to conceptual deficits. Butterworth and his colleagues note that in order to prove a conceptual disturbance is responsible for naming errors (e.g., "cup" produced instead of "bowl"), we need "more than a demonstration that aphasics, as a group, perform poorly on some non-verbal semantic tasks. One needs to show that both the qualitative features of this impairment and its severity are sufficient to account for the verbal semantic difficulties. Otherwise, it may simply be the case that cortical lesions may often damage tissue critical to the performance of purely cognitive tasks at the same time as it damages tissue involved in verbal ones; the association, then is an anatomical accident rather than a functional relationship" (Butterworth, Howard, and McLoughlin, 1984; p. 423).

The combination of deficits in naming and word-picture matching is more likely to result from a disturbance affecting semantic memory when the patient's performance in each of these tasks is consistent with a semantic disturbance (Hillis et al., 1990). These signs include many semantic paraphasias in naming tasks and a comprehension impairment in which the patient has trouble deciding which visual object corresponds to a spoken word if the distractors come from the same semantic category as the target[8] but has little problem in selecting a target among phonologically similar distractors (see chapters 2, 4, and 5). The view that patients with this combination of disturbances have a subtle disturbance in their ability to access the precise meaning of *pictures*, a functional deficit that would account for naming errors as well as errors in matching auditory words to pictures, can be rendered unlikely when adding contextual cues does not improve naming performance in aphasia (Hatfield et al., 1977), and when these patients do not succeed in producing the name of the object when given a verbal definition (Barton, Maruszewski, and Urrea, 1969). In such patients, it is likely that the conceptual description of objects is no longer completely intact or cannot be accessed.

Recent work on semantic deficits in brain-damaged populations has been primarily concerned with two main issues: (1) distinguishing loss of conceptual representations from disturbances in accessing these representations, and (2) identifying partial impairments in the semantic system and its processing. Among the questions posed by contemporary researchers are: Can we establish clear criteria that indicate when a concept has been lost and when it is simply not accessible? Are there different conceptual systems mediating the comprehension of words and visual objects? If such a distinction exists, might there be other forms of semantic descriptions for remaining input modalities—a tactile semantic component, for example? (Cf. Beauvois and Derouesné, 1979.) At what level in the processing sequence that extracts meaning from percepts does the type of material (visual object or word) influence the nature of the conceptual knowledge available to a brain-damaged patient? Are there disturbances affecting semantically defined subsets of concepts, such as living things, animals, objects? These questions motivate the bulk of current research on the semantic disturbance observed in brain-damaged cases and we shall take them up in turn in our discussion of disturbances of semantic representations.

Access vs. Degraded Representation

A combined disturbance in naming and comprehension that has the characteristics mentioned above may reflect a disturbance of the representations of concepts in semantic memory or of accessing these representations. Warrington (1981b), Warrington and Shallice (1979) and Warrington and McCarthy (1973) have attempted to specify a number of criteria that might be used to distinguish the permanent loss of semantic knowledge from impaired access to the underlying conceptual representations. They suggest five phenomena that they believe allow the clinician to make the distinction between these two types of impairments: (1) consistency of performance; (2) preservation of superordinate information; (3) frequency sensitivity of performance; (4) effectiveness of priming; and (5) rate dependency of performance. We shall discuss these in turn.

Consistency of Performance
One fact that emerges quite clearly from the literature is that many aphasic patients are inconsistent in their ability to name objects on different trials. In addition, many aphasics appear as likely to name items which elicit mistakes on a word-picture matching task as those yielding a correct matching response (Butterworth et al., 1984). Inconsistent performance over items has been taken as an indication that permanent representations are not lost, but simply

unavailable on certain occasions: "The accessibility of words may simply vary in an unsystematic way, making a given word inaccessible today but accessible tomorrow" (Butterworth et al., 1984; p. 419).

The impaired comprehension and naming ability of demented patients with Alzheimer's disease, by contrast, reveals a marked specificity of individual items. Huff, Corkin, and Growdon (1986) compared the anomia of a group of mild to moderately affected demented patients with their comprehension of the same items in a word-picture matching test. A strong correspondence was observed between the pictures that could not be correctly named and the pictures that yielded incorrect matching to a spoken word. Pictures that were labeled correctly by the patients were also the items with a correct response on the matching task. Chertkow, Bub, and Caplan (in press) confirmed the item-by-item correspondence between naming performance and the ability to select a picture from a group of semantically related choices when given an auditory word (e.g., LION [word]–ELEPHANT WOLF LION ZEBRA). Further testing indicated that demented patients no longer retained adequate conceptual knowledge of the objects they were unable to name. Presented with questions about semantic attributes of each target picture (e.g., a picture of a shark was presented along with the question, Is it dangerous or not?), the patients made an average of 3.7/6 errors on items they failed to name, a level of accuracy no different from chance. Very few errors occurred, however, to probe questioning of objects that produced a correct naming response (0.44/6 on the average). This evidence points to a central loss of semantic representation in Alzheimer's disease, a deficit that affects the comprehension of both verbal and visual forms of a concept (written or spoken words and pictures or solid objects). The damage may at first be restricted to a subset of concepts, while others remain intact for the patient. Thus, we find that patients with milder symptoms of Alzheimer's disease *consistently* fail to name particular items, because they lack the required semantic description, but have no trouble naming instances of other object concepts which they retain. The item-by-item consistency typical of Alzheimer patients stands in marked distinction to the reported lack of such consistency in many aphasic patients with vascular disease, where, as we have seen, the consistency with which a patient responds to an item on different occasions or on related tests varies quite drastically among individuals.

A simple view is that the presence of fluctuating performance indicates that the patient retains the knowledge needed to carry out the task but cannot always gain access to this information and that consistently poor performance for individual items across tasks or test sessions implies that an item has been lost. Several researchers have adopted this position (e.g., Shallice, 1987, 1988). In fact, Butterworth and colleagues propose a model to explain inconsistent performance in patients with semantic processing impairments. They suggest that a transcoding device, which they call the "semantic lexicon", exists for mapping spoken (and presumably written) words onto meaning and for carrying out the reverse operation from meaning to production.[9] Damage to the semantic lexicon may cause unreliable communication between word forms and their meaning. Their interpretation of the functional disturbance is that the operation of the semantic lexicon has become "noisy"; the meaning of a word will often not be activated precisely enough to determine the correct selection of a picture from semantically confusable alternatives. When the patient attempts to name an object, the code from the semantic lexicon may again be unreliable, leading either to "a total addressing failure, and hence no response, or production of one of the range of semantically related words which match the partial address code" (Butterworth et al., 1984, p. 424).

However, in fact, both of these conclusions—that the presence of fluctuating performance indicates an access disturbance and that consistently poor performance indicates a disturbance of stored representations—depend crucially on the details of the processing model that is assumed. Caramazza and his colleagues (Caramazza et al., 1990) have argued, for instance, that a partial damage to a stored semantic representation may be the basis for consistently incorrect responses (if not enough information is ever available to lead to the correct response on a task) or to inconsistent responses (if the correct response and other responses are both activated). Conversely, Humphreys et al. (1988) have argued that impairment of specific items may occur if there is noise in the access procedure to semantic representations. Certain visual objects, for example, share many attributes with other members from the same category (e.g., sparrow, pigeon, and dove all have very similar properties). When such an item is displayed, the representations for the related members are conjointly activated. They may interfere with the activation pattern of the target item, especially when the operation of the damaged input channel has become noisy, thus preventing correct identification. However, a noisy input channel would not affect a category in which items were perceptually more distinct, such as furniture. Both these arguments undermine the simple correlation between loss of semantic knowledge and damaged entry to the semantic system with consistent and inconsistent responses on semantic tasks, respectively.

Shallice (1988) has questioned the plausibility of the claim that noise in the access mechanism might produce item-consistent impairments. He considers two potential situations where a noisy access routine might produce consistency over items. The first would occur if the amount of information lost through noise does not change very much from trial to trial, so that only the inherent properties of the stimuli (their frequency, structural overlap, etc.) would influence performance. Shallice dismisses this conceptualization of noise as being unrealistic. The second possibility is that the amount of perceptual information needed to categorize a target varies markedly across items, being a very large quantity for one set and a very small quantity for other items. The addition of noise would then affect performance on targets that required much sensory information for categorization but would not prevent items that needed substantially less buildup of information from being identified. Shallice concludes that this outcome may be applicable to the processing of visual objects or pictures, where items may or may not differ strongly in terms of their physical resemblance to other items from the same conceptual neighborhood, as Humphreys et al. (1988) argued. There is no reason to assume, however, that the labels of objects (spoken or written words) would vary in this fashion, so that the explanation cannot suffice for patients who demonstrate item-by-item consistency in the verbal domain (Coughlan and Warrington, 1981). Shallice concludes that consistency with respect to items that are produced over different trials in verbal tasks thus suggests a storage deficit. However, this conclusion still depends upon the premise that noise levels change a great deal from trial to trial, which may not be true. Overall, consistency or inconsistency of responses to particular items over different trials does not necessarily prove that a patient has a storage or an access disorder.

Preservation of Superordinate Information

A striking feature of semantic processing deficits is that the damage rarely entails the complete loss of a concept. Typically, some attributes are missing but others remain available to the patient. Warrington (1975) was the first to document that information about the superordinate category of an object or a word (e.g., that a lion is an animal) may be preserved even though more detailed semantic attributes (e.g., that a lion is a large, carnivorous feline) are missing. The continued existence of partial knowledge accounts for patients' ability to discriminate between exemplars from different superordinate categories (e.g., lion, truck, carrot, boot); finer-grained decisions between conceptually similar items, however, bring out the severity of the disorder.

According to Warrington, the destruction of semantic memory follows an invariant course through a hierarchically organized system, detailed attributes and associations that distinguish related concepts becoming unavailable before their superordinate category. By contrast, impaired access to semantic knowledge (as opposed to the permanent degradation of information) would not conform to this pattern. The recovery of specific elements should be no more difficult than obtaining information about the superordinate category when access to concepts is impaired.

At present, there exists only meager evidence in support of this particular criterion for distinguishing impairment of semantic access from degraded representations. Warrington and Shallice (1979) document a patient who retained partial comprehension of written words he was unable to explicitly identify. The patient (A.R.), whose reading performance appeared similar to a patient with deep dyslexia (see chapter 5), was found to be notably inconsistent in his ability to read aloud the same list of words on repeated testing. A significant number of words that were not read correctly nevertheless were partially understood when A.R. was given probe questions. The authors found no indication that superordinate knowledge was better preserved than attribute information for these words. They concluded that the overall pattern of results distinguished A.R. from cases with permanent damage to semantic memory, and argued that his loss of comprehension reflected impaired access to the full semantic description of a word. However, given the fact that inconsistency does not necessarily imply an access disorder (see above), this argument is not necessarily correct.

Frequency Sensitivity

A third criterion suggested by Warrington and Shallice (1979; see Shallice, 1987, for details) is that lower-frequency items (i.e., less familiar items) should be more susceptible to deterioration of the representations within semantic memory than high-frequency items. When impaired access is responsible for the comprehension disorder, however, "frequency would be expected to be a less important factor as the variability produced by specific access/information retrieval problems would tend to flatten any underlying 'normal' frequency function" (Shallice, 1987; p. 118). A number of patients, including A.R., have been described with putative access disorders who do indeed show absent or weak effects of word frequency on their performance (e.g., see Warrington, 1981a; Warrington and McCarthy, 1983). A contrasting number of cases have been reported with apparent deterioration in semantic knowledge who tend to be more sensitive to frequency variations (Warrington, 1975; Coughlan and Warrington, 1981; Warrington and Shallice, 1984). However, the sample of documented patients is too limited at present to justify any strong claims on the basis of these observations. Both Caplan (1987) and Rapp and Caramazza (1990) have raised questions regarding the analysis of case A.R. In addition, Caplan (1987) pointed out that the same factors that would make frequency an important variable in determining the effects of damage to a stored representation would also affect the operation of the mechanisms that access that representation. The claim that frequency sensitivity is characteristic of damage to stored representations and not of disturbances affecting access to those representations finds no convincing empirical or theoretical support at present.

Effects of Priming and Cuing

A further criterion suggested by Warrington and Shallice (1979) is that an access disorder should be improved by the occurrence of a "priming" item that facilitates the recovery of the target's semantic description. For example, given the word "Egypt" as a cue, Warrington and Shallice found that A.R. had greater success at reading the word PYRAMID (a similar result was observed by Warrington, 1981a, for a patient with concrete word dyslexia). By contrast, these authors maintain that priming should have no effect when information has been permanently lost from semantic memory.

The use of the term "priming" by Warrington and Shallice refers to a procedure where the patient must actively employ a verbal or pictorial cue (or prompt) to facilitate the processing of a conceptually related item. This is more commonly known as "cuing." Cuing is a function that requires some degree of controlled, voluntary processing on the part of the subject. Evidence suggests that damage to semantic representations may in fact abolish sensitivity to cuing, in partial support of Warrington and Shallice. Chertkow and Bub (1990, 1991) have documented that patients with Alzheimer's disease show virtually no improvement on picture naming when given a verbal cue that is associatively related to the target (e.g., picture of a lion; cue: "It's like a tiger"). These patients also demonstrated consistent impairment of the same object concepts over different comprehension tests, a result that according to the consistency of performance criterion indicates damage to semantic representations rather than disturbed access.

A different picture emerges when priming, rather than cuing, is used. Semantic priming usually refers to the passive spread of activation through semantic memory from a word or picture (the prime), and is measured by its effect on the recognition of a subsequent target bearing some relationship to the prime. The word LION, for example, is identified more rapidly if TIGER is displayed a short time—say 500 ms—beforehand (Meyer, Schvaneveldt and Ruddy, 1974). The main point about the phenomenon is that it is largely unconscious; the subject does not have to make any explicit judgment concerning the semantic relationship between the prime and the target, nor to actively use this information when making a response. Indeed, there is good reason to believe that the effect can occur even when little attention is given to the word or picture occurring before the target (Posner and Snyder, 1975), and, more dramatically perhaps, that the influence can persist under display conditions that prevent conscious identification of the prime (Carr et al., 1982; Marcel, 1983a,b).

In a parallel study to that of Chertkow and Bub (1990), Chertkow, Bub, and Seidenberg (1989) examined the effect of semantic priming on the same group of Alzheimer patients. A word-nonword decision task was constructed with paired trials including both related words (TIGER LION), unrelated words (CARPET LION), or nonsense words (FLINK LION). Filler trials were added to the experiment, consisting of pairs of words or a nonword followed by another nonword, to balance the total number of positive and negative responses. The patient's task was simply to indicate verbally—by saying yes or no—whether an item was a legitimate word or not, each response being followed 0.5 second later by the next item of the pair. The critical dependent measure was the time taken by the patient to correctly identify a word that had been preceded by an associatively related item, compared to the reaction time for the same word preceded by an unrelated item. The average difference between the two conditions gives us a measure of passive semantic priming between two words in a recognition task, without requiring the patient to explicitly judge the relationship between them. The results of this study demonstrated substantial priming effects in all the patients. More crucial to the present discussion, Chertkow et al. tested the patients' detailed knowledge of each target word (e.g. LION) by asking a series of probe questions ranging from the general category (animal or object?) to more detailed attributes of the verbal concept (e.g., wild or tame?). For any patient, a number of words were found to have degraded semantic representations, indicated by chance levels of performance on all but the most general probe questions. Responses to these words nevertheless showed a large effect of priming—if anything, larger than the effect observed for items with a more intact semantic description. We have no reason to believe, therefore, that a deterioration in semantic knowledge would generally lead to the complete elimination of associative priming in speeded recognition tasks.

On reflection, the persistence of the priming effect in the face of a major semantic breakdown may not appear too surprising. A typical priming experiment contains many word pairs that are linked on the basis of superordinate category membership (e.g., TIGER LION), and we have already noted that this general level of semantic description can remain available to the patient after detailed attributes of the concept have been lost. If diffuse activation between words from the same category is one basis for semantic priming, then the preservation of superordinate knowledge is presumably sufficient to yield an effect. In the case of priming between words via a more fine-grained relationship (e.g., TUSK ELEPHANT), no relevant data have yet been reported from patients with a well-documented impairment of semantic knowledge.

Milberg and Blumstein (1981; also see Blumstein, Milberg, and Shrier, 1982) have examined the ability of different aphasic patients to explicitly determine whether two words are semantically related (CAT DOG) and have correlated performance on this task with the priming effect obtained for the same pair of items in a speeded word recognition task. The failure to observe any correlation between overt judgments of relatedness and the occurrence of implicit semantic priming·led them to argue that poor comprehension in the aphasic patients must be the result of "a deficit in accessing and operating on semantic properties of the lexicon and not an impairment in the underlying organization of the semantic system" (Milberg and Blumstein, 1981, p. 381).

We believe, however, that the inability of a brain-damaged patient to detect a category relationship between two words does not provide good evidence that the patient has no conscious access to the semantic information tapped by automatic priming experiments. There are many reasons why semantic judgments may be disrupted even when the required knowledge to carry out the task is available, including difficulty at the decision stage of the mental operation, problems in attending to the necessary attributes for the comparison, and defects in working memory. Indeed, Chertkow et al. (1989) found their Alzheimer patients to be particularly bad at determining semantic relatedness, even though the same patients could readily determine the superordinate category of the words they were required to judge. Thus, the patients could indicate, when given a forced choice, that the word LION or TIGER was an animal as opposed to an inanimate object, but could not reliably select the two related words from the triad LION CARROT TIGER. We remain unconvinced, therefore, that semantic priming has been shown to dissociate completely from performance on tasks that probe explicit knowledge of superordinate categorization. However, it is clear that semantic processing may be adequate for a patient to accomplish one task (e.g., determine superordinate classification or show priming effects), but not another quite similar task (e.g., select two related words from a triad) (see Caramazza et al., 1990, for similar arguments).

To summarize, priming evidently occurs in patients who are thought to have damage to underlying semantic representations, as well as in patients who are thought to have impaired access to these representations. It remains unclear how and to what extent the nature of priming is altered by these different functional deficits. As far as cuing is concerned, there is some indication that patients who meet other (disputed) criteria for having disturbed semantic access can use an associated word to successfully complete the recognition process for a target, and that a loss of conceptual knowledge eliminates the possibility of cuing. (See chapter 4 for further discussion of cuing effects on word production.) However, all of these conclusions depend upon the correctness of other criteria for distinguishing access and storage disorders, and are therefore, at best, tentative.

Rate Dependency

A final criterion for distinguishing access and storage disorders, proposed by Warrington and McCarthy (1983), is that a semantic access disturbance is affected by the rate at which the material is presented to the patient for comprehension. These authors documented a globally aphasic patient (V.E.R.) who nevertheless retained a limited ability to understand spoken and written words. In a variety of picture-word matching tasks, the patient's errors were found to be highly inconsistent for repeated items (consistency of performance criterion). Furthermore, Warrington and McCarthy observed that V.E.R. was quite sensitive to the rate of test presentation. When items were administered with a 2-second interval between trials, for example, only 32% of her responses were correct on matching a spoken word to a visual object. With a 30-second delay between each trial, however, performance improved to 57% correct (see Warrington and McCarthy, 1987, for another description of a similar patient).

Warrington and McCarthy interpret the effect of rate as being due to a kind of rapid and pathological fatigue acting within the semantic mechanism. They propose that "the system mediating access to VER's verbal semantic knowledge base becomes refractory. Whether a refractory system is best viewed as an unstable one with an increase in the signal/noise ratio or whether the system itself becomes temporarily inactive is uncertain. . . . In purely operational terms the outcome would be similar, namely, a reduction in the ability to utilize the system efficiently for a period of time following activation" (Warrington and McCarthy, 1983; p. 874). However, rate dependency could be the result of how partially damaged stored semantic representations are used in these tasks, rather than of a disorder affecting access to intact reprecentations. Thus, this feature of performance does not distinguish storage from access disorders.

Summary

Let us summarize the criteria that have been proposed to distinguish storage from access disorders in the area of semantic memory. The fact that there are patients whose responses to individual stimuli on semantic tasks are inconsistent, and others in whom there is item consistency over different tasks, suggests that there are differences among patients that may reflect whether they have lost a concept (or part of one) or cannot access a concept they retain. However, the simple idea that inconsistent performance over repeated testing is a valid marker of disturbed access to meaning and that consistency must imply damage to stored semantic representations themselves, is too simplistic. Inconsistent performance is possible in the face of permanent damage to a representation (Caramazza et al., 1990), and consistent performance may reflect stimulus characteristics that determine performance despite a flawed access mechanism (Humphreys et al., 1988). Only in the case of item consistency over verbal tasks does it seem possible that consistency implies damage to semantic representations (Shallice, 1988). The validity of the other criteria we have described—frequency effects, preserved superordinate information, reaction (present or not) to priming or cuing, and rate dependency—is suspect. More research is needed to refine our theoretical grasp of semantic deficits and to suggest further ways to characterize the differences among these types of patients.

Multiple Semantic Systems

In our earlier discussion, we observed that the data obtained from normal performance offers little clear support for a distinction between verbal and visual semantic codes. More recently, however, the theory of dual semantic codes has gained new momentum from work on brain-damaged patients. This research can be divided into three different categories: (1) The existence of cueing effects limited to verbal as opposed to nonverbal material; (2) semantic memory loss that is specific to words or visual objects; and (3) anomia in one sensory modality instead of the more common naming disorder that affects all modalities. The literature dealing with the implications of these phenomena is hard to assess, because the basic question about what is meant by the term "visual semantics" remain unanswered. "Visual semantics" may refer to semantic properties of objects represented in a visual format—as, say, images; to visual properties of objects represented in a nonvisual format—as, say, a statement that elephants are gray; or to properties that have been associated with objects through visually mediated exposure to instances of the category—as, say, that lions live on the savanna (Caramazza et al., 1990). Most cognitive neuropsychologists who use the term "visual semantics" appear to be referring to semantic properties of objects represented in a visual format and to models of processing that maintain that these features are accessed from presented objects before other properties of a visually presented object are activated (Caramazza et al., 1990). However, other interpretations of the notion are also to be found in the cognitive neuropsychological literature. Keeping these different possible senses of the term "visual semantics" in mind, we now examine the phenomena that have been taken to support one or another model that incorporates the notion of "visual" and "verbal" semantics.

Modality-Specific Cuing

The patient A.R., described by Warrington and Shallice (1979), was impaired in his ability to read aloud or to compute the full meaning of written words, and to retrieve the name of visual objects or pictures. According to the authors' criteria, his disturbance was one of gaining access to the semantic system rather than a deterioration in stored semantic representations. Warrington and Shallice found that verbal cuing increased A.R.'s success at identifying a written word, but that his naming of the correponding picture showed a much smaller benefit from the verbal prompt. On one test, A.R. was given a verbal prompt (e.g., *Egypt*) before he attempted to read a target word (*pyramid*), and his performance was compared to his naming of the pictorial version of the target when given the same verbal cue. The cue helped more in reading than in picture naming. In a further test, the effect of a spoken cue on reading a word (*Egypt*—verbal cue: *Pyramid*—written target) was examined relative to the effect of a pictorial cue that actually depicted the target word (i.e., a drawing of a pyramid). Again, the facilitation provided by a word was much greater than was the case for a picture, leading the authors to conclude that A.R.'s semantic access difficulty for written words could only be aided by verbal information. Warrington and Shallice argued that these outcomes provided evidence for separate verbal and visual conceptual systems. They say that "If a semantic system common to all modalities were being accessed, then verbal prompts would be expected to have equivalent effects on object naming and word reading. . . Similarly, written word reading would be expected to be prompted as well by a picture of the object as by an auditory verbal prompt, since a picture would seem the closest possible cue. . . The prompting experiments, then, support the idea of at least partially independent semantic systems subserving object recognition and word comprehension" (Warrington and Shallice, 1979, p. 59).

We may raise a number of questions regarding the interpretation of these results. First, the observations by Warrington and Shallice concern the effect of cuing (or prompting) on stages of word recognition and comprehension, and therefore, as we have argued above, are more pertinent to controlled retrieval phenomena than passive activation in semantic memory. We do not know whether A.R. would have demonstrated automatic priming effects between pictures and words on a task involving reaction times, such as lexical decision. Evidence from normal subjects indicates that a picture can easily generate semantic priming when displayed for a brief interval before the onset of a verbal target in a word-nonword decision task (Carr et al., 1982; Vanderwart, 1984). Indeed, the complete absence of any change in the nature of priming across verbal and nonverbal forms of an object concept (i.e., the picture of a table or the corresponding word exerts equal facilitation on the time taken to recognize the word *chair*) has been taken as one strong piece of evidence against the idea of dual semantic representations. There are no data from A.R. on a comparable experiment, showing that the effects of a nonverbal prime are not obtained when a word is processed for meaning in an automatic fashion.

A second problem relates to the kind of information that might logically be expected to help A.R. in the controlled recovery of the label for a written word or picture. Warrington and Shallice found that spoken prompts improved A.R.'s reading more than his naming of pictures, and they argue for a dissociation between verbal and visual object meaning systems: "If a semantic system common to all modalities were being accessed then verbal prompts would be expected to have equivalent effects on object naming and word reading" (p. 59). Their assumption, however, requires that A.R.'s semantic deficit be functionally equivalent for picture naming and oral reading: if there is an amodal semantic system common to all forms of input, a verbal cue should have an equally powerful effect on the processing of a word or picture only if the nature of the disturbance was exactly the same for the two kinds of material. Warrington and Shallice claim that A.R.'s reading impairment was due to a problem in gaining access to the meaning of a word; a verbal prompt would exert its influence by making enough semantic information available to the access procedure to enable full comprehension of the target word. His object-naming deficit originated from an entirely different source. A.R. appeared to have little difficulty understanding the meaning of pictures; for example, he attained a score of 89/100 on a spoken version of the Peabody Picture Vocabulary Test, so that his anomia must have occurred after a visually presented object had been identified. Given the completely different kinds of impairment he had for picture naming and reading, there is little reason to assume that a verbal prompt would have the same effect on these two tasks. Our conclusion, then, is that this line of evidence for multiple semantic systems remains ambiguous.

Modality-Specific Loss of Semantic Knowledge

Patients with semantic deficits are not always equally impaired for pictures and words. Warrington (1975), using probe questions to measure the extent of semantic breakdown in three demented patients, noted some discrepancy between their comprehension of words and pictures. One patient, E.M., "was often able to recognize the visual representation of a concept but not the verbal, and AB was often able to recognize the verbal but not the visual representataion of a concept" (p. 655). Other aspects of these patients' performance indicated their agnosia was due to a loss of the detailed attributes of many object concepts, while they tended to retain a grasp of the general superordinate category. Furthermore, "each patient showed a remarkable degree of internal consistency. Their repertoire of known and unknown words or objects hardly fluctuated with time or fatigue" (Warrington, 1975; pp. 655–656).

We have seen that the criteria of consistency and preserved superordinate knowledge relative to attribute information have been taken as evidence for central damage to the semantic system. It follows, then, that the ability to understand a verbal concept when the same concept appears to have been permanently lost in the nonverbal form, and vice versa, must imply a distinction between two different semantic components. According to Warrington (1975), a particular concept "would be represented in two semantic hier-archies, the one primarily visual and the other primarily verbal" (p. 656).

The partial dissociation between verbal and nonverbal (or visual) domains of semantic processing initially reported by Warrington, though suggestive, was based on a small number of observations. Some researchers have questioned the result, arguing that superior comprehension of words relative to pictures or objects in a patient may simply be due to a subtle perceptual impairment affecting the identification of complex visual material (Riddoch et al., 1988). In fact, all cases documented to date with poorer performance in processing of pictures than words have shown this disturbance for categories in which objects are visually similar (e.g., fruits and veg-etables). This reinforces the possibility that poorer performance on pictures than on words is the result of a visual processing im-pairment, because these stimuli may activate several concepts, not just one. The reverse dissociation (better performance on compre-hension tests for pictures than words) may only reflect the existence of perceptual cues in many pictures that can be used by the patient to infer certain attributes of an object. The depiction of a lion, for example, may reveal the fact that the animal has a large mouth and heavy paws, so that a positive response would be reasonable in answer to the question "Dangerous or not?"

Other cases have been documented, however, confirming the pos-sibility of material-specific agnosias that cannot be easily explained in this way. Bub et al. (1988) have analyzed a patient, M.P., who showed very poor comprehension of written and spoken words. In general, M.P., who received a traumatic head injury to the left tem-poral lobe, was only capable of extracting the superordinate descrip-tion of verbal material, and even then with only a modest degree of accuracy. Unlike the Alzheimer patients documented by Chertkow et al. (1989), M.P. failed to produce semantic priming effects in a speeded reading task, an outcome that points to a severe constraint on the passive activation of meaning for verbal material.

Nevertheless, M.P.'s ability to understand pictures was consider-ably better than her understanding of words, both at the level of their superordinate category and when detailed knowledge of attributes was examined. Given the kind of information available to M.P. from pictures (e.g., she had no difficulty indicating the appropriate color for black-and-white line drawings of different fruits and vegetables), it seemed quite unlikely that her superior performance was mediated by guessing semantic attributes from visual cues. Bub et al. concluded that M.P. achieved a level of conceptual representation for pictures and objects that was unavailable to her from words. A similar dissociation between verbal and nonverbal comprehension has recently been observed by McCarthy and Warrington (1988). Perhaps even more startling is the fact that their patient had a selective disturbance in his ability to understand words referring to animals (though not inanimate objects; see the section below on category specificity), but experienced no difficulty understanding and describing the conceptual attributes of these same animals displayed in pictorial form.

An additional source of evidence indicating the lack of a simple correspondence between verbal and nonverbal semantic breakdown derives from the consistency of responses to the same items over different test sessions, presented either as pictures or words. Warrington and Shallice (1984) examined the semantic deficit of four patients who had made a partial recovery from herpes simplex encephalitis, a disease causing bilateral damage to the temporal lobes. They measured the item-by-item consistency of the patients' performance on repeated testing, and found it to be high provided that the format of the concept (verbal or nonverbal) was held constant. Thus, a significant degree of consistency was obtained either for pictures or words across different test sessions, but not across responses to the verbal and nonverbal form of the same concept. Warrington and Shallice commented that "a particular concept can be consistently known from its visual representation and consistently not known from its verbal representation or of course the converse. . . Our inference is that two semantic systems—visual and verbal—are implicated and both are impaired in these patients" (p. 848).

The possibility that pictures and words are not semantically equivalent is hard to dismiss in the face of these rather striking results. The argument based on consistency measures is complicated somewhat by the lack of general agreement regarding their functional significance, but the clear dissociation observed in patients whose intact understanding of an object concept is limited to verbal or nonverbal material is suggestive. While it may be too extreme a position to assume complete modality-distinct duplicate semantic systems, given the evidence from normal subjects that pictures and words ultimately activate the same conceptual representations, different attributes within a single amodal system may be called upon during the comprehension of visual objects and their verbal equivalents. Below, we consider one last piece of evidence pertaining to the issue of multiple semantic codes—the phenomenon of modality-specific anomia— before exploring this idea in more detail.

Modality-Specific Anomia

Typically, aphasic patients with naming difficulties show impaired naming regardless of modality, whether the target object be visual, tactile, a spoken definition, or an auditory event. Rare cases have been described, however, where the naming disturbance is confined to one sensory domain. Patients may be unable to name visual objects, for example, though they easily can produce the label to a verbal definition of the object or when they are permitted to experience the object through another modality (Beauvois, 1982; Lhermitte and Beauvois, 1973). In addition to optic aphasia, as this syndrome has been called, other reports of tactile aphasia (Beauvois et al., 1978) and auditory aphasia (Denes and Semenza, 1975) have also been published. There are no obvious perceptual deficits that can account for these particular forms of anomia. More puzzling still is the fact that the patients appear to identify the objects presented in a modality from which they cannot produce names, because they frequently produce appropriate gestures indicating their correct use. This last point is controversial, and we shall return to it shortly, but assuming it to be correct, how do we then interpret the modality-specific failure to name without giving up the assumption of a unitary, amodal semantic system?

Consider optic aphasia as an example: The patient has no trouble naming through an alternative sensory modality, so the concept of the object and the ability to recover its pronunciation must be intact. The object encountered in the visual modality is apparently categorized and understood, at least according to the gestures supplied by the patient. If a single, modality-neutral semantic component holds the knowledge responsible for labeling an object, why can't the patient name through vision, when naming through audition or touch is performed without difficulty?

The answer given by some theorists (e.g., Beauvois, 1982; Shallice, 1987) is that multiple semantic systems must exist, mediating object categorization in different sensory domains. Optic aphasia, in terms of this framework, would involve the preservation of visual semantics (i.e., the patient understands the object he sees), but its disconnection from verbal semantics, the component holding the verbal label and verbal associates of the object.

An alternative viewpoint, developed by Riddoch and Humphreys (1987), begins by questioning the claim that comprehension of visual objects is adequate in optic aphasia. The fact that patients can provide the appropriate gesture for a visual object, they argue, need not always imply that meaning has been correctly accessed. Many objects have properties that allow one to infer a reasonable gesture by analyzing the physical characteristics of their parts without identifying and categorizing the entire structure. For example, an unfamiliar object with a wedge-shaped blade on the end and a handle might lead us to make a scraping movement should we be forced to guess how to use it, and given that the function of many objects is necessarily linked to their structure (Bransford and McCarrell, 1977), we might have a reasonable chance of producing the correct gesture.

To be certain that patients understand a visual object, Riddoch and Humphreys contend, we need to examine more than the appropriateness of their manual gestures. Patients with optic aphasia may not achieve a complete semantic record of an object they cannot name, despite the impression given by their gestures, so that we need not assume the existence of a modality- specific, visual semantic system to account for the syndrome. In these patients, visual objects may not gain reliable access to a single semantic system from their perceptual description, but semantic knowledge remains intact and can be contacted through other sensory channels (e.g., touch) to mediate the categorization and naming of objects. Thus, optic aphasia may represent a particular and subtle form of visual agnosia.[10]

As support for their explanation, Riddoch and Humphreys (1987) document a patient whose modality-specific anomia fits the general description of optic aphasia (i.e., a marked visual anomia unrelated to any obvious perceptual disorder, with a relative sparing of tactile naming and naming to definition). While the patient (J.V.) often produced correct gestures to the objects he was unable to name, further testing by means of probe questions revealed that his comprehension of these same visual objects was far from intact. Riddoch and Humphreys concluded that access to meaning via the structural description of an object was disturbed in J.V., and that his gestures were the result of a preserved ability to infer a correct movement from physical attributes.

The interpretation of optic aphasia as a variety of semantic access disorder in the visual domain may explain some of the reported cases, but there are a number of other instances that are unlikely to fit this account. First, we need to ask just how specific are the gestures produced by a patient. It is reasonable to doubt the adequacy of comprehension if the gestures, though technically correct, are rather vague and insufficient to disambiguate the function of the object from other related or unrelated objects. For example, on seeing a tennis racquet, the patient may perceive that the object has a long handle for grasping and a round head for striking something. He may then indicate the general act associated with any object that fits the description <handle plus striking surface>, but the gesture would be roughly the same for a carpenter's hammer, tennis racquet, sledgehammer, sword, etc. Thus, vague gestures that fail to give one a precise idea of the mimed object's identity cannot be taken as evidence that the patient has understood its specific function. More detailed gestures, however, are not so easily dismissed; consider, for example, a patient who consistently uses her left hand to gesture when shown a fork, but switches to her right hand on seeing a spoon. Here, it is difficult to argue that knowledge specific to each object has not been contacted, particularly if other findings lend additional support to the argument that comprehension has taken place. Some optic aphasic patients appear to produce such gestures (Shallice, 1988), maintaining the viability of the interpretation of optic aphasia as a dissociation between visual and verbal semantics.

An Alternative Account of Modality-Specific Effects

There is an alternative formulation of optic aphasia, modality-specific semantic disturbances, and modality-specific cuing effects based on the notion that visual objects recruit specialized identification procedures containing a subset of the knowledge dedicated to the processing of object concepts. We discussed the possibility that identification procedures play a role in semantic tasks earlier in this chapter. Suppose that recognizing and naming an object is mediated only by activating the appropriate identification procedure, without requiring any contribution from additional semantic information not directly relevant to perceptual categorization. We have to know, for example, that a leopard has spots and that it has the form of a large cat, to identify particular exemplars of the concept, but the basic act of categorization would presumably not require us to also know that the animal is nocturnal or that it stores its kill in trees. Many of the modality-specific effects we have described could reflect a patient's processing of identification procedures or core concepts, but not both, and/or disturbances in linking these processing components with each other and with other processors.

For instance, naming of visual objects in optic aphasia is very poor, as we have seen, yet the name of the same object concept presented as a verbal definition is easily produced. One possible explanation of this dissociation is that the semantic attributes tapped by the definitions that researchers generally give to optic aphasic patients differ qualitatively from the knowledge that is needed to identify visual instances. The categorization of a physical object as an instance of a concept always involves the problem of translating a perceptual structure into meaning. A verbal definition commonly includes associative and functional properties of the object, which may not place the same demands on the semantic encoding mechanism. Consider the problem facing the perceptual system when we encounter a big, tawny catlike animal with big paws and a ring of shaggy fur around its neck. Now compare the definition of a LION supplied by *Webster's Ninth Collegiate Dictionary* (1986): "A large carnivorous chiefly nocturnal cat of open or rocky areas of Africa and Southern Asia" (p. 696). Clearly, the task of finding the concept that matches the input differs fundamentally in the verbal and visual examples. Optic aphasic patients are impaired in their ability to obtain the labels for visual objects after a relatively high-level stage of visual processing has been reached. We assume that a valid identification procedure has either been fully contacted or is partially available, but that the patient is often unable to map the resulting conceptual entity onto the form of a word. By contrast, the naming routine activated by more abstract semantic properties not directly linked to perceptual categorization remains unaffected, and the patient readily produces the correct label when given a suitable definition.

It is far too early in the investigation of modality-specific effects in semantic tasks to know if these effects are entirely explicable by invoking the notion of an identification procedure. However, it is possible that at least some of the effects we have described reflect the existence of modality-specific identification procedures as well as core concepts. Whether this is correct, and whether this would correspond to the notions of "visual" and "verbal" semantics developed by some theorists, is as yet unknown, but it seems a possible account that ties together many separate lines of reasoning and evidence.

Category-Specific Breakdown of Semantic Processing

Remarkable evidence has recently emerged from study of adult brain-damaged patients to support the claim that different classes of objects are processed differently at the semantic level. Some patients demonstrate a striking loss of comprehension for objects that is restricted to only a few superordinate categories, while performance on other categories remains much more intact. Warrington and Shallice (1984), for example, have reported a selective agnosia for living things and foods, along with relative sparing of inanimate objects, in patients with herpes simplex encephalitis. On a variety of measures—naming of line drawings, carrying out the gestures appropriate to foods or other objects, and word- picture matching—patients were found to be considerably more accurate for nonliving things than living things and foods (e.g., naming of objects, 80% correct; foods, 20%; and living things, 6%). Similar cases have been documented by Sartori and Job (1988) and Silveri and Gainotti (1987).

The failure of these patients to identify animal and food exemplars is unlikely to be the outcome of an incidental property like structural complexity or confusability shared by the members of each category , a possible explanation that a number of authors have raised (e.g., Riddoch et al., 1988). There is no indication that patients have any subtle disturbance in their perceptual abilities. For instance, they may show normal accuracy when asked to name photographs of man-made objects taken from unconventional viewpoints, a difficult task requiring efficient contact with the shape of an object in three dimensions. Furthermore, the existence of other brain-damaged cases showing relatively greater loss of comprehension for man-made artifacts, as opposed to living things and foods, rules out an explanation based simply on the claim that certain kinds of object are intrinsically harder to identify than others. Thus, Warrington and McCarthy (1983) have described a patient with left hemisphere damage and aphasia who was much worse at performing word-picture matching (with five response alternatives) for objects (58% correct) than foods (88% correct), and worse on a second version of the task (with two pictures as choices) for objects (63% correct) than flowers (96% correct) and animals (86%). An additional report showing a comparable advantage for members of biological categories has been described by Warrington and McCarthy (1987).

The demonstrations of category-specific agnosias in the neuropsychological literature offer powerful evidence that classes of objects with different semantic properties have their meaning derived by different functional mechanisms in the brain.[11] The nature of the categories represented in the mind and the brain, and the extent to which they mirror the formal distinction between natural kinds and man-made artifacts raised by philosophers remains unclear, however. Warrington and Shallice (1984), in their study of herpes encephalitis patients, adopted a broad classification of items into living things and foods on the one hand and objects on the other, a division that only approximates one that philosophers have emphasized between natural kinds and artifacts. Food exemplars used as test material by these authors included fruits and vegetables but also manufactured products like ice cream, beer, and chocolate. In one patient, a more detailed breakdown was provided of the categories yielding significant impairment relative to normal performance on a task requiring the patient to supply a definition for each exemplar (presented in the form of a word referring to the object). The categories reliably affected (i.e., on which the patient's scores deviated statistically from those of a control subject) were vegetables, trees, fruit, flowers, precious stones, fish, diseases, metals, and insects (all natural classes), but also musical instruments, clothes, and drinks. The patient was also found to be reasonably accurate in supplying definitions of another biological category, listed as "animals" (presumably mammals), indicating that neither the spared nor the affected categories in this particular agnosic disorder could be entirely classed as natural kinds or man-made artifacts.

Additional questions arise when further details of category-specific impairment are considered. The patient described by Warrington and McCarthy (1987), who was poorer at matching words to pictures of man-made objects than biological items, showed greater difficulty for small manipulable objects (e.g., "brush": 58% correct) than large objects like "tank" (78% correct). Obviously, the relevant distinction here cannot be described simply in terms of a dissocation between artifacts and natural categories. The explanation offered by Warrington and McCarthy for a dichotomy between man-made artifacts and natural categories was that artifacts are discriminated from one another within a given superordinate set more by their functional properties, whereas biological categories are differentiated more are differentiated more by their physical properties. It is not clear that this explanation is correct, or whether it will account for finer-grained dissociations such as the one reported between small and large artifacts.

Another issue concerns the locus of the functional impairment in the system responsible for the disturbed comprehension. In some cases (e.g., the patients described by Warrington and Shallice, 1984), the deficit concerns both the identification of visual instances and the understanding of their corresponding words. Other patients have a disturbance that primarily affects the mapping between word forms and the conceptual identity of an object, so that while naming or word-picture matching are impaired (the patient may label a peach an apple), the visual object itself is perceived and understood correctly (cf. Hart, Berndt, and Caramazza, 1985). This latter type of deficit would appear to affect the operation of the processing routines that translate between meaning and word units rather than the structure of the semantic mechanism itself. According to Hart et al., their findings suggest "that the lexical/semantic system is organized categorically and specifically at the level of the input and output processes to and from the system" (p. 440).

We may summarize our brief discussion of categories and the question of their psychological validity as follows. Recent analyses of brain-damaged patients who are impaired in their ability to process the meaning of visual objects or name them, or both, have pointed to interesting dissociations between categories that may in part correspond to the widely held distinction between natural kinds (or perhaps more conservatively, biological kinds) and artifacts. Patients have been described who fail to identify different animals, fruits, and vegetables, but who are much better when dealing with nonbiological objects. Other patients show the reverse dissociation, performing more accurately when required to understand referential terms for man-made objects as opposed to biological exemplars. There are ambiguities in the existing results, however, that limit us from drawing any strong conclusions regarding the nature of the categories represented in the functional organization of the semantic mechanism. Additional questions concern the variable locus of the processing deficits in the cognitive system responsible for different varieties of category-specific semantic impairment. Some patients clearly have sustained damage to processing components that are required to classify both words and visual objects as conceptual instances for selected sets of concepts. For other patients, the deficit would appear more limited in scope, affecting the comprehension (and production) of words referring to particular classes of objects, but leaving their identification of actual physical exemplars intact. These cases of selective "verbal" semantic impairments appear to result from disorders of the procedures that map certain classes of concepts onto lexical forms and spare the operations involved in the semantic processing of visually presented objects.

SUMMARY

We have described the classical theory of what concepts are, and several modern alternatives to that theory. We have seen that many patients have disturbances affecting the structure of concepts and the abilities to access concepts from verbal and nonverbal stimuli and to map concepts onto linguistic forms. These disturbances can be selective: they can affect processing of linguistic forms at the semantic level more than processing in the nonverbal sphere and vice versa; they can affect certain classes of concepts and not others. These disorders must be distinguished from disturbances that affect the processing of the linguistic forms of words themselves, which are discussed in chapters 2, 4, and 5.

NOTES

1. I use the terms "concepts" and "semantic representations" indistinguishably in this chapter to refer to representations in what has been called "semantic memory" (Tulving, 1972, 1983). Semantic memory is the store of knowledge that a person has about items and events. It is distinguished from "episodic memory"—memory for experiences in a person's own life. Semantic memory is also different from what is often called "long-term memory". Long-term memory is a system in which representations of stimuli are maintained for periods of time longer than a few seconds or

minutes. Long-term memory contains semantic representations, but is not itself the repository of a person's knowledge about items and events. The relationships between these memory systems—semantic memory, episodic memory, and long-term memory—are not hard-and-fast. It is also not trivial to differentiate these systems from other memory systems, such as those responsible for performance on some short-term memory tasks (like free recall and span tasks) or for unconscious memory effects seen in priming tasks. We will not attempt to clarify these distinctions further here, since this book is about language, not memory.

2. Biologists, for example, have tended to move away from essentialist definitions of individual species toward "polythetic" classifications—subdivisions based on individuals that share a large number of properties but do not necessarily all have any one property. Sokal (1977) points out that "adoption of polythetic principles of classification negates the concept of an essence or type of any taxon. No single uniform property is required for the definition of any group, nor will any combination of characteristics necessarily define it" (p. 190).

3. Alfonso Caramazza (personal communication, 1990) has pointed out that the speed of accessing an instance of a concept might contribute to a subject's judgment of its prototypicality, rather than the other way around.

4. These dimensions are often highly influenced by specific features, so the multidimensional view can overlap with the feature view.

5. Many exemplars of the concept must be stored, rather than one, because these exemplars differ in many properties relevant for perceptual identification.

6. The consequences of a semantic deficit can show up on tasks that do not involve language. Some authors have demonstrated that as a group, patients with aphasia perform abnormally on semantic judgments that require no explicit understanding of linguistic material; Cohen, Kelter, and Woll (1980), for example, reported that aphasic patients made many errors when asked to match two pictures on the basis of common attributes or actions (e.g., FROG matched to KANGAROO or SNAIL). Caramazza, Berndt, and Brownell (1982) found that a certain percentage of anomic patients (6/20) were impaired in their ability to judge the perceptual similarity between pairs of cuplike drawings relative to a normal and right brain–damaged group. The affected patients demonstrated a lack of sensitivity to the relationship between the diameter and the height of each object, a dimension that normally plays a crucial role in the perceptual differentiation of CUP from BOWL (Labov, 1973). The conclusion reached by Caramazza et al. was that certain anomic patients cannot reliably identify and label objects because they have lost their complete semantic description. Perceptual analysis of these objects will no longer be adequately guided by underlying conceptual factors (cf. our comments on identification procedures), and judgment of the visual similarity between exemplars will therefore be disturbed. This book focuses on language, however, so these nonverbal consequences of semantic deficits will not be explored here.

7. Any damage to object concepts would interfere with the comprehension of both verbal and nonverbal material, given the assumption that words and pictures make contact with the same underlying semantic representations. We discuss this assumption at various points in this chapter.

8. Patients do not generally have trouble matching words to pictures when the foils come from different semantic categories than the target.

9. The semantic lexicon is considered to be totally distinct from the orthographic and phonological lexicons discussed in chapters 2, 4, and 5.

10. There have been other suggested interpretations of modality-specific anomias designed to preserve the idea of a unitary semantic store. Ratcliff and Newcombe (1982) argue that two possible naming routes may exist for visual objects: one requires categorization of the object as a concept; the other is the direct (nonsemantic) translation of the physical structure of an object into a pronunciation (i.e., the second routine is analogous to the direct translation of print into sound). Ratcliffe and Newcombe maintain that the semantic naming route operating alone is inherently unstable, and therefore cannot be used to support an accurate naming response without the simultaneous operation of the nonsemantic procedure. Optic aphasia, according to these authors, is caused by a disruption of the nonsemantic route from perception, leaving naming dependent on the error-prone semantic mechanism.

The interpretation suggested by Ratcliff and Newcombe has a number of weaknesses (cf. Shallice, 1987). First, there is at present no justification for the reality of a nonsemantic naming route to visual objects, despite the evidence that such a route does exist for written words. Second, we have no reason to believe that the normal operation of the semantic pathway cannot deliver accurate responses. The motivation for this idea originally came from attempts to explain semantic errors in deep dyslexia (see chapter 5) by making a similar assumption; i.e., the nonsemantic reading route was assumed to be inoperative, and reading aloud was thought to be based on intact semantic translation of words into pronunciation (Marshall and Newcombe, 1973). Evidence since then has revealed that the paralexic errors in deep dyslexia must in fact be due to a partial impairment of the semantic route (Beauvois and Desrouesné, 1979; see also chapter 5).

The hypothesis of an unstable semantic naming route also appears unlikely on intuitive grounds. We normally have little trouble producing the correct label for an object when conversing: semantic errors, though they may occur, are few and far between. The explanation for optic aphasia given by Ratcliffe and Newcombe, then, does not appear very plausible.

11. Shallice (1988) has suggested that there may be "a giant distributed net [for semantic representations] in which regions tend to be more specialized for different types of processes" (p. 302).

4   Production of Spoken Words

A very common problem that aphasic patients have is an inability to produce the form of a word correctly in spoken language. There are several reasons why a patient may be unable to produce a word appropriately. He or she may have inadequate information about the concept related to the word, leading to an inability to specify the word semantically and thus to activate the word that is appropriate in a given context. He or she may be unable to access the form of the word, even if the patient knows a great deal about the word's meaning. He or she may have a disturbance in converting the stored sound pattern of the word to a form needed to use to send messages to the motor neurons. Finally, the patient may have a variety of disturbances in the actual production of the sounds of the word he or she wishes to produce. Disturbances of semantic and conceptual representations were discussed in chapter 3. In this chapter, I describe the processes involved in accessing lexical phonological representations, changing stored phonological representations into a form suitable for articulation, and articulating speech, and then describe disturbances of these processes.

ORAL PRODUCTION OF WORDS

Accessing Lexical Entries

When we speak, we convert thoughts into linguistic form. One crucial step in this process is activating the words that correspond to elements of thought. Most researchers assume that this process involves matching aspects of a concept to some part of the representation of the meaning of a word. We discussed the basic nature of nominal concepts in chapter 3. Concepts serve to divide the world into units, some of which make contact with words. For instance if a speaker wishes to convey the information that a dog is eating a bone, he or she must first divide the thought into elements that correspond to the meanings of the words *dog, eat,* etc., in order to match each of these parts of the complete thought with words. It would do an English speaker no good to divide the thought into units like *dog is eating* and to search his or her store of words for the lexical item corresponding to this thought, because this thought unit does not correspond to a word in English. The process of matching concepts to words is likely to differ in some ways for different sorts of words. The concepts corresponding to common nouns are quite different from those that correspond to abstract nouns; the former, but probably not the latter, can activate visual images that may become part of the mediating procss between concepts and words. Logical connectives such as *and, but, if,* and *or* are different again, as are prepositions, articles, and other vocabulary elements.

In addition to semantic facts relating to the items, actions, and properties a speaker has in mind, other factors also are relevant to the choice of words in speech. Syntax is one of these factors. When a speaker is looking for a word during sentence production, he or she often knows that the word must be of a certain grammatical category (noun, verb, adverb, etc.) to fit into the sentence that will be (or has already begun to be) constructed. Other factors, such as whether an item has been mentioned in the discourse, will affect a speaker's choice of a word, a pronoun, or even whether to delete an item (see chapter 9). Speakers use different words when talking to different listeners (e.g., children vs. adults). Thus, the search for a word is usually based upon syntactic, discourse, and pragmatic, as well as intrinsic semantic information.

Many theorists maintain that what is initially activated by concepts and other information sources is only part of what we ordinarily mean by the term *word.* A word includes at least four different types of information, depicted in figure 4.1. Two of these information types—the meaning of a word and the syntactic information associated with it—have been thought to be separable from the others. Together, these information types have been called a word's "lemma" (Kempen and Huijbers, 1983 Levelt, 1989). The activation processes we have are considering are those that activate a lemma.

We been focusing upon retrieving words (lemmas) that correspond to what we may call single concepts, such as *dog, eat, scratch, hit,* etc. As indicated above, not all concepts are related to simple words (e.g., the concept THE DOG ATE cannot be expressed as a single

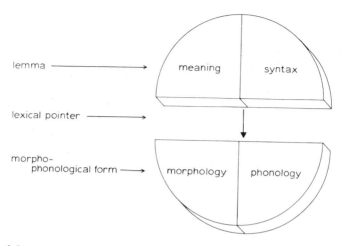

Figure 4.1
A lexical entry consisting of a lemma and a morphophonological form. (Reproduced with permission from Levelt, 1989, p. 188.)

word in English). But the opposite is also true: not all words correspond to simple concepts. The word *eating* refers to the action of eating going on over time; it contrasts with the meaning of the word *eaten*, which refers to eating that has been completed. This means that some words are selected on the basis of the combination of several concepts (such as whether the action specified by the intrinsic meaning of *eat* is ongoing or completed). Languages differ significantly as to whether single or combined concepts are expressed as single words, or as derived or inflected words, or as both of the latter. It is an open question whether all morphologically complex words (such as *eating* or *eaten*) are listed and accessed in the same way as simple words (see chapter 6).

Several models have been proposed of how word selection happens. One model that has been frequently cited in the aphasia literature is the logogen model proposed by Morton (1969, 1979a, b), which we reviewed in chapter 2 in connection with word identification. As the reader will recall, this model postulates the existence of units that are sensitive to a variety of different sorts of information, and which "fire" when their resting thresholds are elevated by the presentation of that information. For instance, the logogen corresponding to the word *dog* will have its threshold raised by the concept DOG, the syntactic category noun, etc. The logogen theory makes several predictions. One is that more frequent words are more easily activated. Some studies of pauses in speech bear this out, inasmuch as they show that pauses are more frequent before low-frequency words than before high-frequency words (Levelt, 1983; but see Beattie and Butterworth, 1979, for contradictory data). Other models include the use of discrimination nets (in which words are accessed by a process that checks for the presence or absence of features of the concept in a binary branching tree: Goldman, 1975), decision tables (in which words are selected by pairing conceptual features with the semantic features of lexical items in a pair of matrices: Miller and Johnson-Laird, 1976; Steedman and Johnson-Laird, 1980), and spreading activation models (see discussion of word form activation, below). An excellent review of these models is found in Levelt (1989).

This brief description of some of the factors involved in accessing the conceptual and syntactic aspects of words indicates how complex the process is. Despite its complexity, the process of accessing lemmas is accomplished extremely quickly. Normal speech is produced at a rate of between 100 and 200 words per minute. It has been estimated that the normal speaker has a "production vocabulary" of about 20,000 words. Based on speech error data, it seems that the wrong word is chosen only about once per million. No matter how words are activated, the only way for words to be correctly selected at this rate is for the search through the entries in a mental lexicon to occur in parallel, at least in part. Not surprisingly, all the models described above include some parallel search.

There is experimental evidence that indicates that this stage of word activation—accessing the lemma of a word—is separate from the next stage of word activation—accessing the phonological form of a word. Levelt et al. (1991) presented subjects with pictures of objects to name, and measured the effects of this task on the ability to make a lexical decision for a word presented at various time intervals after the onset of the picture. The words could either be semantically or phonologically related to the picture. These authors found that there was no overlap between the time period in which there were priming effects on recognition of semantically related words and that in which there were priming effects on recognition of phonologically related words (the latter came after the former). This suggests that activating a lemma does not overlap in time with activating the phonological form of a word. Levelt and his colleagues rationalize this organization of processing stages in terms of efficiency considerations for the word production system as a whole.

Accessing Lexical Phonological Representations

Once the meaning and syntactic form of a word are activated, the sound pattern corresponding to these features of the word must be activated. In chapter 2, I described the phonological structure of words, emphasizing linguistic analyses that postulated a variety of levels of phonological structure within a word. The questions I consider here are: (1) What is the form of a word that the speaker accesses in his mental dictionary (lexicon)? and (2) What stages does that form go through, if any, before it is actually uttered as the sound pattern of that word? I shall then discuss the question of whether the form of a word that is accessed in speech production is the same as that activated during auditory comprehension—i.e., whether there are two phonological lexicons (one for output and one for input) or only one (that is used in both output and input processing).

Several everyday observations indicate that a speaker must access a representation of the sound pattern of a word that is modified before it is actually articulated. Words can be uttered with various intonation contours, at different loudness levels, in whispered form (i.e., without any voicing), and in many other ways that lead to very different articulatory gestures being associated with their constituent sounds. The level of formality of speech, the rate of speech, and other factors also lead to different realizations of the same phonemes in a given word. Though we do not know the storage capacity of the human brain, it is unlikely that all these articulatory forms are permanently stored for each word in a speaker's vocabulary. What is much more likely is that a speaker accesses a standard (or "canonical" or "citation") form of a word, which is then modified as a function of speech loudness, speed, etc. The minimal phonological information that must be lexically specified is that which allows the speaker to assign the surface forms of each of the segments in the word in any discourse context. Aside from the nonlinguistic factors just mentioned that change the citation form of a word before its actual production, the citation form may also be affected by language-universal and language-specific phonological processes that make it unnecessary for every feature of each segment to be lexically specified (see the discussion of phonological structure in chapter 2).

Researchers have studied the representations involved in word production using a variety of sources of data. Evidence regarding the phonological form of words in a speaker's lexicon has come from data about subjects' knowledge of aspects of the sound patterns of words whose exact form temporarily eludes them. This "tip-of-the-tongue" (TOT) state occurs naturally, and can be induced in normal subjects by asking them to produce a low-frequency word from its definition. Brown and McNeill (1966) and other researchers have shown that subjects in the TOT state can frequently indicate the word's onset, the number of syllables in the word, which syllable was stressed, and sometimes the final segment of the word. These findings suggest that the TOT state arises after a subject has activated enough semantic information to specify a particular word (as would be expected in TOT states induced using the experimental technique described above), but when only part of the form of the lexical item has been activated. This partial information includes a specification of the first (and possibly last) phoneme, the number of syllables in the word, and the location of stressed syllables.

Additional evidence that these features of word form play important roles in speech production and are all accessed as a unit comes from the study of another type of speech error called a "malapropism" (Fay and Cutler, 1977). Malapropisms have three characteristics: (1) the error is a real word; (2) the error and the target are unrelated in meaning; and (3) the error and the target are closely related in pronunciation. Malapropisms are of particular interest because they presumably reflect a process of mis-selection of a word based upon the phonological similarity of the uttered word (the error) and the target word, and are not due to any semantic relationship between the error and the target. Fay and Cutler found that the target and the error had the same grammatical category in over 99% of malapropisms, the same number of syllables in 87% of cases, and the same stress pattern in 98% of cases. They also tended to share their first few phonemes. Fay and Cutler suggested that malapropisms arise when the words "nearest" a target are inadvertently activated instead of the target word.

The co-occurrence of information regarding the first phonemes of a word, its number of syllables, and the location of its stressed syllable in both TOT states and malapropisms suggests that this information is activated as a unit at a single stage of processing. The most likely stage of processing at which these aspects of phonological form are activated is when the form of a word is initially accessed, since they can be accessed when other phonological features remain unavailable and they are the basis for activation of inappropriate words. Obviously, information about the beginning of a word and its syllable content cannot be the entirety of the information in a word's lexical entry, since it is not enough to specify the correct word. There are many trisyllabic words that start with /f/ and have stress on the first syllable, and only one of them is the correct form for the word associated with the concept of "movable objects in a room or establishment that render it fit for living or working" (Morris, 1969, p. 534). Something more has to be specified for a speaker to use the word *furniture* to refer to this concept, rather than *fuselage*, *fugitive*, *funeral*, or some other word. If the interpretation of the converging data from TOT and malapropisms is correct, however, this additional phonological information—though lexically specified—is activated at another point in processing, or in a separate fashion, from that which is available in TOT and which forms the basis for malapropisms.

Another source of evidence that researchers have used to study the representations involved in word production is to examine naturally occurring speech errors. Fromkin (1971), Garrett (1976, 1978, 1980), Shattuck-Hufnagel (1986), Dell (1984), Levelt (1989), and others have shown that these slips of the tongue often affect only a portion of the sound structure of a word. This indicates that particular sound elements are separated out from the remainder of the sound structure of the word and are subject to an error-producing process. In turn, this shows that some part of the speech planning process involves just these selected aspects of the sound structure of a word. Slips of the tongue have been been said to show that a variety of units of phonological structure—distinctive features, phonemes, syllable components (onsets, rimes, nuclei, codas), and syllables—are all separately activated by the speech production process. We shall consider the evidence for the separability of each of these units in turn.

The errors in (1) and (2) below are taken as evidence for the role of distinctive features in speech planning. Fromkin (1971) argued that errors such as these could best be described as involving the exchange of the features [±nasal] or [±voiced] between the affected consonants. In (1), the feature [−nasal] of the /p/ is exchanged with the feature [+nasal] of the /n/, and in (2), the feature [+voiced] of the /b/ is exchanged with the feature [−voiced] of the /f/.

(1) *p*ity the *n*ew teacher → *m*ity the *d*ue teacher.

(2) *b*ig and *f*at → *p*ig and *v*at.

The error in (3) has been taken as evidence for the role of phonemes in speech production.

(3) you *b*etter stop for *g*as → you *g*etter stop for *b*as.

This error could arise through the exchange of multiple features, but this is unlikely. Shattuck-Hufnagel and Klatt (1979) have shown that exchanges involving several distinctive features are as common as exchanges that only involve single features, as in (1) and (2). This makes it likely that there is another phonological unit involved in errors such as (3). That unit is likely to be the phoneme.

In fact, slips of the tongue provide strong evidence for the phoneme as a unit of speech planning. Errors such as (4a) and (4b) indicate anticipation of later phonemes, (4c) and (4d), perseveration of a phoneme, (4e) and (4f), metathesis (exchange) of a consonant, and (4g) and (4h) metathesis of a vowel:

(4a) John dropped his cup of coffee → John dropped his cuff of coffee.

   b) also share → alsho share.

   c) I am not allowing any proliferation of nodes → . . . proliperation of nodes.

   d) John gave the boy → . . . gave the goy.

   e) Keep a tape → Teep a kape.

   f) The zipper is narrow → The nipper is zarrow.

   g) ad hoc → od hac.

   h) Wang's bibliography → Wing's babliography.

It may be possible to reanalyze these errors as reflecting the "next phonological structure up"—syllable components such as onsets, rimes, nuclei, or codas. Examples (4a–f) can reflect abnormal interactions of syllable onsets or codas, and examples (4g) and (4h), exchanges of syllable nuclei. But there is evidence that phonemes, not just syllable constituents, do exchange and otherwise affect each other. The critical fact is that individual phonemes within consonant clusters are subject to similar errors, as in:

(5a)   fish grotto → frish gotto.

b)   split pea soup → plit spea soup.

c)   brake fluid → blake fruid.

In (5a) and (5b), one phoneme from a consonant cluster has been moved and in (c) a phoneme from one cluster has been exchange with another. Individual phonemes can also be omitted from clusters. The clusters in which these errors arise occur word-finally as well as word-initially. It thus appears that the speech planning mechanism activates the phonemes of words at some stage of speech production.

Additional research has added to our understanding of the nature of the phonemes that are computed in the production process. Stemberger (1982, 1983b) has suggested that speech error data supported the existence of so-called archiphonemes—segments that are specified for their essential, underlying, distinctive features only (see chapter 2, note 2). Consider the error in (6):

(6)   in your scruffy clothes → in your gruffy clothes.

The word-initial segment /s/ has been dropped from *scruffy*, leaving a now word-initial velar stop consonant. In the intended utterance (*scruffy*), this stop consonant is in second position and is unvoiced. However, this consonant does not have to be marked as [−voiced] in the lexical representation of *scruffy*, because all English stops in this environment (after a word initial /s/) are phonetically realized as [−voiced]. The fact that this segment was produced with the feature [+voiced] in the error suggests that it was unspecified for voicing in the intended word and that it could become voiced in word-initial position. Stemberger argued that this indicates that features that are redundant in a given context are not represented lexically.

Errors involving phonemes also provide evidence regarding the phonemic inventory of a language. Fromkin (1971) argued that an important negative finding in her corpus was that the segments /č/ and /ǰ/, which can be split into a stop consonant and a fricative consonant—/č/ being pronounced as /ts/ and /ǰ/ being pronounced as /dz/—do not show splitting of these two component articulatory elements. Thus, errors such as the hypothetical example shown in

(7), in which the "d" portion of the /ǰ/ is split off and duplicated, do not occur:

(7) "In St. Louis," John said → In St. Douis," John said.

Similarly, diphthongized vowels (*ey, uw, aw,* as in *hay, who, how*) are always treated as a single vowel, as would be expected from a phonological analysis of English. These data thus indicate that segments such as /č/ and /ǰ/ or diphthongized vowels are single segments at the level of processing at which these errors arise. On the other hand, the sound of /ŋ/, in words like *sing,* can give rise to errors involving either the /n/ or the /g/ part of this complex sound. This corresponds to the underlying representation of this consonant in English, which linguists say consists of two segments. It appears that the sound pattern accessed and/or processed by the speech production mechanism includes a representation of the phonemes of a word, and that these phonemes are quite close to those described in linguistic theory in terms of their nature.

Facts regarding the distribution of certain types of errors indicate that syllable components are also processed in speech production. Syllable onsets and the two components of the rime—the nucleus and the coda—can be separately affected by error processes (8a–c). MacKay (1972) found that word blends (8d) were more likely to involve the onset of one word and the rime of another than to break up the rime between the nucleus and coda [as in the very rare errors of the form (8e)]. Shattuck-Hufnagel (1986) reported that 76% of exchange errors occurred between vowels in stressed syllables (8f). Exchanges between onsets and codas are very uncommon, either within or between words.

(8a) *space food* → *face spood.*

   b) *clip peak* → *cleap pik.*

   c) *do a one-step switch* → *do a one-stetch.*

   d) *grizzly + ghastly* → *grastly.*

   e) *grizzly + ghastly* → *gristly.*

   f) *debate focused on* → *debote feik.*

If the only phonological elements that entered into errors were phonemes, and if these errors were not subject to any constraints, we would not expect these patterns in the data. Two accounts of these findings are possible: errors affecting phonemes might be constrained by the position of a phoneme in a syllable, or syllable components can become involved in errors. Either way, the conclusion is that higher-order phonological structures are available to the production mechanism, since they affect the pattern of errors found in speech. This is confirmed by experimental results. Treiman (1983, 1984b) found that subjects were better at adding an additional syllable to a nonword after its onset than between the consonants in its onset (i.e., it was easier to change *skef* into *skazef* than into *sazkef*) and at adding a syllable between the nucleus and coda than between the two consonants of a coda (i.e., it was easier to change *isk* into *itask* than into *istak*). This indicates that onsets and rimes are units that are hard to separate during speech production.

There are other constraints on errors that are not easily related to the structure of particular words involved in the error, but appear to be due to the availability of phonological information about the sound structure of a language during the speech production process. We noted in chapter 2 that languages specify particular constraints upon sequences of phonemes in particular syllabic contexts. English, for instance, requires that the liquid that follows word-initial /st/ be /r/, not /l/; Italian requires that most morpheme-final syllables be open (i.e., end with a vowel). Errors obey these language-specific rules, even if segments have to accomodate to new environments to do so. The error in (9), for example, shows a change of the initial cluster /sf/ in sphinx to /sp/ when that cluster is interchanged with an /m/ (Fromkin, 1971). Word-initial /sf/ only occurs in a few loan words; it cannot appear in English in syllable-initial position. Therefore, when the first sounds of these words are exchanged, phonological rules further change the /sf/ into /sp/. The operation of phonological rules that are conditioned by morphology is illustrated by the examples in (10). In (10a), the /b/ of tab is interchanged with the /p/ of *stops*. In English, when a word ending in a voiceless stop consonant such as /p/ is pluralized , the plural marker takes the form of unvoiced /s/, but when a word ending in a voiced stop such as /b/ is pluralized, the plural takes the form of the voiced /z/. In (10a), the word-final stop consonants interchange, and the phonological plural marker accomodates to the newly created "word," demonstrating the automatic application of this phonological rule. Similarly, the plural marker in (10b) is corrected for the new consonant that it follows after /d/ has been changed to /t/ in the word *seeds*.

(9)   sphinx in the moonlight→ minx in the spoonlight.

(10a) tab stops→ tap stobz.

   b) plant the seed/z/→ plan the seet/s/.

Fromkin (1971) and others have argued that these constraints involve phonological and morphophonological rules of English, and have therefore concluded that the speech production mechanism has access to these rules. However, these accomodations may have a different origin: they may reflect a set of articulatory constraints that preclude the production of illegal allophones. Phonemes in errors adjust allophonically to their new syllabic positions, and most investigators believe that this is due to articulatory factors. The adjustments in (9) and (10) may have a similar origin. We should, however, note that allophonic variation is language-dependent. This carries with it the implication that, even if these accomodations are due to articulatory, not abstract, constraints on word sound production, they are still due to learned articulatory patterns that are specific to individual languages. They are not due to general motoric factors that determine ease of articulation.

In summary, the data from speech errors and experimental studies of word production indicate that the word production system computes distinctive features, phonemes, and syllable components. Interestingly, other phonological units that are important in linguistic theory, such as entire syllables, do not seem to enter into slips of the tongue. This does not mean that these aspects of phonological form are not computed during the speech production process. We have argued that the data from the TOT state and malapropisms indicate that the syllabic structure of a word is part of the lexical phonological representation that is initially accessed when a word's sound pattern is activated, and that syllable structure is one of a number of features of phonology that constrain errors. Apropos of the relative frequency of different error types, we might mention that distinctive feature errors are also very rare. This, too, however, does not imply that distinctive features are not computed: errors affecting distinctive features have been noted, and allophonic accomodation in errors reflects the operation of constraints on distinctive feature realization that arise at the articulatory level of processing. The conclusion that can be drawn from these studies of slips of the tongue is that different aspects of phonological form are computed at different stages of processing.[1]

The idea that different aspects of the lexical phonological representation of a word become available sequentially has been suggested by Levelt (1989), who has developed a model in which lexical phonological information is "fleshed out" in three stages. The first is the stage of "morphological/metrical" spellout and converts lemmas (specifications of the semantic and syntactic features of a word) into representations of the morphological and metrical (i.e., syllable) structure of the word. This stage would take the features INGEST THROUGH THE MOUTH TO GAIN NUTRITION and PAST and yield the information that the lexical item had a single morpheme and was monosyllabic (the word in question is *ate*), or the features INGEST THROUGH THE MOUTH TO GAIN NUTRITION and PROGRESSIVE and yield the information that the lexical item had two morphemes, was bisyllabic, and had stress on the first syllable (the word in question is *eating*). The second stage—"segmental spellout"—adds information regarding syllable constituents (onset, rime, nucleus, coda) and the segments found in each. The final stage—"phonetic spellout"—addresses actual phonetic plans that specify articulatory gestures. The data described above broadly support the division of word sound processing into the stages outlined by Levelt (1989). Levelt (1989) appears to think of these three stages as all being part of the process of activating lexical phonological representations and their phonetic values. Most other researchers think of at least the third as part of the speech production process that occurs after lexical phonological representations have already been activated. The important point is that the production of the phonological forms of words is "incremental," that it involves a sequence of operations that apply to various phonological structures—segments, syllable components, syllables,—and error-generating mechanisms affect each of these operations in normal subjects.

How are these phonological representations actually activated? Two basic types of models have been proposed. One involves a series of "productions" (Newell and Simon, 1972), in which a position in a frame is filled with a representation, and this activates a procedure that replaces or adds new information to the frame. For instance, a syntactic frame in a sentence may specify that a verb is needed and the semantic frame may specify that the verb should refer to the act of eating; the procedure triggered by this filled frame would then begin to activate the form of the word /eating/, beginning with the "morphological/metrical" spellout operation. The second type of model postulates the existence of units with certain features that match input specifications. These units have resting thresholds, are activated by appropriate features in the input, and fire when activated beyond a certain threshold. For instance, the lexical entry [eating] is specified as a verb, meaning the act of ingesting for nutrition, in the progressive aspect; when these features are present in the mental representation of an utterance, they all activate [eating] which then fires. Logogen theory (Morton, 1969, 1979a, b) and other "spreading activation" theories are of this type. As we have seen before in connection with word recognition, the main difference between these two types of theories is that spreading activation theories imply that many different words are all simultaneously active to varying degrees, since many words are compatible with parts of the information in a slot, while procedure-type theories tend to lead to the activation of only a single lexical item for a given slot. Spreading activation theories tend to be less sequential and less specific in what they activate than procedure-based theories. It is beyond the scope of this text to compare these models in detail with respect to how they account for data regarding the activation of word forms in speech. They both may play roles in activating lexical phonological representations. The reader is referred to Levelt (1989) for discussion of this matter.

Time Course of Activation of Lexical Phonological Representations

Speech production develops over time, and several researchers have suggested that some aspects of the phonological representation of a word are held in a memory system during the temporal development of an utterance. This temporary storage system has been called a phonological "buffer." Several pieces of evidence have been taken as indications that speech production involves a phonological buffer. One is the idea, discussed above, that different aspects of the phonological form of a word become available or are changed over time. However, though the incremental nature of lexical phonological realization could make use of a buffer, it is also possible that each phonological representation is simply transformed into its successor and that none are maintained for any signficant duration in a buffer. Another reason that is often advanced to believe a phonological buffer exists in the speech planning system is that many errors involve phonological units in different words (e.g., blends, exchanges, duplications; see the discussion of words in sentences below). This, too, is not a reason to believe that the production of single words involves a buffer. Perhaps a buffer is only needed when words are uttered in sentences and other higher-level linguistic structures (see below).

However, there is experimental evidence that a buffer is involved in single word production. The evidence is based on the finding of a "syllable latency effect" in single word production. The time it takes to read a word aloud increases with the number of syllables in a word (Eriksen, Pollock, and Montague, 1970), even when the number of letters in the words are the same (Klapp, Anderson, and Berrian, 1973). The syllable latency effect disappears when subjects are instructed to make a semantic judgment about the stimulus, suggesting that it is not due to input-side processing. In a related series of experiments, Sternberg et al. (1978) found that, when subjects were asked to recall lists of words as soon as they saw a visual signal, recall of lists of two-syllable words began later than recall of lists of one-syllable words. In this situation, the subjects already knew the words. The difference between one- and two-syllable words thus must reflect processes involved in accessing, planning, and beginning the articulation of the longer words. If the form of a word were simply activated from the beginning to the end, and articulation began as soon as the first sound of a word was activated, none of these results should occur.

These results thus indicate that the phonological form of a word is partially planned before articulation begins. However, the amount of time involved in this preplanning is very small for single words—10 ± 5 ms per word according to the experimental results just cited. Since most consonants occupy about 80 ms and most vowels about 200 ms of the waveform, this would not be enough time to utter more than a small part of a single consonantal phoneme. The mental specification of the preplanned aspects of the phonological forms of words is carried out much faster than the articulation of these aspects of a word's form. Many authors do not use the term "buffer" to refer to this very short-duration storage system, reserving the term for a slightly longer-duration store that may be related to articulatory codes and that may play a role in the production of words in connected speech.

The Number of Phonological Lexicons

Both the processes of recognizing spoken words and of producing words in speech involve activating representations of the sound patterns of words—a phonological lexicon. Do humans have one phonological lexicon that is used in both tasks, or separate lexicons for input and output phonological processing?

Considerations of a very general nature argue in favor of a single lexicon: it would seem a priori that such a system would take up less space in the brain and facilitate tasks like repetition and possibly learning a language. The argument for a single lexicon is also based upon the observation that patients often have disturbances affecting both the input and output sides of phonological processing. The first argument in favour of a single lexicon based on co-occurring deficits was presented by Wernicke (1874).[2] Caramazza, Berndt, and Basili (1983) described a patient of this sort. J.S. did poorly on tests of phoneme discrimination, in tests of matching written nonwords that sound like words ("pseudohomophones," such as *leef*) with pictures, and on tests of detecting rhymes in a set of printed words. He also made many phonemic paraphasias in speech and naming. Caramazza et al. concluded that J.S. had a disturbance in his phonological processing system, and that the co-occurrence of the impairment in both input- and output-side processing implied that there was only one such system. Though the authors do not explicitly say so, they imply that they conceive of this single system as one that includes the phonological lexicon.

Shallice (1988) has criticized both these theoretical and empirical arguments—the first for being entirely theoretical and hypothetical, and the second because researchers who postulate a single phonological lexicon on the basis of co-occurring input and output phonological processing impairments have not ruled out the possibility that these are separate deficits. As we discussed in relationship to semantic deficits in chapter 3, what is needed is the demonstration that the input and output deficits are similar, either in qualitative or quantitative terms, and no case study has shown this to be the case.

On the contrary, neuropsychological evidence appears to point to dissociations in processing aspects of lexical forms in recognition and production tasks. The most striking dissociations documented to date occur with written words and are discussed in chapter 5. These show patients who spell by a sublexical route but who read by a lexical route, and thus whose reading and writing deficits affect partially complementary sets of items. No such dramatic dissocations have been found in the neuropsychological literature for auditory processing, but other cases favor the two-lexicon model. Two patients (Michel and Andreewsky, 1983; Howard and Franklin, 1987) have shown an unusual disturbance, in which they make semantic paraphasias in repetition (e.g., *Eisenhower* → *Krushchef*) and cannot repreat nonwords. This pattern indicates that repetition in these patients cannot proceed via a nonsemantic route, but requires the activation of semantic representations (which give rise to semantically and associatively related words on the output side). Since both comprehension and naming were much better than repetition, the disturbance cannot be located in either an input or an output lexicon, but must be located in the connection between the two. It follows logically that, if there can be a deficit in the connection between an input and an output phonological lexicon, both must exist.

Data from normal subjects also support the two-lexicon model. Shallice, Mcleod, and Lewis (1985) showed that subjects can simultaneously read random words aloud very quickly and detect a given name in a list of auditory words randomly presented. This contrasted with the marked interference that occurred when subjects had to detect a spoken name while they were repeating auditorily presented words. The first task makes use of output and input processing of word sound patterns and the second makes use of input processing twice. The results suggest that the operations involved in output and input processing of word sound patterns are separate, since so little interference arose when both were in use.

Like many other questions raised in this field, the question of whether there are two phonological lexicons or a single phonological lexicon used in both production and recognition tasks is not settled. However, the evidence favors the two-lexicon model.

Word Production in Context

Although humans occasionally name objects and repeat single words, the predominant situation in which they access and produce the phonological forms of words is in connected speech. Indeed, much of what we have learned about the mechanisms involved in word sound production comes from errors made in connected speech that involve more than one word.

There are several similarities between the task of producing words in isolation and in context. Words are produced in isolation in two basic situations: when a subject activates a word on the basis of its meaning (naming objects, providing words from definitions, translation of individual words, etc.) and when a subject produces a word on the basis of its form (repetition and reading single words). In either case, the speaker can use semantic and syntactic information (the word's lemma) to activate a word's form, just as is done in discourse situations.

There are also differences between tasks of producing the sounds of words in isolation and in context. Though the same basic type of information is presented to the word form production system in the two cases, the way this information is presented to the mechanisms that activate word forms is different. The semantic stimulus for producing a word in isolation is usually a picture or a verbal definition (or some combination of the two when pictures are semantically cued); in discourse situations it is usually a mental representation of a concept. The form and content of such a mental representation is likely to be different from the semantic values activated by both pictures and definitions (see chapter 3 for some discussion of this point). Moreover, the concept that must be actualized in a word develops in the context of producing a discourse, and parts of it may unfold over time and become available to the word form production system in a different fashion than occurs when a speaker views a picture or hears a verbal definition. Finally, the basis for establishing the syntactic category of a word differs in typical single word production tasks and in producing words in context. For all these reasons, it is likely that the process of accessing the lexical phonological representations of words in context differs to some degree from producing words in isolation.

Aside from these differences, producing words in context differs from producing single words because words must be inserted into syntactic and intonational structures in context. Garrett (1980), Shattuck-Hufnagel (1979), and others have suggested that this process involves copying over lexical phonological representations into syntactic structures. However lexical phonological representations are inserted into sentences, the process provides the opportunity for errors to arise, both in normal speech (as we have discussed above) and in language disorders.

In addition to these differences in the processes involved in activating word forms, the development of the specific phonological form of a word differs in isolation and in context because of the effects of supralexical phonological factors. To this point in this book, we have only discussed the phonological structure of single words. However, the phonological structure of a single word is not the sole determinant of how a word is actually pronounced. Words always are pronounced with intonation contours; even when they are pronounced in isolation or in a list, they are assigned some intonation contour. In phrases, sentences, and discourse, intonation contours convey semantic values such as illocutionary force (whether an utterance is a statement, a question, etc.), focus and presupposition (whether an item is emphasized or assumed to be part of the discourse structure), and others. Because our present focus is on the production of word sound patterns, we will not go into the structure of intonation contours here (but see chapter 8). However, as we indicated in chapter 2, intonation contours interact with word sound patterns to determine the actual articulatory gestures of speech. As Mark Liberman (personal communication, 1988) has put it, both lexical and supralexical phonological structures make claims upon the same vocal tract.

One major effect of supralexical phonological structure upon lexical phonology is to reorganize lexical phonological boundaries. (See the discussion of Church's model of speech recognition in chapter 2.) Consider, for instance, the question:

(11)   Who do you want to see?

In casual speech, this can be pronounced as either (12a or b):

(12a)   Who do you /wɑnтɑ/ see?

   b)   Who do you /wɑnɑ/ see?

In (12), *to* has been cliticized in (a), creating a flap for the /t/, and it has been cliticized and contracted in (b), eliminating the /t/ altogether. The two lexical words, *want* and *to*, have been reduced to a single phonological word, with important consequences for how their phonological segments are pronounced.

The effects of supralexical phonological structure upon lexical phonology are profound, and are not limited to obvious cases such as cliticization, flap formation, and segment reduction. The absolute value and ratio of the first and second formant frequencies of a single vowel can vary through more than half the range of values for the entire set of vowels, as a function of the prosodic context of the vowel (M. Liberman, personal communication, 1988). We produce the segmental and syllabic phonological features of words within a prosodic envelope.[3]

At least parts of the prosodic envelope of an utterance are probably planned before an utterance begins. Gee and Grosjean (1983), Van Wijk (1987), and others have shown that naturally occurring pauses in speech are strongly related to phonological phrases, suggesting that they are planned as units. The initial height of the fundamental frequency of an utterance (F_0) is related to the length of the utterance, suggesting that a speaker sets initial F_0 as a function of utterance length (Ohala, 1978; Cooper and Sorensen, 1981).[4] Vowel duration is a function of the number of syllables in a phonological phrase (Nooteboom, 1972). These and other phenomena suggest that some features of prosody are planned in advance of articulation. This provides a rationale for inquiring as to whether some lexical phonological representations are planned ahead when planning at the intonation level is going on. Because of the interactions between supralexical and lexical phonological structures in programming the articulators, we might expect that this will be the case, and several lines of evidence indicate that it is so. For instance, in a variant of an experiment we discussed above, Sternberg et al. (1978) added function words to lists of words to be recalled (e.g., *bay and rum or cow*). These added words had no effect on the latency of initiation of repetition. Sternberg et al. concluded that the units of articulation planning were phonological phrases that were based upon stress patterns. Function words did not bear stress and were amalgamated into larger phonological phrases.

How far ahead of the utterance are segmental values of words' phonological forms specified? Levelt (1989) has argued that segmental and phonetic spellout (see above) can proceed on a phonological word-by-phonological-word basis (i.e., a stress-bearing group of lexical words). The fact that most exchanges of phonemes in slips of the tongue affect words in the same phonological phrase is consistent with this model. Anticipations tend to occur over phonological phrase boundaries and thus provide evidence that the phonological structure of lexical items is at least occasionally planned more than one phonological phrase at a time. Given the relative rarity of anticipations compared to exchanges, this may be an exceptional occurrence. Preplanning of the phonological forms of words appears to be limited to a few lexical items in most speech settings.

Two basic mechanisms have been proposed for how lexical phonological forms are activated in context. These follow the procedural and spreading activation models of lexical form activation discussed above, and can be diagrammed as in figures 4.2 and 4.3.

The procedural model replaces one type of representation by another. The spreading activation model also has this effect, but it does so by passing on activation from one item to its constituents. As we have seen several times, the differences between the models are that the spreading activation model activates more representations than the procedural model, because activation spreads "upward" from lower to higher nodes and then "downward" again to lower nodes. For instance, in the activation of the word *reset* in figure 4.3, activation spreads downward to the first syllable /re/, and then back upward to other words starting with this syllable, such as *resell*, and then downward again to the sounds in these words. In most models of this type, each node inhibits all other nodes at its own level in proportion to its own level of activation. In this way, the spreading activation in the up-and-down direction is damped out by inhibition spreading laterally within each level.

The spreading activation type of model can account for several features of speech errors, some of which are not directly explicable in the procedural type of model. Among these features are:

- Lexical biases in errors (Dell and Reich, 1981; Baars, Motley, and Mackay, 1975). Errors affecting phonemes are more likely to result in words than nonwords (e.g., *darn bore*→ *barn door* is a more likely error than *dart board*→ *bart doard*). This occurs because of the activation of lexical items by upward spreading activation.
- The repeated phoneme effect (Wickelgren, 1969, 1976; Nooteboom, 1973; MacKay, 1970; Shattuck-Hufnagel, 1985; Dell, 1986, 1988). Exchanges of consonants in syllable onsets are more common when the vowels or consonants in the following rimes are

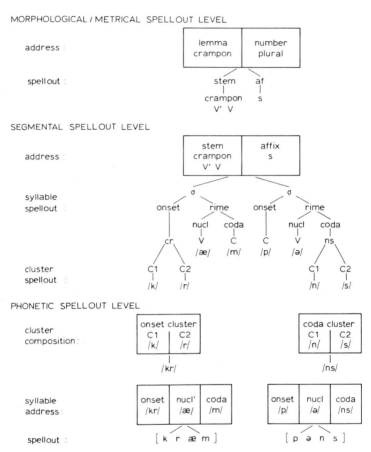

Figure 4.2
Levels of processing in the generation of the phonetic plans for the word "crampons," according to Levelt. (Reproduced with permission from Levelt, 1989, p. 345.)

FRAME   NETWORK   STRATUM

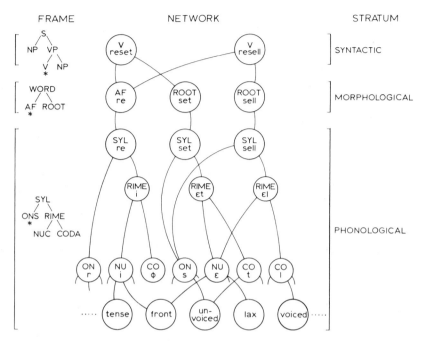

Figure 4.3
Example of strata, frames, and connected network in activation spreading
theory. (Reproduced with permission from Levelt, 1989, p. 352.)

the same (e.g., *fit to kill* → *kit to fill*). This occurs because of upward activation of syllables in the network.

- Rate dependency of errors. Dell (1986, 1988) has drawn attention
  to the fact that several features of speech errors are different in
  speech that is produced quickly or slowly. Both the lexical bias
  and the repeated phoneme effects, for instance, decrease substantially when speech is produced quickly. The spreading activation
  model accounts for this, because spreading activation takes time
  and, at fast rates, there is not enough time for all the up-and-down
  spreading activation that is needed to have higher-level nodes
  (e.g., words and syllables) influence errors.

The spreading activation mechanism thus has several features of
considerable interest, some of which we will see are relevant to
aphasic sound-production errors. Note that the spreading activation
mechanism does not necessarily conflict with the older serial-stage
procedural model. Both postulate sequences of representations that

are activated. The spreading activation mechanism enriches the older model by adding feedback from later to earlier levels of activation and lateral inhibition of items at each level of processing. The questions that we have been discussing—what types of representations are activated and what the basic downward flow of activation of these representations is—must be addressed by both types of models.

Articulation

The final stage of word sound production is the actual movement of the vocal tract to produce linguistically appropriate sounds. The structures involved in speech sound production include the lungs and the muscles that move them (the intercostals and, to a lesser extent, the diaphragm), the trachea, the larynx, the pharynx, the nasal cavity, the palate, the tongue, the jaw, and the lips. The subglottal parts of the system provide the source of air and the energy to move it. The larynx acts as a resonator, with the vocal cords vibrating between 100 and 200 times per second during normal voiced speech in an adult male. This determines the fundamental frequency (F_0) of the sound produced. Air necessarily passes through the pharynx and oral cavity, where its resonances are changed as a function of the shape of these cavities and the position of structures such as the tongue within them. The nasal cavity provides an additional resonating source when the palate is lowered. Resonances of the vocal tract, called "formants" and numbered consecutively from F_1 as they ascend the frequency scale, are systematically related to the positions of the articulators and the energy coming from the subglottal source. (See chapter 2 for additional discussion.)

The articulators are an unusual group of structures from the point of view of the motor system. The number of structures whose movements must be coordinated and the rapidity and precision with which they are coordinated probably surpasses that involved in any other naturally developing movement that humans make. There are several structural features of the vocal apparatus that make the system suited to this task, including the metabolism of the muscle fibers in the articulatory muscles themselves, the multiple sources of innervation of key structural elements such as the tongue, and the balance between moveable and fixed structures in the system. There are probably also features of the motor control processes involved in speech production that have the effect of allowing this system to function as it does (Stevens, 1983; Kent, 1986; Kelso, Tuller, and Harris, 1986; see Levelt, 1989, chapter 11, for a review). The system as a whole has two important operating characteristics: (1) it has a movement capacity such that transitions between the end points of articulatory gestures are not absolutely sharp, and (2) it is capable of rapidly adjusting itself to produce linguistically relevant sounds using different articulatory gestures. The first of these operating characteristics leads to the phenomenon of co-articulation. Co-articulation refers to the blending of the articulatory gestures associated with several single linguistic segments at a given point in the articulatory process (see also chapter 2). The same process is relevant to the articulatory system's ability to integrate lexical and supralexical phonological information in a single articulatory gesture. The second operating characteristic allows the system to accomodate to both exogenous and endogenous changes in its physical environment (such as speaking with a pipe in one's mouth or speaking in a totally nasalized voice).

The neural structures that control the articulatory system must receive information about the lexical and supralexical phonological structures that are to be realized physically in an utterance. Many theorists have concluded that the lexical phonological information sent to the neural control system is coded at the level of allophones. Levelt (1989) has argued that this information is coded on a syllable-by-syllable basis, in which phonemic segments are represented as allophones. Levelt takes several findings as evidence for this theory. The first is that allophonic variation is largely determined by the position of a phoneme in its syllable, and it therefore makes sense for these two pieces of information to be coded together. The second is that the articulators involved in producing vowels and consonants tend to differ. Production of consonants mostly involves articulators other than the tongue and involves the intrinsic tongue musculature when the tongue is involved; vowel quality primarily depends upon the position of the tongue body in the vocal tract and is thus achieved through the extrinsic tongue muscles (primarily the genioglossus). Thus, it is possible to program the articulators efficiently by separately regulating these two sets of structures on a syllable-by-syllable basis.[5]

Final Remarks

We have reviewed the highly structured and efficient processes that
are involved in activating the representation of the sound of a word
in a speaker's mind, and preparing that representation to be usable
in connected speech. The process begins when lemmas are activated. We have divided the process of producing the sound pattern of
a word itself into at least three operations: (1) accessing the permanent lexical phonological representation of the word, (2) inserting
that representation into a sentence, and (3) preparing that representation for articulation. We have seen that, though experts disagree as to the details of each of these operations, there is good
agreement on the idea that a word's lexical phonological form becomes available in a series of stages, rather than all at once. It is not
surprising that these complex processes frequently break down in
disease states. Nor is it surprising that there are different patterns of
breakdown that arise from impairments of different aspects of this
process, or that the effects of breakdown are constrained by the characteristics of the normal system.

DISTURBANCES OF WORD SOUND PRODUCTION

Disturbances of the ability to produce the phonological forms of
words are ubiquitous in aphasic patients. They take different forms.
Consider the following four performances:

• A patient is shown the picture of an octopus on the Boston Naming Test, and says: "Oh . . . I know what that is . . . that's an animal that lives in the sea . . . it's good to eat . . . the Japanese eat
  it a lot . . its name . . . oh . . . its name has something to do with
  a part of its body . . . maybe the legs . . . let's see [the patient
  then counted the number of tentacles] . . . eight . . . eight
  . . . octo . . . octopus."
• A French-speaking patient is describing the receipt of several
  packages. He says: "On entrait dans cette /gras/ dans cette salle
  /pɛRpadidylɛRma/." [We went in this /gras/ in this room
  /pɛRpadidylɛRma/; /gras/ and /pɛRpadidylɛRma/ are not French
  words].
• A French-speaking patient is asked to name a picture of a pencil
  (the French word is crayon, pronounced /krE jɔ̃/). He says "/krava/,

/krəbɛ/, /krevɔ̃/, /krɛjɔ̃/," pronouncing the segments in each of these utterances perfectly from the point of view of a trained listener (Joanette, Keller, and Lecours, 1980).

- A Japanese patient, whose speech sounds abnormal, is asked to repeat the word /deenee/ as part of a larger phrase. Using x-ray microbeam measurements, it is shown that the relationship of velar lowering at the point when the /n/ is pronounced varies in relationship to the movements of the lips and dorsum of the tongue in three successive utterances, indicating that the mechanisms responsible for nasalization and those responsible for the configuration of the oral part of the vocal tract are not coordinated as they are in normal speakers.

These four clinical observations seem to indicate different types of disturbances in word sound production. The first patient seems to have a block in activating the word he wishes to utter. We might guess that he cannot use the concept of OCTOPUS to access the form of the word. He attempted to activate the word by successively enumerating features of the object he wishes to name. Ultimately, he used the fortuitous fact that a physical feature of the object is related to the name of this particular object to activate the word he is looking for. Having once accessed the word, the patient immediately and unhesitatingly produced its phonological form without the slightest phonological disturbance. The second patient also does not seem to be contacting words, and produced very unusual phoneme strings instead of lexical forms. The third patient seems to know the word he wants to pronounce. However, in the process of producing the form of the word, he somehow mixed up aspects of its phonemes. His problem does not seem to be one of articulation itself: trained observers could not detect any abnormality in the sounds of the phonemes that are produced. What seems most likely is that the process associated with converting the lexical phonological representation into the form used by the articulators—the various incremental specifications of word sound discussed above—has gone wrong, leading to phonemic paraphasias. The fourth patient has a disturbance in programming the articulators.

These four performances seem to exemplify disturbances of different stages of word form production described above. The first patient has a problem activating the lexical phonological form of a word. The second patient may have difficulty accessing lemmas or the lexical phonological representation of a word, or both. The third patient has trouble preparing a lexical phonological representation for articulation. The fourth patient has trouble with articulation. Our review of disturbances of word sound production will try to relate these disturbances to these stages of processing of lexical forms, exploring the nature of the errors that arise at each stage.

Disturbances in Accessing Lemmas and Lexical Phonological Forms

The clearest sign of disturbance in accessing lemmas and lexical phonological forms is an inability to produce a word from a semantic stimulus (a picture or a definition), coupled with intact processing at the semantic level and at the phonological level when it is activated by a nonsemantic means. Intact semantic processing can be determined by a patient's ability to answer questions about pictures, and by other tests (see chapter 3). Intact phonological processing ability can be ascertained by seeing if a patient can repeat or read aloud. If a patient can answer questions about a picture, and can repeat or read words that are comparable to those needed in a picture naming test, failure to name a picture is most likely due to a disturbance in accessing lemmas or lexical phonological forms (though other possibilities do exist, as we shall see).

Disturbances in accessing word forms may appear in a variety of ways. Some semantic paraphasias may be the result of patients' compensating for an inability to access a particular lemma or phonological form (semantic paraphasias may also have other causes—see chapter 3). If a patient fails to access the form of a word, he may produce a synonym, a semantically associated or related word, a superordinate term, or a phrase. When these forms are produced in picture naming or other production tasks, they are usually considered to be semantic paraphasias or periphrases, and are frequently attributed to disturbances affecting semantic or conceptual representations. However, they could reflect disturbances of accessing phonological forms, along with the compensatory strategy of shifting to a synonym.

The phonological form of the errors a patient makes has also been related to whether he or she has a disturbance affecting accessing lexical phonological representations. Kohn (1984) argued that disturbances of accessing the phonological output lexicon would result in a series of random omissions, substitutions, and reordering of phonological features of a word. She identified a group of patients (all with Wernicke's aphasia) in whom errors contained abnormal numbers of syllables (in particular, extra syllables that were unrelated to the target word), scrambled phonemes within the target, relatively few target phonemes, and a large number of nontarget phonemes. All of these features of speech output suggested to Kohn that these patients did not access the complete phonological specification of a word in the phonological output lexicon. A similar analysis was presented by Butterworth (1979), who distinguished between two types of neologisms made in the spontaneous speech of one aphasic patient. One type of neologism was separated from the preceding words in the utterance by pauses of 450 ms or longer, and showed a random selection of phonemes in its first segmental slot. Butterworth argued that these neologisms resulted from the failure of the patient to access a representation in the phonological output lexicon, and the use of a random phoneme generator to produce a form that would allow the patient to retain his place in the conversation.

These analyses are not definitive, because similar errors can occur in situations where lexical phonological access is not needed. For instance, Lecours (personal communication, 1973) described a patient who said /aplagɛ̃dəplɔtis/ for the French word for "policeman" (agent de police) in a repetition task. This error has more syllables than the target and shows many rearrangements of target phonemes; by Kohn's criteria, it would be taken as a failure to access the phonological form of the word. However, the error has much in common with the target (all its phonemes are found in the target, for instance), and it arose in repetition, where the target is given to the patient. For these reasons, it is hard to use the form of an error (whether semantic or phonological) as an absolute guide to whether or not the form of an intended word has been accessed for production, and researchers have tried to apply more direct tests to see if patients access phonological forms of words.

When a patient fails to name an object, or produces an incorrect name, it is possible to investigate his knowledge of the phonological form of the correct word. Some aphasic patients are able to indicate the number of syllables in a word, or the first syllable, or the syllable that bears main stress, despite an inability to produce that word on a naming task (Goodglass et al., 1976). These features of word forms are those that are accessible in the tip-of-the-tongue state and that

form the basis for malapropisms. The ability to retrieve them suggests that the patient has processed word forms to the point at
which they become available, e.g., the morphology/metrical spellout stage in Levelt's model. Patients may also be tested for their
abilities to select from an array of pictures two pictures whose
names rhyme or share other phonological features. Again, good performance indicates that a patient has access to at least some features
of word form. Not enough research of this type has been undertaken
to know if the features of word form that are accessed under these
task conditions can be easily related to aspects of phonological representations postulated to be activated at specific stages of word
output processing in models of this process in normals. In addition,
though positive results of these tests clearly indicate that a patient
has at least partial access to lexical phonology, the opposite
performance—an inability to produce or indicate these aspects of
word form—cannot unequivocally be taken to imply a failure to access the phonological form of a word. A patient may fail on these
tasks for a variety of reasons other than an inability to access lexical
phonological forms.

Is it possible to distinguish disturbances in accessing lemmas
from disturbances in accessing lexical phonological representations? If a patient has some knowledge of the form of a word (as seen
in some resemblence between the phonemic paraphasia and the
target or good performance on picture homophone- or rhyme-
matching tasks), we would be able to say that some portion of the
word's form has been activated. If a lemma must be activated before
a word's form can be accessed at all, this would imply that the patient has accessed the lemma and is failing to access word form.
However, if the patient makes no response or produces sound sequences that have no relationship to the target (or to any word), and
cannot demonstrate knowledge of aspects of word form, we cannot
tell whether he or she is failing to access lemmas or is accessing
lemmas but no part of the form of a word.

Cuing is frequently used in an effort to improve aphasic patients'
performances. Many researchers have suggested that the response of
a subject to phonological prompting or cuing also indicates whether
or not he or she has accessed word forms normally. The logic behind
this approach is that, if a patient has lost the permanent representation of a word in the phonological output lexicon, he or she will not
benefit from cues or prompts based upon phonological form, but if a

patient has trouble activating a representation that is still present in the phonological output lexicon, cuing with aspects of the phonological form of a word could lead to improved performance. Thus, the effectiveness of phonological cuing is said to be of help in distinguishing between the total loss of the phonological representation needed for speech production and a disturbance of accessing a representation that is still present. However, the interpretation of the results of cuing is not straighforward. Cuing may fail to improve performance even if some part of a lexical phonological representation is retained (for instance, if the cue simply provides information about phonological form that the patient already has, it would not be expected to improve performance), so we cannot unequivocally associate failure of cuing to improve performance with loss of lexical phonological representations. Also, phonological cuing may improve performance if a patient's problem arises at the planning stage (see below). Goodglass and his colleagues (Goodglass et al., 1976) have demonstrated that there is considerable variation in the effectiveness of phonological cuing in aiding patients who cannot name objects. However, whether this variation is systematically related to subjects' knowledge of phonological aspects of the words they wish to pronounce remains unknown.

The effects of semantic cuing may also help in determining the locus of a deficit in the word production process, though, again, the patterns we see are not always immediately interpretable. It is intuitively understandable that semantic cuing might help a patient find a word for a concept if he or she had an inadequately precise specification of the concept (see chapter 3 for further discussion of semantic cuing and priming in patients with semantic disorders). However, semantic cuing sometimes appears to help patients who know a great deal about a concept and whose problems arise at the stage of lemma or lexical phonological access, as in the case of the first patient we described. In that particular instance, the patient found the name of the item because of a peculiarity of its phonological form—that it partly reflected a physical feature of the animal. In most cases, phonological form is arbitrarily related to word meaning, but clinical experience indicates that there are instances in which patients appear to cue themselves regarding an item by enumerating its characteristics or are helped by an examiners' semantic cues. Thus semantic cuing, by the patient or an examiner, does seem to be effective in helping access phonological representations. Semantic cuing would not be expected to be helpful if a phonological representation were lost or if a patient had a planning disturbance.

Taken together, phonological and semantic cuing can thus be helpful. Positive effects of either indicate that phonological representations have not been lost. Positive effects of semantic cuing are most consistent with the view that a word production disturbance lies at the level of concepts or lexical phonological access, whereas positive effects of phonological cuing suggest a disturbance in lexical phonological access or planning. Thus, positive effects of both types of cuing suggest a disturbance in lexical phonological access; positive effects of semantic cuing and no effects of phonological cueing suggest a conceptual or semantic disturbance; and positive effects of phonological cuing and no effects of semantic cuing suggest a planning disturbance. These interpretations are not hard and fast but, coupled with other aspects of performance, they may help in deciding where a subject's word production problems lie.

It is quite clear that all of these criteria—the nature of a patient's output errors, the ability of a patient to indicate the phonological features of a word through picture matching or other means, and the ability of a patient to benefit from phonological and semantic cuing or prompting—are individually and collectively inadequate to prove absolutely that a patient cannot activate the lemma or lexical phonological representation of a word. In each case, there are other explanations for these performances. Nonetheless, a convergence of performances would make it quite likely that a patient suffers from a disturbance at the level of activating lemmas or the phonological forms of words, or of both.[6]

Disturbances of Word Sound Planning

Phonemic paraphasias have classically been thought to reflect a patient's inability to "plan" the sound pattern of a word. In terms of the stages of processing described above, this refers to the conversion of the representation of the sounds of a word into a form appropriate for articulatory production. Before we discuss these errors, we should consider a potentially confusing aspect of nomenclature. The term *planning* has traditionally been used to refer to errors that arise after a lexical phonological representation has been accessed and before articulation begins. Most aphasiologists have not been very specific about what processes apply to lexical phonological representations between these two end points. The model that most aphasiologists seem to work with maintains that lexical phonological representations consist of a specification of the phonemes of a word, possibly organized into syllables. However, we have seen that most psycholinguists are working with a second type of model in which different aspects of the phonological structure of a word become available at different stages. There is more processing associated with lexical phonological activation in the second than in the first type of model. Consequently, an error can be ascribed to a stage of activation of lexical phonological representations in the second type of model that does not exist in the first type. For instance, exchanges of phonemes within a word can be ascribed to the phonemic spell-out stage of lexical phonological activation in Levelt's model, but can only be ascribed to a stage of postlexical phonological processing (such as inserting lexical items into syntactic frames) in the first type of model, because no intralexical stage of phonological processing exists in that type of model. We might want to say that, in the second type of model, this is an error of a part of the lexical phonological access process, not "planning."

The real issue is not terminological, however, but scientific. We cannot ascribe errors to different stages of processing until we are sure of what the stages are. Since models of these processes are only now being developed, we will have to live with some uncertainty for the present. In the discussion to follow, I use the term "planning," attempting as best I can to ascribe errors to disturbances of stages of activation of lexical phonological forms or processes related to inserting these representations into sentences and integrating them with prosodic and other aspects of sound in preparation for articulation. To the extent possible, I try to indicate the model that individual researchers use as I present results.

The evidence for the existence of disturbances in word sound planning comes from three sources. First, some phonemic paraphasias are related to target words in ways that suggest that they are due to disturbances in planning word sounds. Second, some patients indicate that they appreciate that they have difficulty in getting the right sounds and sound sequences in a word, by making multiple attempts to produce the correct form of a word. Third, some patients show a pattern of performance across tasks that suggests that this is the stage of processing at which phonemic paraphasias arise.

Table 4.1
Examples of Word-interaction Errors*

---

1. Nancy sold the table→/Ne*i*lsi/sold/dʌ/table.

C.M.'s attempt at "Nancy" contains two complete anticipatory copies involving substitution. Two vowels with main stress interacted in the copying of the /ei/ from "table" into the slot for /æ/ in "Nancy." Also, the /l/ from "sold," and possibly from "table," is copied into the coda slot that should have contained an /n/.

2. Tim flies planes. → /Tʌmz/, Tim*s* plane, planes, planes.

The /z/ of "flies" and/or "planes" is added to the end of "Tim" as an anticipatory copy in coda position.

3. Jane rode her bike to the store. → Jo*a*n. /dʌ. dʌ/—

The vowel from "rode" interacted with "Jane" in an anticipatory copy. The copy is incomplete because the target word that was the source of the copied phoneme (i.e., "rode") was not produced.

4. Nurses tend patients. → /N*ei*, N*ei*/—

This example is another incomplete anticipatory copy in which vowels of the same stress level interacted (i.e., "nurses" and "patients").

5. Children wear mittens. → /tʃIld/.children/wIl.wi. wi. iwItən. wItəpn/.

This example contains two perseveratory copies involving substitution: The /l/ from "children" is copied into the /r/slot in "wear," and the /w/ from "wear" is copied into the initial slot in "mittens."

6. She grows tomatoes and broccoli. → She grows /p-/. bananas. no. /təma*k*. tawa*ti*. towa*ti*z/ and /tamatos/ and. uh—

The /k/ and /i/ in "broccoli" are copied into his attempts to say "tomatoes." These are perseveratory copies, with the consonant copy preserving

---

The first source of evidence that phonemic errors arise during planning processes comes from the observation that certain errors are closely related to their targets. Examples taken from Kohn and Smith (1990) are listed in table 4.1.

A second source of evidence that aphasic patients have disturbances in planning the sound patterns of words whose phonology they have accessed comes from the observations made on successive phonemic approximations in naming tasks. Examples are given in table 4.1. Joanette et al. (1980) noted that about half the successive attempts to produce a word made by some aphasic patients became progressively closer to the target in terms of the number of distinctive features separating the utterance from the target. In these cases, it must be the case that the patient knows the target representation and does not produce it properly. In the cases in which successive

Table 4.1
Continued

syllabic position. Notice that the possible copy of the /o/ from "grows" to /towatiz/ was not considered because it can also be considered to be a within-word copy.

7. Dan hates milk. → Dan/*hæn*/—

There is perseveratory copy of both the vowel and coda in "Dan" to "hates."

8. Matthew broke his ankle. → Mæ*k*u. Mæ*k*/.Matthew—

The /k/ from "broke" was copied into "Matthew" into an ambisyllabic slot.

9. Joe took his dog on a walk. → l*og*, /dzorg/.he/tUrk.tʌ/—

The /ɔg/ of "dog" was copied into "Joe." /Dzorg/ was not analyzed becuase the target word is unclear: perhaps he was trying to say "Joe" or "dog."

10. Tom baked the cookies. → Tom /bei/. baked /dʌ.t*ʌ*./Umi./Uk*ə*./Uk./ Uki/.

The /t/ in "Tom" was perseveratively copied into the initial slot of "cookies," preserving position insofar as the interacting consonants were both syllable (and word) onsets.

11. William plays the organ. → Willian /r-r/-plays the /kʌ. wɔr-.wɔrg/.

The initial phoneme of "William" is perseveratively copied in front of the initial phoneme of "organ," thus involving addition, as opposed to substitution.

Reproduced with permission from Smith and Kohn, 1990, p. 145.
* Only the copied (i.e. incorrect) phonemes are in italic.

productions were progressively more distant from the target, patients often stopped producing a sequence of approximations, and sometimes produced semantically related words or synonyms (a so-called synonymic shift, mentioned above). These shifts provide evidence suggesting that the patient knew he or she was progressively deviating from the target word, and therefore knew the sound of the target.

A third argument, that some phonological disturbances occur in the planning of the sounds of a word, is based upon the comparison of a patient's performance across multiple tasks. Caplan et al. (1986a) reported a patient, R.L., who made similar phonological errors in word repetition, word reading, and picture naming, in each case producing errors closely related to the target word and showing a strong word length effect (see below). Since the form of the word was given to the patient directly in the repetition task and indirectly (through its orthographic form) in the reading task, errors in these tasks could not have been due to R.L.'s inability to access the form of the word from semantics. Rather, they must reflect some disturbance of processing the word. Since the errors were similar in the three tasks, they are not likely to have been due to disturbances affecting input processing: the input processing is different in reading and repetition and no input-side linguistic processing is needed at all in picture naming. The errors were not low-level articulatory in nature. The errors thus most likely arose in the process of planning the form of the word that is suitable for articulation. Other patients (sometimes termed "reproduction conduction aphasics") with similar patterns of performance have been described by other researchers (Ellis, 1982; Miller and Ellis, 1987; Bub et al., 1987).

These three sets of observations and lines of reasoning all suggest that some disturbances resulting in the production of phonemic paraphasias occur after a word's form has been accessed, and before that form is actually articulated. These disturbances thus all fall at the stage of production that we have been calling the sound planning stage. What determines the likelihood of producing a phonological error at this stage of processing? An obvious factor is the complexity of the sound structure of the word that must be produced. Though there are many aspects of word form that might make one word harder to produce than another (e.g., the nature of the consonants or vowels in the word), one factor dominates the list of those that make for phonological errors: the number of syllables in a word. In many cases, patients who make phonemic paraphasias show an effect of word length. Words of three or more syllables are particularly difficult for many patients. Other aspects of word form do affect this process, as well as length, though their effects are less marked and more variable. Consonant clusters are often harder to produce than single consonants. Beland, Caplan, and Nespoulous (1990) have argued that words that are hard to syllabify (e.g., words with adjacent vowels in French, which require special syllabification rules) are harder than words that follow the simpler syllabification rules of a language. The full range of aspects of form that affect patients' abilities to plan the sound structure of a word are not yet known.

In contrast to the strong effects of length and the weaker but sometimes discernible effects of other aspects of word form upon the frequency of phonemic paraphasias, many other aspects of words have variable effects, or do not affect the occurrence of phonemic paraphasias, as far as is known. Word frequency, for instance, has a variable effect upon the occurrence of these types of errors: in some patients (e.g., Pate, Saffran, and Martin, 1987) the effect is minor, while in others (McCarthy and Warrington, 1984) it is more pronounced. Semantic features such as abstractness and imageability have not been shown to determine whether or not phonemic paraphasias arise. Grammatical class is an interesting parameter in this respect. There is no documented case of a patient who made increased numbers of phonemic paraphasias with one or two of the major grammatical categories (nouns, verbs, adjectives) compared to the remaining major grammatical categories. However, in most patients, phonemic paraphasias do not occur in function words, or only rarely affect function words, compared to these major grammatical categories. This may reflect the increased frequency of the function words in the language. However, it may be that the processes of accessing and planning the sound values of function words are different from those for content words, and less subject to the disturbances that produce phonological errors than the latter (see chapter 8).

Phonemic paraphasias that arise at this stage of processing are extremely unusual in normal subjects in tasks that involve single word production. The slips of the tongue we discussed above all occur in discourse, not in naming objects or in repetition or reading of single words. In this respect, aphasic patients make errors that are only very infrequently seen in normals. The errors themselves are similar to those seen in normals in certain respects—they involve exchanges, substitutions, and deletions of segments, and do not violate the phonotactic rules of the language. However, many phonemic paraphasias have properties that are very different from normal slips of the tongue. Exchanges and duplications of consonants in onsets and codas, and exchanges and duplications of entire syllables, are quite common in aphasic phonemic errors, and virtually nonexistent in normal slips of the tongue. It is tempting to conclude that most normal sound errors occur after a speaker has accessed the form of a word, and when he or she integrates that form into a sentence and prepares the resulting form for articulation, while many aphasic sound-based errors arise during the process of accessing or planning the form of a word. Phonemic paraphasias arising in single words—especially complex ones—have in fact been cited as an example of a type of error that does not occur in normals, and the question of whether they arise because of new psychological operations that arise after brain damage has been raised. It is not necessary that this latter view be correct; these errors could arise because a process that rarely goes wrong in normals (accessing the entire form of the word) is disrupted in aphasia and mechanisms already present in the brain are used to compensate for this new disturbance with new resulting error types.

Several models of the error-generating mechanisms involved in producing phonemic paraphasias have been proposed. An early contemporary paper by Lecours and Lhermitte (1969) developed a broad framework for viewing these errors. The authors suggested that phonemic paraphasias could be seen as additions, deletions, displacements, and replacements of either phonemes or distinctive features of words. Words were considered to consist of sequences of phonemes each of which had a distinctive feature composition; higher-order organization of phonemes into syllables and other structures was not considered. The authors hypothesized that substitutions would be more likely to involve phonemes with minimally different distinctive feature compositions, and that replacements would be more likely among phonemes that shared many distinctive features and were minimally separated in the word. They thus predicted that many phonemic paraphasias would be influenced by neighboring phonemic context (e.g., /probité/ → /propité/, in which the substitution of /p/ for /b/ may have been affected by the presence of another /p/ in the word). In addition, the authors argued that the basic phonemic errors they postulated could be additive, as in /agriculteur/ → /agructulgure/. Lecours and Lhermitte suggested that phonemes activate their distinctive features and that the time course of this activation is such that a phoneme begins to become active prior to its actual production and remains active for some time thereafter. The authors believed that these activated patterns of distinctive features interfere with each other to yield phonemic paraphasias. The authors provided examples of the operation of these error-generating processes.

Many aspects of this model are likely to be incorrect. The most obvious problem with the model is that the error-generating mechanism can generate any phonological error at all. For instance, as it stands, the model predicts that movements of phonemes to create impossible consonant clusters or vowel sequences are just as likely to occur as movements that create legal sequences. However, actual errors are reasonably highly constrained; for instance, illegal clusters hardly ever occur. These constraints appear to be due to the tempering of phonemic error generation by higher-order phonological structures. This implies that these structures are available to the speech production system, possibly because they are lexically represented or because they reflect the operation of general phonological rules that apply during word sound production (as in the Beland et al. model discussed below). The first of these possibilities implies that Lecours and Lhermitte's model of lexical phonological representations is inaccurate, and the second, that their model of phonological processing is incomplete. A second problem is that some of the model's predictions are not true of all aphasic patients. For instance, Nespoulous et al. (1984) found that single consonantal substitutions in word repetition were closely related to the target phoneme in terms of distinctive features in only some patients. Despite these problems, the Lecours-Lhermitte model made the clear statement that phonemic errors could be due to disturbances that arose after lexical phonological representations were accessed and before they were converted to articulatory plans. The problems with the model simply illustrate that the error-generating processes that arise in these mechanisms are subject to constraints and differ in different aphasic patients.

Another model of lexical phonological processing that has been applied to phonemic paraphasia has been developed by Beland and her colleagues (Beland et al., 1990). The authors based their theory on the observation that phonemic errors respect relationships between three different levels of phonological structure: segments, syllables, and stress contours. In the vast majority of phonemic paraphasias, however complicated, syllabification is appropriate for the phonemic content of an utterance, and stress contour is appropriate for both syllabification and phonemic content. Beland et al. relied on phonological theory to model the intricate interaction between segmental phonology, syllable structure, and word stress contours in phonological errors. They argued that the preservation of these relationships would be accounted for if phonemic paraphasias were due to changes in segmental representations that were then subject to the rules of word-level phonology, including syllabification and stress assignment. An abnormal segment would trigger a set of syllabification and stress-assignment rules (not those triggered by the original segment, but those rules that were appropriate for the erroneous segment). Striking examples of this mechanism were given by Schnitzer (1972) in a study of a dyslexic patient. For instance, Schnitzer's patient read the word *reconcile* as /raykan'sil/, providing three changes of vowel quality and a change in the location of main stress. Schnitzer pointed out that all these changes would occur if the patient changed the final long /i/ in *reconcile* to a short /i/, and then applied the syllabification and stress-assignment rules appropriate for the new segment. Beland et al. took their analysis one step further, arguing that particular aspects of the syllabification process are particularly complex and themselves make it likely that segmental errors will occur. Analyses such as those provided by Beland et al. and Schnitzer begin to apply phonological theory to the notion of "planning" the sound pattern of a word. In essence, they claim that the phonological derivation of a word suggested by linguists corresponds to the process of planning the sound pattern of a word. This model thus differs from Levelt's in detail, but is similar in the sense of postulating that a series of phonological representations are constructed during the process of lexical activation.[7] The model is explicit in claiming that planning errors arise because these operations go astray.

We have emphasized that phonemic paraphasias are subject to many constraints. Lecours and Lhermitte were forced to constrain their error-generating mechanism to stop it from producing illegal sequences of phonemes. We can view the models of Beland et al. and Schnitzer as claiming that errors in underlying representations or in the derivation of a phonological representation are constrained by normal phonological processes such as syllabification, stress assignment, vowel reduction, etc. There are also constraints that arise at more peripheral levels of sound production. For instance, Nespoulous et al. (1984) found that single consonantal substitutions in word repetition were closely related to the target phoneme in terms of distinctive features in only some patients and not others. In the first group of patients, articulatory factors were significant determinants of error type. Unvoiced stop consonants tended to become dentals (i.e., /p/ and /k/ became /t/) and voiced stop consonants tended to lose their voicing. These errors were not obviously due to disturbances at the level of articulation itself: they had none of the characteristics associated with these errors, to be described in the next section. They appear to be errors affected by the relationship between the articulation of one phoneme and a minimally different phoneme. It is reasonable to argue that these errors are planning errors that are subject to articulatory constraints. These articulatory factors did not constrain the errors made by the second group of patients. Thus, phonemic paraphasias are subject to different constraints in different patients. This also suggests they arise at different stages of word sound planning in different persons, or at least are constrained by factors that apply at different levels of sound planning in different cases.[8]

The models of "planning" errors we have been describing so far all are relevant to the production of single words. Another model of the generation of phonemic paraphasias claims that they arise during the process of inserting lexical items into sentence structures. Buckingham (1980) has championed this model. This model cannot account for the presence of phonemic paraphasias in single word production tasks such as picture naming or word repetition. It does account for the presence of phonemic paraphasias in discourse, especially if these errors can be clearly shown to be different for single words and words in context. Kohn and Smith (1990) have described a patient of this sort. C.M. made more errors with vowels than consonants in sentence repetition, but equal numbers in word repetition. C.M.'s most common error in sentence repetition was to copy a vowel from a neighboring word onto a target vowel, an error that cannot arise at all in single word production. Fifty-five percent of sentences with errors had between-word phonemic copies; only 13% of single words with errors had phonemic copies. This case argues for an error-generating process related to sentence production; Kohn and Smith consider it to be an inefficient removal of phonological information from a speech planning buffer.

Not all phonemic errors that occur in sentence production are due to mechanisms of this sort. Pate et al. (1987) conducted a series of experiments with one conduction aphasic patient who made a significant number of phonemic paraphasias. They had the patient read single words, words in phrases, words in blocks that did not correspond to syntactic or semantic units, and sentences, as well as recall sentences that had been presented visually. The percentage of phonological errors did not change in these different conditions (except for the memory condition, which added some complexity). Nor did the errors themselves change; for instance, omissions of unstressed syllables occurred far more frequently than omissions of stressed syllables in all presentation conditions. When phrases and words were matched for number of syllables, the patient did much better in reading phrases than words. When he read phrases, he hardly ever made exchanges of consonants from adjacent words, but did so reasonably often with consonants within each of the words in the phrase. Pate and her colleagues concluded that these errors arose in the process of planning the phonetic values of the sounds of words, largely independently of context. It thus appears that phonemic errors can arise both during planning the phonological form of single words and in integrating the phonological forms of single words into their sentential context.

In summary, there is good evidence that many word sound errors arise after a lexical phonological representation has been accessed (or, in a model such as Levelt's, at late stages of the access process). The errors of this sort that have been most carefully studied are phonemic paraphasias. They arise both during single word phonological planning and during the integration of single word forms into context. They apparently consist mainly of elementary operations on phonemes—deletions, insertions, exchanges, and copies—constrained by both higher-order lexical phonological structures and articulatory considerations. It is likely that other types of errors will be described and analyzed. It may be that all "phonological planning" errors result from error-generating mechanisms found in normal speakers, though this is not yet clear. Some of these errors can become very complex (see above), and it remains unclear whether these complex errors, in particular, arise through normal error-generating mechanisms. The exact details of the process of planning lexical phonological representations are still being debated, and the analysis of these errors may well change as more is learned about the speech production process.

Disturbances of Articulation

Aside from disturbances in accessing and planning phonological representations, patients often have disturbances in the physical production of the sounds of words. The evidence that the speech production process is interrupted at the point of the actual production of sounds in some patients consists of measured abnormalities in the acoustic waveform produced by a patient and in the movement of the articulators themselves in sound production. There are many studies of the acoustic abnormalities found in aphasic speech (Blumstein et al., 1980; Shewan, Leeper, and Booth, 1984; Shinn and Blumstein, 1983; Ryalls, 1986; Kent and Rosenbek, 1982; Gandour and Dardaranda, 1984, etc.) For instance, as discussed in chapter 2, the distinction between voiced and voiceless stop consonants, consisting of the onset of voicing relative to stop consonant release, is categorical in speakers of a given language. In English, periodic voicing begins approximately 40 ms earlier in voiced stop consonants than in unvoiced stops. Though there is a range of VOT associated with voiced consonants and another range associated with unvoiced consonants, there is also an intermediate range in which voicing never begins in normal subjects. Blumstein and her colleagues (Blumstein et al., 1977a, 1980) found that some patients with Broca's aphasia did not respect this basic constraint on the production of voiced and unvoiced consonants, but frequently produced intermediate forms in which voicing began during this "illegal" portion of consonant production. These abnormal productions must reflect a disturbance at the actual articulatory stage of speech programming, and cannot be due to abnormalities in speech planning. Some authors have argued that errors that respected VOT boundaries might also reflect disturbances at the articulatory level that are so severe as to produce a misarticulation that falls into a completely different phoneme or feature acoustic range. MacNeilage (1982) pursued this possibility in analyzing a subset of the errors reported for patients with "apraxia of speech" (Trost and Cantor, 1974)—devoicing errors in morpheme-final stop consonants. These errors are easily understood in terms of the complexity of the articulatory gestures needed to produce voicing in stop consonants in morpheme-final position, but would be hard to attribute to a disturbance at the stage of planning more abstract phonological representations if they do not also occur in other syllabic positions. Thus, acoustic data are sufficient, but arguably not necessary, to establish the presence of a disturbance affecting the execution stage of speech production.

Direct physiological measurements of the movement of the articulatory mechanism also have revealed disturbances in patients with Broca's aphasias that reflect abnormalities of the articulatory process. Itoh et al. (1979, 1980, 1982) used fiberoptic techniques to examine velar movements in these patients, and found abnormali-

g of various articulators (for instance, the lowering
a nasal dental was not properly coordinated with the
ent for apical closure in the Japanese word "deenee").
ations were confirmed by x-ray microbeam analysis of
nts of multiple articulators in a subsequent study (Itoh,
Sasanu. and Hirose, 1980). These observations, and others made
in patients with Broca's aphasia, apraxia of speech, and dysarthria,
clearly indicate that some patients have disturbances affecting the
articulation of particular phonological segments (Schonle et al.,
1987).

From the clinical point of view, it is important to be able to identify dysarthria and apraxia of speech without recourse to these
diagnostic instruments, which are not available in most clinical
settings. Dysarthria is marked by hoarseness and slurred articulation and, at least in its most typical form, is not hard to recognize,
though distinguishing different types of dysarthria is very difficult
and controversial. Dysarthria is not significantly influenced by the
type of linguistic material that the speaker produces or by the
speech task (naming, repetition, reading, etc.). It appears to result
from a neural disturbance that affects either lower-motor neurons
(those that activate muscle cells directly) or neurons in the basal
ganglia, brainstem, and cerebellum that coordinate the activity of
these neurons. Some cases of dysarthria result from disturbances to
the white matter tracts that synapse on lower-motor neurons, usually fairly close to the lower-motor neurons themselves. Though these
white matter lesions do affect the output from upper-motor neurons
to lower-motor neurons, it may be that such white matter lesions
exert their effects by depriving the lower-motor neuron of input that
originated in the coordinating structures (brainstem nuclei, basal
ganglia, cerebellum). Dysarthria following purely cortical lesions is
rare, though reported.

Apraxia of speech is also partially distinguishable from other
phonological output disorders. In very severe cases, patients with
apraxia of speech can be almost totally unable to utter any speech
sounds. In most cases, however, some speech production is possible.
Clinically, apraxia of speech can be told apart from dysarthria by its
variability as a function of linguistic material and task, and from
planning disorders by virtue of the slower rate and greater effortful-
ness of speech in this condition. More detailed analyses of speech
errors show that apraxia of speech is also associated with somewhat

different types of phonological errors, on average, than conduction aphasia (the typical syndrome with planning disturbances). Trost and Canter (1974), Darley, Aronson, and Brown, (1975), Alajouanine, Ombredane, and Durand (1939), and others provide classic descriptions of apraxia of speech. A summary of the major differences between apraxia of speech and conduction aphasia is presented by Cantor et al. (1985): increased errors in word-initial consonants; strikingly more difficulty with consonant clusters; more substitutions that differ from the target phonemes by only one distinctive feature (rather than more than one feature); audible distortions of the sounds of phonemes; few additions and interchanges of segments; frequent articulatory hiatuses, which sound like epenthetic schwa (/sətar/ for /star/); prolongations of segments (/f:laᵂr/ for /flaᵂr/ (flower)); and syllable omissions in polysyllabic words. These types of errors seem to reflect difficulty in initiating words and in producing more complex phonological forms, and a consequent attempt to simplify phonological structure while keeping the segmental phonological values of the speech that is produced as close to those of the target word as possible.

Word and Nonword Repetition: Different Routes and Their Disturbances

Repetition is a simple means of assessing a patient's single word output: it is easier to say words and ask that they be repeated than to draw pictures and ask that they be named. It also serves as the basis for a major distinction between aphasic syndromes in the standard clinical taxonomy of aphasia. It is therefore worthwhile to digress to discuss repetition briefly. My focus is on impairments of repetition that are potentially useful in diagnosing the stage of processing that is impaired in a patient's word sound production.

We have been modeling the word sound production process in three stages: lexical phonological access, phonological planning, and articulation. Repetition can bypass some of these stages. The production of a word in spontaneous speech or a picture-naming task requires a subject to access the phonological representation of that word from a conceptual or semantic representation. If a subject is asked to repeat a word, however, this stage of processing may be bypassed since the subject is given a representation of the surface form of the word. The fact that normal subjects can repeat nonwords indicates that it is possible to bypass this processing stage. Similarly, there may be a different sort of phonological planning involved in repetition than in word production from semantics, since the surface form of a word is presented in repetition but has to be planned on the basis of a lexical phonological representation in word production from semantics. However, it is important to keep in mind that, though the lexical phonological access stage may be avoided, and the phonological planning stage avoided or simplified in repetition, it need not be the case that these stages are in fact bypassed. Much research suggests that normal subjects automatically analyze auditorily presented utterances as words (if they are in fact words of the listener's language) and extract their meaning (see chapter 2). Repetition of words and sentences can proceed via a "deeper" route that activates semantic representations through input-side processing and then goes through the normal output-side processes to produce an utterance. McCarthy and Warrington (1984) have documented a double dissociation between good performance on repetition tasks that maximize semantic processing and those that minimize such processing (see also Morton, 1980, for a description of a patient who repeated words via a semantic route). This double dissociation indicates that repetition may be based upon either a semantic or a nonsemantic route. A model of the different processing routes that underlie repetition is shown in figure 4.4.

Repetition can be impaired at several levels. Disturbances affecting input-side processing will show up in two ways: input-side tasks (phoneme discrimination, lexical decision, etc.) will be disturbed or a repetition disturbance will exist despite good picture naming and reading, or both these patterns will manifest. Output-side disturbances affect all output tasks (picture naming and reading as well as repetition), and are not associated with disturbances of input-side tasks such as phoneme discrimination.

A more complex issue that is relevant to speech production disturbances is whether it is possible to distinguish disturbances on the output side affecting the activation of entries in the phonological output lexicon from those affecting the operation of a "phoneme output buffer." We have discussed the role of a buffer in planning the production of the sound patterns of words uttered in isolation and in connected speech. We have concluded that there is very little look-ahead in planning the sound patterns of single words, and that look-ahead is likely to be also quite limited in connected speech.

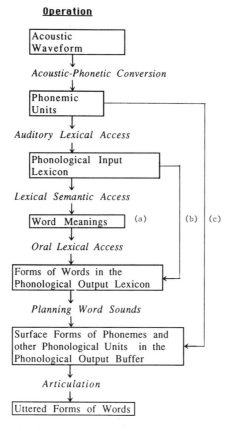

Operation

Figure 4.4
A three- route model of repetition. The three routes specified in this model
are: (a) from whole word input phonological representations to semantics
and then to whole word output phonology; (b) from whole word input phonological representations directly to whole word output phonology; and (c)
from sublexical phonological units to sublexical output phonological units.

Despite these considerations, some theorists in aphasiology have postulated the existence of a "phoneme output buffer," whose role is to maintain sequences of phonemes in memory while articulation is being planned. Certain types of phonemic errors have been ascribed to malfunctions of this buffer. According to the model depicted in figure 4.4, the phonological representations in the phoneme output buffer can come from words that have been transferred from the phonological output lexicon, or they can be transferred from auditory and written input on a sublexical, segment-by-segment basis. According to this model, the latter route must be the source of elements in the phoneme output buffer when nonwords are repeated or read aloud.

According to the model in figure 4.4, a disturbance affecting the operation of the phonological output buffer would affect the production of both words and nonwords on all tasks that require spoken output—naming, spontaneous speech, reading, repetition. In contrast, a disturbance of the phonological output lexicon should have a much more selective effect. The phonological output lexicon is required for spontaneous speech and naming, in which phonological entities must be activated from semantic representations, and these activities should be impaired when the phonological output lexicon is disturbed. Repetition and reading of words *can* proceed by either a lexical or a nonlexical route, and therefore may not be affected when the phoneme output lexicon is disturbed by itself. Repetition and reading of nonwords do not involve the phonological output lexicon, and should not be affected by its disruption.

These expectations must be modified, however, if the model in figure 4.4 is incomplete and there is some interaction between lexical and nonlexical phonological processing. We have discussed spreading activation theories of wordform production above. In these theories, nonwords activate words by reverse spreading activation from phonemes to words. This activation of lexical entries reverberates back down through the production system to activate phonemic segments not present in the target, and thus can cause phonological errors. Words activate other words by the same mechanism, but these additional activated lexical entries are subject to lateral inhibition coming from the word that the speaker intends to pronounce, and thus cause less interference at the level of phonemes. These models thus predict that repetition of nonwords should be more difficult than repetition of words. Disturbances of the phonological output buffer may thus be more apparent in repeating nonwords than words, despite the fact that this buffer is involved in repeating both these classes of stimuli.

Data from patients' repetition performances appear to confirm the interactive nature of lexical and nonlexical phonological processing. The most striking pattern was reported by Caramazza, Miceli, and Villa (1986). Their patient performed virtually perfectly on repetition tasks when required to repeat words, but extremely poorly when required to repeat nonwords.[9] Miller and Ellis (1987), Caplan, et al. (1986a), and Bub, Black, and Behrmann (1986) also describe patients whose performances suggest an interactive model of the buffer and the output lexicon. These patients made qualitatively similar phonological errors in reading and repetition of both words and nonwords and in naming pictures, thus indicating a problem in the buffer in terms of the model in figure 4.4. However, all these patients also showed effects of lexical status upon performance in repetition and reading tasks. The patient of Caplan et al. performed better for words than nonwords in these tasks, and the patients described by Miller and Ellis and Bub and his colleagues both showed an effect of word frequency. The reverse pattern—better nonword than word repetition—has not been described. These observations suggest that the phonological output buffer interacts with the phonological output lexicon.[10]

A final interesting challenge to any model of repetition is that there are some patients who do not appear to have either input- or output-side disturbances but who nonetheless have difficulties repeating single words. I have seen patients whose abilities to perform phoneme discrimination, lexical decision, auditory comprehension, picture homophone matching, and picture naming tasks were all normal, but who made errors in single word repetition. In such cases, it appears that the combination of processes involved in repetition overloads the capacities of the patient. Strub and Gardner (1974) have made a similar suggestion. However, Shallice and Warrington (1977) have criticized this suggestion and have proposed an alternative analysis of this pattern of performance in terms of a short-term memory deficit. More research is needed to know if overload of a "repetition" mechanism does occur (see Caplan and Waters, in press, for discussion).

Phonological Errors and the Classic Aphasic Syndromes

Many authors claim that the disturbances found in the production of the phonological forms of words differ in different clinical aphasic syndromes. Patients with Broca's aphasia are said to have a low-level disturbance of sound production—dysarthria or apraxic of speech. Those with Wernicke's aphasia are said to have disturbances in accessing the forms of words. Conduction aphasic patients are said to have disturbances in some aspects of the planning of word forms because of an impairment in transmitting the phonological form of a word from one cortical area to another. However, there are problems with this account.

It does seem that dysarthria and apraxia of speech are most likely to occur in Broca's aphasia; as we have noted, both direct measurements of speech production and acoustic analyses of spoken speech suggest that these patients often have motor execution disturbances. However, disturbances of motor speech production have been found in less severe forms in fluent aphasic patients. It may be that these disturbances differ in different syndromes, when they are examined in detail. For instance, Baum et al. (1990; Baum and Blumstein 1987; see Blumstein, 1988, for review) have suggested that, though both Broca's and Wernicke's aphasia patients have trouble with producing the correct duration of aspects of articulation, the former have trouble with aspects of duration that affect the distinctive feature content of phonemes (such as VOT) while the Wernicke's aphasia group have trouble only with those aspects of duration that do not affect the distinctive feature content of phonemes (such as the duration of voicing in voiced fricatives, which differs in different fricatives). However, these differences are only statistical regularities and both types of patients produce both types of errors. More recently, Blumstein (1990) has argued that patients with Broca's aphasia have difficulty producing speech sounds that require the coordination of two or more separate articulators, while in fluent (Wernicke's) aphasia patients have trouble with speech sounds even if they only require the correct regulation of a single articulator. For instance, voicing requires the coordination of vocal tract closure with vocal cord vibration, each of which involves a quite separate part of the vocal tract, and patients with Broca's aphasia have been found to produce stop consonants with abnormal

VOTs. In contrast, duration of frication in fricative consonants requires regulation of only one aspect of the vocal tract—the maintenance of a configuration of articulators required for this feature of sound—and patients with Wernicke's but not Broca's aphasia have been found to have difficulty with this feature. However, again, only a very small number of patients have been studied for these effects. Moreover, it is somewhat surprising and counterintuitive that patients who are thought to have motor output problems (Broca's aphasia) are those whose articulatory troubles are thought to arise only with more complex articulatory tasks (coordinating two articulators), whereas patients who are usually thought to have no or minor disturbances of articulation and whose lesions are generally farther away from the motor tract itself (Wernicke's aphasia) are those with disturbances affecting production of even single articulatory gestures. Clearly, the issue of whether particular aphasic syndromes or lesion sites, or both, are associated with particular articulatory disturbances will require more investigation to resolve.

Disturbances of phonological output that are more removed from speech production itself also appear to be similar in different aphasic syndromes. In one of the first investigations of phonemic paraphasias in spontaneous speech that compared different syndromes, Blumstein (1973 a, b) found that patients in all categories made very similar errors. In a similar vein, the study by Nespoulous et al. (1984) cited above, that indicated that there are differences among aphasic patients with respect to the degree to which their errors are influenced by production factors, showed that these constraints could either occur or not occur in both fluent and nonfluent patients. It appears that, at best, differences between the speech production impairments found in different syndromes are statistical matters. One cannot infer what aspect of word sound production will be intact or impaired simply by knowing the traditional clinical class of aphasia to which a patient belongs.

CONCLUDING REMARKS

I have presented a fairly simple model of the process of producing the sounds of words, dividing this process into several stages: accessing the word's lemma; accessing the lexical phonological representation of a word; developing the entirety of the lexical

phonological representation of a word; inserting a lexical phonological representation into a sentence; coordinating the lexical
phonological representation with supralexical phonological structures such as intonational contours; preparing the resulting sound
pattern to activate neural commands to the articulatory muscles;
and actually articulating the sounds of words. I have indicated that
this simple model needs to be expanded in a considerable amount
of detail. Though much of the detail remains to be determined,
and though aspects of the model itself are still being investigated
and debated, it is possible to allocate disturbances of word form
production to these different stages of processing.

NOTES

1. These errors arise in normal speech, and their characteristics may reflect
the insertion of words into phrases. However, they still provide evidence for
the existence of differential processing of different aspects of word-form in
oral production.

2. A note regarding historical aphasiology is of interest here. Shallice
(1988, pp. 7–9, and chapter 7) uses the term "center for auditory word-
representations" and "center for motor word-representations" to describe
the two classic centers in Wernicke's model and thus seems to take this
classic model as one with two phonological lexicons. However, most aphasiologists have understood Wernicke's "motor" center to be one that is involved with speech output processing that occurs after word forms have
been activated, and have considered this model to be a single-lexicon theory
(e.g., Caplan, Vanier, and Baker, 1986a; Caplan, 1987c). The moral seems to
be that reconstructing the thoughts of researchers who lived over a century
ago, and who used different terms that were less specific than those in use
today, though interesting, is difficult.

3. Conversely, the details of the prosodic envelope are affected by the segmental values and stress contours of single words (see chapter 8).

4. Levelt (1989) points out that the relationship may be reversed—speakers
may set F_0 and then adjust utterance length accordingly—but this seems
intuitively unlikely.

5. A third piece of data cited by Levelt is that neither syllables as whole nor
allophones are involved in slips of the tongue. Syllables and allophones
would be exempt from the error-generating mechanisms responsible for
slips of the tongue if they become available to the speech production system
only after the point at which these mechanisms operate. This, however, is a
weak argument if syllables are computed prior to the point in processing at
which slips of the tongue arise (see text above).

6. The question of whether lexical phonological representations have been lost or are inaccessible could be investigated using the criteria that distinguish loss and access disorders established by Warrington and Shallice (1979; see chapter 3). Warrington and Shallice argue that disturbances of access are characterized by lack of item specificity on repetitions of a task, failure to show frequency effects in performance, sensitivity of performance to rate of stimulus presentation, and effectiveness of prompting or cuing; disorders of storage (i.e., loss of representations) are characterized by the opposite pattern of effects of these variables. We have questioned the appropriateness of some of these criteria (see chapter 3 and Caplan, 1987c, chapter 12), but they could be explored in relationship to activation of lexical phonological forms (they have not yet been investigated in this domain).

7. A sidelight is that this model claims that the underlying form of a lexical phonological representation is simply a sequence of segments. This is very much like the Lecours-Lhermitte model that we have just criticized for being underspecified. In fact, in the model of Beland et al., the stored phonological representation of a word is even more underspecified than in Lecours and Lhermitte's, because the underlying segments in their model have incomplete distinctive feature content. The model of Beland et al., however, maintains that syllable structure, stress contour, and surface distinctive feature content of segments are all computed on the basis of language-universal and language-specific rules. The constraints on phonemic paraphasias are due to the way error-generating mechanisms interact with these rules. Thus, unlike the Lecours and Lhermitte model, Beland's model does provide for (at least some of) the needed constraints on error-generating mechanisms.

8. It is difficult to know at what level of processing a constraint arises. For instance, Beland et al. claimed that certain sequences of segments (such as two adjacent vowels) are hard to syllabify because the syllabification rules of French do not usually deal with these sequences. However, it is possible that these seqences are hard to syllabify because of articulatory factors. It is equally hard to know where "phonotactic" constraints "come from"; that is, what level of processing is responsible for their existence. It is likely that constraints arise at multiple levels of processing and have complex effects on errors. The nature of constraints and their consequences is just beginning to be explored.

9. Caramazza et al. argued that this dissociation was so extreme as to suggest that fundamentally different mechanisms mediate the activation of articulatory representations in words and nonwords, nonwords utilizing a buffer mechanism of the sort described above and words utilizing a "direct," "lexico-articulatory" conversion process that maps the entirety of a word's phonological form onto an articulatory code. However, it seems more appropriate to try to model this dissociation by varying the parameters in spreading activation models.

10. More extremely interactive models, such as that advanced for reading by Seidenberg and McClelland (1989) and discussed in chapter 5, would not

separate word and nonword processing at all. Lexical effects arise in these models because words are more familiar to the system than nonwords.

It is not clear whether interactions that affect performance in repetition extend to the level of semantic representations, or just word form. Semantic values (e.g., abstractness) have been shown to affect some patients' ability to read words aloud (see chapter 5), but no such effects have been found to date in the production of *phonological* errors in either reading or repetition.

5   Reading and Writing Single Words

In this chapter, we are concerned with the procedures that determine the ability to read and write single words.[1] The chapter is organized as follows. I first describe the nature of orthographic representations—the ways that languages are represented in written form. I then present a brief summary of the processes that are involved in reading and writing single words. The processing model that we develop is used to provide a theoretical framework for interpreting a variety of reading and writing disorders observed in brain-damaged patients.

ORTHOGRAPHIC REPRESENTATIONS

Writing systems for language vary considerably in how they represent a language. They can be as different as Chinese characters and English letters. An important feature common to all orthographic systems, however, is that they all represent words of a language. There are no known orthographic systems in which the only units of representation depict phrases or sentences and not words, although there are frequently aspects of an orthographic system that indicate the beginnings and ends of sentences and some aspects of their internal structure (as the punctuation marks , . ; : do in English). Words are thus the basic units of representation in orthography. However, orthographies represent words in a variety of quite different ways.

Some orthographies represent words in quite direct phonological fashion. Italian and Serbo-Croatian, for instance, are languages in which each sound of a word is represented by a letter or a sequence of letters. The term for a letter or combination of letters that represents a particular sound is a "grapheme." Languages like Italian and Serbo-Croatian have very simple "grapheme-to-phoneme conversion" rules. With only a few exceptions, there is a single phoneme for every grapheme and there is a single grapheme for every phoneme in these languages. We say that graphemes and phonemes stand in a one-to-one relationship to one another when going from print to sound and vice versa. French, on the other hand, is a slightly more complicated language with respect to how words are represented orthographically. French has a one-to-one system for conversion of graphemes to phonemes, but a set of one-to-many correspondences between phonemes and graphemes. That is, any given grapheme in French only receives one pronunciation, but a given sound of French—particularly the vowel sounds—can be written in many ways. For instance, the forms *o*, *au*, *eau*, *aux*, *eaux*, and many others all represent the sound "o" in French. English is yet more complicated. In English, the correspondences between graphemes and phonemes are many to many in both directions. A single sound of English, such as the sound of "long i," can be written in a variety of fashions—*i consonant e* (as in *pike*), *y* (as in *my*), *ie*, (as in *pie*), just as it is true of the sounds of French. In English, however, graphemes are also ambiguous. The sequence of letters *ea*, sounds like "/ɛ/" in *bread* and *head*, like "/ee/" in *heat* or *beat*, and as the sound "/ɚ/" in a word like *search*.

These examples also demonstrate another way in which the orthography of English is more complicated than that of Italian or French: the sound associated with a particular grapheme depends to some extent upon the graphemes that occur near the grapheme in question within a word. For instance, the sound of "ea" in the word *search*, depends upon the grapheme *ea* being followed by the letter "r"; the particular sound that "ea" represents in the word *search* only occurs for the grapheme "ea" in this particular "context." It is not the case that every time the grapheme "ea" is followed by "r," it is pronounced as it is in the word *search*; in the word *ear*, for instance, "ea" is pronounced as it is in the word *beat*. However, the only time that "ea" *is* pronounced as it is in the word *search* is when it is followed by the grapheme "r." In other words, the system of grapheme-to-phoneme correspondances in English is many to many and context-dependent.

Despite these differences, Italian, Serbo-Croatian, French, and English all have one important characteristic in common. Each of these languages has an alphabetic script. However complex the relationship between graphemes and phonemes, the orthographies in these languages are such that the smallest unit of representation is an individual phoneme and almost all the phonemes of a word are somehow represented in the orthography. Other orthographies do not have these properties. Hebrew and Arabic orthographies, for instance, are consonantal scripts, which do not represent the vowels of a language. In these languages, skilled readers determine what the vowels of a word must be. They do this partly through recognition of the word itself and partly because many or all of the vowels are determined by rules of word formation and syntactic agreement and therefore can be deduced from the context in which a word appears. Another type of orthography is a syllabary. In languages such as the Indian language Kanaada, the elementary orthographic units represent syllables, not phonemes. There are approximately 60 syllables in the language Kanaada, and there are about 60 elementary orthographic signs, each representing a different syllable.

Consonantal and syllabic orthographies obviously contrast with the alphabetic, phonemic-based orthographies of English, French, Italian, and most European languages. However, all of these orthographies also have one important feature in common: they all represent some aspects of the sounds of words. These types of orthographies all stand in contrast to writing systems such as Chinese and one form of written Japanese (Kanji), which are "ideographic." In an ideographic script, words are not represented phonologically. Rather, they are represented through a set of symbols, each of which corresponds to a particular word (or a portion of a word in a compound or morphologically complex form). In a language like Chinese or a script like Kanji, a skilled reader must memorize the visual forms of thousands of words in his language, and can never deduce the sound of a character without knowing what word the character represents. To be more accurate, ideographic orthographics usually have a few "diacritic" markers that indicate a few phonological features of each symbol, but these at most represent a few aspects of a word's sound.

PROCESSING WRITTEN LANGUAGE

What kind of transformation do visual words undergo as they are recognized and understood? Many theorists assume that reading and writing are skills demanding the prior activation of speech-based (phonological) codes. These theories maintain that the initial stage of word recognition consists of extracting a pronunciation from sublexical spelling units, and that there is no reason to view subsequent aspects of the recognition of spoken and written words as being fundamentally different. The opposite point of view maintains that entire written words are recognized prior to being understood or transformed into sounds. The question of the relationship between spoken and written language has remained controversial for almost a century.[2]

The literature contains many speculative discussions about why one or the other model of written language processing must be correct. We briefly review these speculations, only to conclude that none of these a priori considerations are definitive. We then turn to experimental studies and models that shed more light on the issue, though they too are inconclusive at present. Fortunately, though still under development, these models provide enough of a framework to approach disturbances of reading and writing.

There are several basic facts about language that favor the view that reading and writing involve mapping written forms onto phonological representations. These facts amount to the observation that orthographies are man-made forms of language representation, secondary to the naturally occurring forms that are involved in auditory-oral language use. Though all normal humans exposed to spoken language learn to speak and comprehend auditory language, many people do not learn to write or read, and many languages have never developed a written form. Normal children learn to use spoken language before they learn to use written language, and clearly map written language onto spoken language (i.e., a child learns that the printed word DOG sounds like the spoken word /dog/ and discovers its meaning via its sound, rather than mapping the printed form DOG onto the concept of a dog directly). These facts favor the view that processing of written language is phonologically mediated.

These considerations are far from definitive for many reasons. First, the implication, if any, of written language being a secondary form of representation compared to spoken language is not necessarily that sublexical orthographic units be mapped onto sublexical phonological units while a written word is being recognized. It is sufficient that orthographic representations be mapped onto phonological representations before being *understood*, even if the orthographic representations are whole words. This is a separate issue from whether phonology is required for written word *recognition*.

Thus, it is entirely consistent with the observation that written language is a secondary form of representation, that there be systems for recognizing written words from orthographic representations and generating orthographic representations from sound that do not involve mapping sublexical orthographic units onto sound units and vice versa. Second, we can look at the development of reading and writing as a form of skill acquisition. Skills may originally depend on a process that is later discarded as the skill becomes more efficient and automatized. This point of view allows for the development of skilled processing of written language without phonological mediation, either in recognizing or understanding words, even if the early stages of developing this skill do involve phonological mediation.

A consideration of the demands incurred by the variability of the orthographic correspondences in English and many other languages also appears to place certain constraints on a possible architecture of the reading and writing mechanism. Many researchers have argued that our ability to translate novel patterns like FLORP into sound indicates that there must be a means of recognizing printed forms by assembling a pronunciation of a letter string through the application of general correspondences between spelling units and sound. On the other hand, such a procedure can reliably obtain the pronunciation of legitimate words only when they have a predictable relationship between orthography and phonology. As we have seen, this condition does not apply to many items in some alphabetic orthographies, either in reading or writing. These considerations provide *a priori* grounds for assuming that the normal reader must have access to the spelling of at least some whole words. Thus, some researchers have argued that reading and writing must involve both a phonologically mediated subword translation process (to deal with nonwords) and a whole word recognition and production process (to deal with words with regular spellings). These two routes are depicted in figure 5.1.

Though both a phonologically mediated and a direct, whole word–based route are possible ways to read and write single words in languages with alphabetic scripts, the fact that both routes are possible does not prove that both routes are actually used. A great deal of psychological research into reading is directed toward the question of whether both routes are used and the subsequent question of how both routes operate (Humphreys and Evett, 1985). We

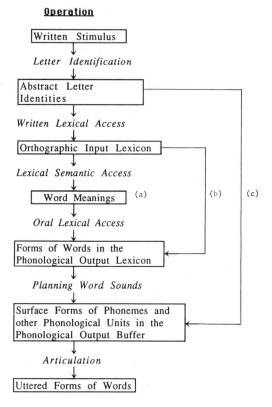

Figure 5.1
The "two-route" model of the reading process. There are really three routes from written input to sound in this model: (a) from whole-word orthography to semantics and then to whole-word output phonology; (b) from whole-word orthography directly to whole-word output phonology; and (c) from sublexical orthographic units to sublexical output phonological units.

shall briefly review some of the complex literature on this topic here, dealing entirely with the reading process (about which more is known).

Let us start with evidence for the phonologically mediated route. If the phonologically mediated theory is right, we would expect there to be a difference in reading those words that can be directly accessed in their entirety through a prelexical phonological media- tion process and those words that cannot be accessed through this process. Though there are several suggestions about the units in- volved in orthographic-to-phonological translation, most researchers agree that these transformations must map graphemes onto their most common phonological values.[3] Thus, when a grapheme, such as *ea*, is ambiguous, the most common phonological value for that grapheme is produced by the phonologically mediated route. We therefore would expect that, if the sublexical phonological mediation theory of written word recognition is correct, words with regular grapheme-phoneme correspondences (or GPCs) would be easier to recognize than words with irregular correspondences.

The data bearing on this hypothesis are complicated. Several experiments in which words are read aloud seem to show that this is in fact true. Baron and Strawson (1976) and Coltheart (1978) found a so-called "regularity effect" in reading word lists, demonstrating that subjects read lists of regular words faster than lists of irregular words. Several investigators have questioned the importance of the Baron and Strawson results because they were obtained with lists rather than single words, and others have suggested that the regularity effect might reflect the time it takes to pronounce a word rather than the word-recognition stage of reading. However, these potential interpretive problems were answered by Gough and Cosky (1977) who found a regularity effect in reading single words aloud but discovered that this effect disappeared if subjects were instructed to wait a variable amount of time (until a signal appeared) to report the word they read. Gough and Cosky argued that delaying the motor response emphasized the importance of the time it took to prepare for articulation or to articulate a word, because enough time passed between the presentation of the word and the signal to respond for any word to have been recognized. Any increase in reaction time (RT) in the "delayed report" condition must therefore reflect the difficulty a person has in saying a certain type of word, not in recognizing that type of word. Since delaying the response had the effect of abolishing the RT advantage for regular words, Gough and Cosky concluded that regular words were read faster in the normal situation without a delay because they were recognized faster, not because it was easier to pronounce them.

Coltheart (1978) nonetheless argued that any reading-aloud task, with or without a delay between the presentation of a word and speech, involves more than simply accessing the lexicon; it involves speaking as well. Therefore, he argued that reading aloud is not a good task with which to measure lexical access, and, therefore, not a good task with which to assess the role of GPCs and phonological mediation in the basic aspect of reading—accessing the lexicon from print. He claimed that the lexical decision task, in which a subject must say whether a letter string is a word or not, is a much better task, since it is very close to being a task that requires accessing the lexicon and nothing more. Coltheart (1978) therefore reviewed the literature dealing with regularity effects in lexical decision tasks.

In these tasks, there is an effect of regularity, but Coltheart (1978) pointed out that it only affects subjects' appreciation that nonwords are not words, and does not affect the speed with which a subject recognizes real words. These results suggest that nonwords are recognized in part by a GPC-based system. Rubenstein, Lewis, and Rubenstein (1971) also reported that so-called pseudohomophones, stimuli such as *burd* or *blud* which are orthographically nonwords but are pronounced like real words (*bird, blood*), take longer to reject as nonwords in a lexical decision task than nonwords that are not pseudohomophones. These results also suggest that nonwords are recognized in part by a GPC-based system and that the fact that these nonwords sound like words temporarily interferes with a subject's ability to appreciate that they are not real words of the language. However, the results are quite different for real words. Coltheart (1978) reviewed the literature on regularity effects for real words in lexical decision tasks and found that there are no such effects. Coltheart's conclusion is that phonologically mediated reading based upon regular GPCs is not a important method by which subjects recognize a real printed word. Since the results with pseudohomophones show that normal readers can and do use GPCs to read nonwords, the conclusion Coltheart drew was that phonologically mediated reading is so slow that normal reading is based upon the direct, whole word recognition route simply because it is faster. The pseudohomophone effect for nonwords arises because a subject keeps searching his lexicon when he is presented with a nonword in a lexical decision task, and does so for a long enough period of time for the GPC system to yield a phonological representation of the presented stimulus. Since this is, in fact, a phonological word, a subject must check this phonological word against the printed stimulus to appreciate that the actual stimulus is incorrectly spelled. This takes time, making pseudohomophones longer to reject than "normal" nonwords.

More recently, regularity effects have been reexplored in both reading-aloud and lexical decision tasks by Seidenberg and his colleagues (Seidenberg et al., 1984; Waters and Seidenberg, 1985). They presented several types of words to normal subjects in these tasks, including regularly spelled and exception words, matched for frequency and length. Seidenberg and his colleagues found an effect of regularity upon reading-aloud latencies, as other authors had reported, but they found that this effect was almost entirely confined to words of low frequency. They too found no significant effects of regularity upon lexical decision RT. Seidenberg and his colleagues conclude that high-frequency words are recognized directly by the whole word recognition route and that their subsequent pronunciation makes use of the lexical entry so accessed. For infrequent words, pronunciation may use this route but also is based on synthesizing the pronunciation of the phonemes in a word, which are yielded by the operation of GPCs. This model is a variant of the two-route model depicted in figure 5.1, which also introduces the idea of the rate at which the whole-word and subword recognition processes occur in the model.[4]

If most words are recognized as whole units and their pronunciation is based on their entire form, we may inquire as to how word forms are activated visually. There is good evidence that visual word forms are largely activated on the basis of their constituent letters; that is, a reader identifies the letter in a word and then matches a representation of the word in memory against these letters. The overall shape of the word plays little role in this process of recognition of visually presented words. The evidence for this is that distortions of overall word form that do not affect the form of individual letters, such as writing word in aLtErNaTiNg case, do not affect word recognition very much (McClelland and Johnston, 1977; see Henderson, 1982, for review). It thus appears that the most skilled oral reading and word recognition consists of identifying letters from a visual stimulus, using those letters to activate visual word forms stored in memory, and then accessing the pronunciation associated with the visual word from.

The role of phonology in accessing the meaning of written words may be different, however. Van Orden and his colleagues (van Orden, 1987; van Orden, Johnston, and Hale, 1988) have reported experiments that indicate the visually presented words activate their meanings via their sounds. Van Orden (1987) had subjects say whether a printed word was a member of a particular category (e.g., to say whether ROSE is a flower). They found that homophones were often misclassified (e.g., subjects responded "yes" incorrectly when asked if ROWS is a flower). This misclassification occurred even when words were displayed for very short periods of time and then replaced with a pattern-mask (a pattern that interferes with the retention of the retinal image of the previously presented word). Further experiments (van Orden et al., 1988) showed that the same effect arose for pseudohomophones (e.g., SUTE for article of clothing). These results strongly suggest that reading for meaning is phonologically mediated. If the phonological forms of pseudohomophones are obtained by a process of converting sublexical orthographic spelling units to their corresponding sounds, these results further suggest that this process plays an important role in reading for meaning.

Van Orden (1987) suggested that the way printed words activate their sounds is more complex than that proposed by the two-route model we have been considering. He suggested that this process consists of "covariant learning," which is "sensitive to a statistical regularity . . . between orthographic features and phonological features" (p. 193). We can explore this mechanism by considering the finding that properties of orthographic-to-phonological correlations other than the regularity of GPC correspondences in a word affect subjects' performances in reading aloud and lexical decision tasks. For instance, some words in English, though themselves regular, contain letter sequences that are pronounced differently in different words. Consider, for example, the sequence of letters *ave*. In most words, this sequence is pronounced with a long "a" (*pave, rave, shave*, etc.). However, there is one very frequent word in the language, *have*, in which *ave* is pronounced with a short "a." We say that *gave*, though regular, is "inconsistent," because the set of "neighbors" of *gave* is not totally regular. Glushko (1979) found that both lexical decision and reading latencies for "regular inconsistent" words were longer than for completely regular words with no inconsistencies in their sets of orthographic neighbors. Bauer and Stanovich (1980) also found an effect of regularity in lexical decision tasks using Coltheart's materials (Coltheart et al.,1979), when the regular inconsistent words were removed from the original set, leaving only regular consistent words. These results suggested to the authors that something other than lexical access via the direct whole word route was taking place during the process of reading real words in these experiments, but that this additional process did not consist entirely of the use of GPCs or any other sort of simple phonological mediation. A word like *gave* is completely regular if considered in isolation. Glushko's results suggest that, despite this intrinsic regularity, a word like *gave* is recognized by a system that is sensitive to the existence of similarly spelled words with irregular pronunciations. This process is one which makes use of knowledge of similar *lexical entries*, not spelling-sound correspondences.

One account of these lexical analogy effects has been developed by Seidenberg and McClelland (1989). They developed a computer-implemented model, based on the parallel distributed processing (PDP) framework alluded to in earlier chapters, that learns to read. The way this learning is accomplished is complex and important. The model was presented with the written forms of all the four-letter simple words of English, in repeated exposures, and developed a pronunciation for each word. The orthographic forms of words were represented as letters, each word activating all the letters it contains in a set of units devoted to letter recognition ("the orthographic system" in the model). The representation of each word thus consisted of a set of activation levels for its constituent letters, and was distributed over the entire set of units in the orthographic system. This set of activation levels was passed on in parallel to a set of processing units, known as "hidden units," where it set up another pattern of activity. The strength of activation of each hidden unit was determined by the input to that unit (itself determined by the pattern of activation set up in the orthographic system by the presentation of a particular word) multiplied by the strength of the connection between the hidden unit and each unit in the orthographic system. Finally, the activation in the hidden units was passed onto units in the "phonological system," where a third pattern of activity emerged, determined in the same way as the pattern that emerged over the hidden units (the strength of activation of each phonological unit was determined by its input—the pattern of activation in the hidden unit system induced by the presentation of a particular word—multiplied by the strength of the connection between the hidden unit and each unit in the phonological system). This final pattern was taken to represent the phonological values in the word. The difference between these computed phonological values and the real phonological form of a presented word was calculated and used to adjust the weights of the connections in the set of hidden units.

The first few times a word was presented to the model, the computed pronunciations were wildly erroneous, but slowly the system began to perform very much the way humans do. It simulated over two dozen results in the experimental literature, producing both the regularity-by-frequency interaction effect and many experiment-specific effects of regular inconsistency. It also produced reasonable pronunciations for nonwords, and could do lexical decision tasks.

This model is very different from the two-route model we have been discussing. It does not have either a whole-word or a subword process for transforming orthographic representations into phonological forms. In this model, there is no place where either the phonological form or the orthographic form of a word is represented in a dictionary-like entry. Both the orthographic and the phonological forms of a word are represented as a set of activation levels of units that are involved in representing all the words the system has been exposed to. Moreover, the model has neither GPC rules nor direct mappings between the orthography of a word and its pronunciation. Rather, everything the system knows about the correspondence between orthography and phonology is represented in the pattern of activation of the units in the orthographic system, the system of hidden units, and the phonological system. One and the same set of weighted units represents the facts that the usual phonological value of "i" is short /i/, that "i" is usually pronounced short when it is part of the word ending "int" (*mint, hint, tint,* etc.), that "i" is nevertheless long in the word *pint,* that "i" is usually pronounced long when it is part of the word ending "i-consonant-e," that "x" is always pronounced /ks/, and that *yacht* is pronounced /yɔt/.

Despite its considerable success, the Seidenberg-McClelland model has its limitations. The representation of phonological form used in the model is unrealistic (see Pinker and Prince, 1988), and the extent to which this representation contributes to the success of the model is unclear (see Lachter and Bever, 1988, for general comments on the role of representations in determining the success of PDP models). The model does not perform as well as normal subjects in reading aloud nonwords, and it may not be possible to improve this aspect of its performance without compromising its ability to make lexical decisions (Besner et al., 1990). The model does not actually produce a pronunciation, and it may not perform as well when its computed phonological forms are actually produced. These and other problems are perhaps not insurmountable (Seidenberg and McClelland, 1990). Fortunately, we do not have to resolve all the questions that come up regarding normal reading mechanisms to begin the linguistic and psycholinguistic characterization of acquired disturbances of reading.

The mapping procedure between words and their orthography raises the same issues as apply to reading. Only the direction of the mapping is reversed. Theorists have defended the same positions as in the case of reading. Most theorists assume that there are mappings from both semantics and phonology to orthographic representations. The former is likely to be used in writing words spontaneously, while the latter is likely to be used in writing-to-dictation tasks. We shall consider the evidence for these mappings in turn.

Evidence for a mechanism that converts lexical semantic representations into orthographic forms without activating phonological representations comes largely from the existence of patients who can produce the names of objects in written but not spoken form. In some cases, these patients have been shown to have very little knowledge of the spoken form of a word, if any at all (Bub and Kertesz, 1982b). We discuss these cases when we take up the topic of phonological agraphia later in this chapter.

What is the evidence for the existence of a phonologically mediated route from word meaning to a word's orthographic pattern? Analysis of writing errors in normal performance ("slips of the pen") reveals that a significant proportion of responses are connected to the underlying sound of the target words. Hotopf (1980, 1983) has examined a corpus of such errors taken from a variety of sources, and reports the occurrence of homophone confusions (*weight* instead of *wait, write* for *right*), word substitutions for items that are phonologically similar (28 instead of 20A, 3 instead of C), and even occasional responses like QUES for *cues*, which suggest a reliance on phoneme-grapheme translation. Since there is good reason to assume that the writer actually knew the correct spelling of each target, the mistakes indicate that the spoken form of a word can exert an influence on the orthographic mechanism.

Though suggestive, these results need not imply that speech-based codes play a direct functional role in skilled writing. Many different codes are automatically activated by the language mechanism during the recognition or production of words and sentences. Information present at one level may affect the course of events at another level in the system without being crucially involved in the performance of the task. Seidenberg and Tanenhaus (1979), for example, have reported that normal subjects carry out rhyme judgments of *auditory* words more slowly when the pairs have different orthographic endings (e.g., *pie sky*). While this result indicates that the spelling of a word can automatically enter into the phonological judgment, we would surely not conclude that it forms an essential part of the auditory word-recognition process. Similarly, phonological forms of words may be activated in writing and may influence errors without being part of the process that activates the orthographic form of a word from its meaning. Perhaps the sound pattern of a word is activated *after* its orthographic form has been accessed from semantics but nonetheless it influences the writing process.

Despite these considerations, observations such as those made by Hotopf raise the possibility that the phonological form of a word may become active in the process of activating the orthographic form of that word from its meaning. Evidence for a spelling route that transforms the phonological form of a word to the orthographic description of a word without any reference to its meaning comes from the performance of brain-damaged cases (Goodman and Caramazza, 1986) We review this evidence below. It, too, raises the possibility that the phonological form of a word can be accessed in the route from lexical semantics to orthographic forms of words.

How does the phonologically mediated spelling mechanism work? Do sublexical sound-spelling correspondences play a role in spelling words derived from concepts or in spelling words or nonwords to dictation? Is a single-route model viable, in which lexical and sublexical phonological-to-orthographic mappings are combined in a single mechanism?

One view of the mechanism for deriving spelling from sound (termed "phonological spelling," because the response is based directly on the spoken elements composing the target), is that it functions by converting each phoneme into a corresponding letter (e.g., B, D, F) or group of letters (e.g., PH, CK, OO) that determines its pronunciation (Coltheart, 1978). Phoneme-to-grapheme translation has been considered to occur independently of a whole-word phonological-to-orthographic conversion procedure (Morton and

Patterson, 1980; Ellis, 1982). However, the assumption that phonological spelling occurs by mapping phonemes to graphemes has been called into question by a number of experimental results. Campbell (1983), for instance, has demonstrated an influence of an auditory word on the spelling of a dictated nonsense word that is similar to the Glushko effect in reading and lexical decision tasks. This kind of evidence is not compatible with the standard version of the dual-route model and has led to a number of alternative proposals. Patterson and Morton (1985) have modified the standard model to include both phoneme-grapheme correspondences and correspondences based on the endings (vowel plus consonant or consonant cluster) of monosyllabic words. A similar theoretical approach has been taken by Shallice, Warrington, and McCarthy (1983) who consider the visual word form system to be hierachically organized into a number of distinct levels—graphemes, subsyllabic units, syllables, and morphemes. Another theory eliminates the assumption of distinct routines for spelling words and nonsense words. Rather, the stored visual form of each word can be actively divided into smaller units ranging from the initial or terminal segments to individual graphemic elements, which then provide the basis for the transcoding of nonwords (Marcel, 1980).

At present, these different formulations have not been tested in sufficient detail to permit a clear statement of their relative worth (but see Patterson and Morton, 1985; Shallice and McCarthy, 1985, for valuable steps in this direction). In general terms, the distinction between them rests on the origin of the correpondences used to spell phonologically—either generated actively from whole-word exemplars (Marcel, 1980) or obtained directly from more analytic units existing independently of whole word representations (Shallice et al., 1983; Patterson and Morton, 1985). All these models can account for the tendency to employ orthographic units larger than the grapheme (though they make different assumptions about the nature of these units), and for the biasing effect of a word on the probability of using a particular mapping option (see Kay and Marcel, 1981, and Patterson and Morton, 1985, for details). Whether all these spelling-sound correspondences can be included in a single PDP-type model of written word production remains uncertain. For our purposes, we need only note that phonologically mediated spelling can yield orthographic segments of varying magnitude.

An interesting question concerns the functional role of the writing routine that allows for a mapping of the phonology of a word onto its spelling. If the meaning of a word can provide direct access to its description in the visual word form system, why should there be any need for an additional entry point from the spoken representation? The answer most frequently given is that smooth written production of sentences depends on the temporary storage of words in a buffer that maintains information while the response is organized and executed. Many theorists consider whole-word phonology to be the most suitable code for this kind of storage device. The following comment, taken from Hotopf (1983), illustrates the general point of view: "If the words, having been accessed, have to be held in a buffer store for a few seconds, as is likely to be the case in writing, then acoustic, as opposed to visual, coding will, according to the evidence from studies in short-term memory, be the more durable" (p. 166; see also Patterson, 1986; Barnard, 1985; Caramazza, Berndt, and Basili, 1983).

We will be working with a model of writing in our analyses of acquired agraphia that incorporates three procedures for activating written forms. The first procedure accesses the orthographic pattern of an entire word directly from its meaning. The second maps the sound of the word as a whole onto its orthographic form. The third uses a knowledge of the correspondences between sublexical phonological units—mostly phonemic segments—and their permissable orthographic values to assemble a written form. The processing modules that comprise these routines and the flow of information between them are depicted in figure 5.2. This model is sometimes called a two-route model because it includes a whole-word and a sublexical mechanism for converting phonology to orthography. In fact, it incorporates three routes for written word production: semantic→ orthographic whole word; phonological whole word→ orthographic whole word; sublexical phonology→sublexical orthography.

In summary, though the two-route model of reading has been challenged, and the comparable model of writing is likely to be challenged, the functional architectures described in figures 5.1 and 5.2 can serve as the basis for analyzing acquired disorders of written language processing. Where pertinent, we shall refer to how PDP models treat acquired disturbances of the written language system.

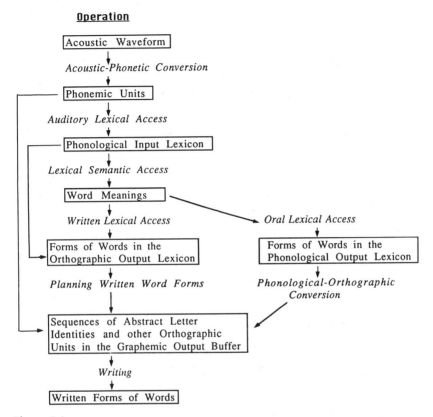

Operation

- Acoustic   Waveform
  - *Acoustic-Phonetic Conversion*
- Phonemic   Units
  - *Auditory Lexical Access*
- Phonological Input Lexicon
  - *Lexical Semantic Access*
- Word   Meanings
  - *Written Lexical Access*   *Oral Lexical Access*
- Forms of Words in the Orthographic Output Lexicon   Forms of Words in the Phonological Output Lexicon
  - *Planning Written Word Forms*   *Phonological-Orthographic Conversion*
- Sequences of Abstract Letter Identities and other Orthographic Units in the Graphemic Output Buffer
  - *Writing*
- Written Forms of Words

Figure 5.2
The "two-route" model of writing. The model specifies two routes from meaning to spelling—a route that accesses the spelling pattern of a word directly from its meaning, and one that that accesses the spelling pattern of a word from its phonological form (which has been activated on the basis of meaning). The model specifies many ways to convert spoken words into orthographic patterns. These include routes (a) from whole word input phonological representations to semantics and then to whole word output orthographic representations; (b) from whole word input phonological representations to semantics, then to the phonological form of a word, and then to the word's orthographic form; (c) from whole word input phonological representations directly to whole word output orthographic representations; and (d) from sublexical phonological units to sublexical output orthographic units.

ACQUIRED DYSLEXIAS

In the past decade or so, there have been intensive efforts to describe acquired alexia in terms of deficits in components of the written language processing system. Most of these studies deal with how reading aloud breaks down, and this is the focus of our presentation. The following summary of this research deals only with what are now thought to be primary deficits affecting this system, omitting discussion of acquired alexias due to other language disorders, to visual processing deficits that affect the recognition of stimuli other than words, and to attentional disturbances (as seen, for instance, in attentional dyslexia). The reader is referred to Shallice (1988) for a discussion of "peripheral" dyslexias.

Phonological Dyslexia

Patients with phonological dyslexia are very impaired in their ability to read even simple nonsense words but nevertheless can attain a high degree of accuracy in their recognition and pronunciation of written words (Beauvois and Derouesné, 1979; Shallice and Warrington, 1980; Patterson, 1980). In one case described by Funnell (1983), the dissociation between legitimate words and pseudowords was virtually complete; W.B. was completely unable to read nonwords (0/20 correct) but could read aloud 85% of words varying in a wide range of different attributes (imageability, orthographic irregularity, morphologically complex words, and grammatical morphemes). None of these variables had any effect on his performance, so that the only determining factor was the lexical (whole word) status of the written target.

The interpretation of phonological dyslexia is that the patients have sustained damage to the procedure for translating orthographic units smaller than whole words into a pronunciation, required whenever a spelling pattern is read that does not have a permanently stored description as a whole word (i.e., a nonsense word). The routine that translates orthographic whole words into a response remains largely intact, however, and performance is vastly superior for these items. Referring to figure 5.3, we see that the orthographic lexicon, holding the representation of real words, can directly contact their meaning, *without* the intermediate step of accessing the pronunciation. A *second*, whole-word routine bypasses the compo-

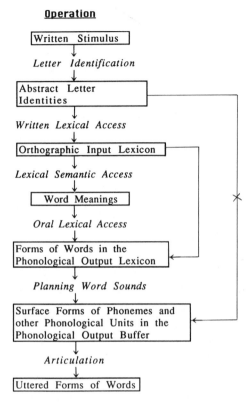

Figure 5.3
The reading model showing the location of the deficit in the route from sublexical orthographic units to sublexical output phonological units characteristic of phonological dyslexia.

nent that delivers the semantic description, and translates the orthographic form of the word directly into a spoken representation. Finally, subword units are converted to sound by assigning phonemic correspondences to them and assembling a reponse; it is this last procedure which is damaged in phonological dyslexia. Severely impaired phonological dyslexic patients have lost the ability to translate nonlexical orthographic patterns to sound and can only read via the semantic and whole word phonological routines.

While the ability of phonological dyslexic patients to read words is largely intact, many cases are noted to be impaired in their reading of morphologically complex words (derived or affixed words) and grammatical function words (words like IF, BUT, THEN, etc.). Some authors have argued on the basis of this assocation of deficits that the procedure mediating the translation of subword units into sound is needed for accurate identification of bound morphemes (e.g., ING, ENT, ION) and function words (Patterson, 1980). The disturbance giving rise to these errors, however, appears to be independent of any deficit in the subword routine from print to sound. Patients with phonological dyslexia have been documented who have no trouble reading and comprehending a full range of words (including morphologically complex and function words; Funnell, 1983), refuting the claim that pronunciation assembled from subword orthographic units is needed for processing affixes or function words. We review the nature of impairments affecting morphological processes in chapter 6 and function words in chapter 8.

Surface Dyslexia

Patients with surface dyslexia demonstrate the opposite of the dissociation observed in phonological dyslexia. Nonsense words are read aloud quite accurately, but the patient is impaired in the ability to recognize whole words and translate them into a pronunciation. We have indicated that the subword routine will not deliver a correct pronunciation if the target word violates regular correspondences between spelling and sound. Thus, the patient makes numerous errors when asked to read these items aloud, and the response is typically a pronunciation obtained by inappropriately applying the subword procedure to the translation process. Thus, LOVE would be pronounced "LOAVE" (consistent with the most general correspondence for OVE), HEAD as "HEED," STEAK as "STEEK," and so on.

In the early descriptions of surface dyslexia, the reading of regularly spelled words (e.g., FREAK, GROVE) was never completely intact (Marshall and Newcombe, 1973; Shallice and Warrington, 1980), and the lack of a clear difference between regular words and exception words led some authors (e.g., Marcel, 1980) to doubt the possibility of dissociable procedures for whole word and subword units. A case (M.P.) described by Bub, Cancelliere, and Kertesz (1985), however, demonstrates that the dissociation can occur. M.P., a normal reader before suffering a closed-head injury, was found to demonstrate excellent reading of both regular and nonsense words, but made numerous regularization errors when reading exception words. Like all other surface dyslexic patients (e.g., Coltheart et al., 1983; Shallice et al., 1983), M.P. was not completely unable to read any exception word correctly; Bub et al. found that correct performance depended crucially on the word's frequency. The interpretation of this patient's performance, then, is that the subword procedure remained completely intact whereas the whole-word routine had been damaged in such a way that it could only deal reliably with higher-frequency words (see our discussion of the Seidenberg and Waters results, above).

Surface dyslexic patients usually have no trouble understanding words they can read aloud correctly, though their comprehension of irregular words is severely disturbed. Since many words no longer make contact with a permanent representation in the orthographic lexicon, they can only gain access to meaning indirectly, via their pronunciation assembled through the subword routine. Thus, words are understood as they are pronounced, and irregular items will either be considered nonsensical (e.g., *steak* might be rendered "steek," a nonword) or misunderstood if their regularized translation happens to match a real word (e.g., the written word *bear*, would be pronounced "beer" by the typical surface dyslexic, and would then be defined as "an alcoholic drink"). A few rare cases have been described, however, who continue to understand irregular words, despite the fact that their pronunciation is based on a regularization error (Kay and Patterson, 1985; Kremin, 1985; Margolin, Marcel, and Carlson, 1985). The patient will indicate, for example, that the word *yacht* refers to a kind of boat, even though he or she has just translated it from print as "yachet." The interpretation of the deficit in these cases is that accessing the orthographic representation of words and using it to activate meaning has *not* been affected; instead, the disturbance involves the ability to access the pronunciation of words in the phonological output lexicon (figure 5.4). The patient, knowing the meaning of a written word but lacking access to its spoken form, is forced to assemble a response from subword units and therefore produces a regularization.[5]

An alternative account of surface dyslexia has been developed within the PDP framework. Patterson, Seidenberg, and McClelland (1989) "lesioned" the hidden unit level in their model by setting different numbers of the weights in these units to zero. In one experiment, 20% of the weights were "removed" in this fashion. The lesioned model was then presented with a list of high- and low-

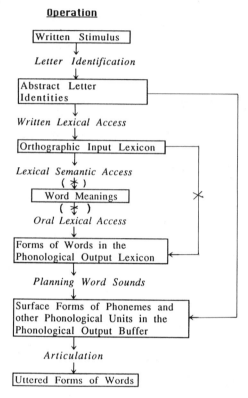

Figure 5.4
The reading model showing the location of the deficits in the routes from
lexical orthographic representations to lexical output phonological units
characteristic of surface dyslexia.

frequency regular and exception words to "read." The model's performance, averaged over ten tests, was compared with two patients
with surface dyslexia: M.P. and T.R. The model performed very
much like M.P., reading irregularly spelled words poorly if they
were of lower frequency. It did less well in simulating the performance of T.R., who showed a more pervasive effect of regularity
that affected high- as well as low-frequency words. The lesioned
model did produce many regularization errors (about 50% of its
erroneous responses were of this sort), but this was a lower rate of
production of these errors than that found in either of these patients
(both made about 85% regularization errors). The performance of
this model, when lesioned, thus mimics certain aspects of surface

dyslexia, though it is not yet clear whether it can provide a close match to all of the details of this disorder.

Nonsemantic Reading

The failure of the whole-word reading procedure without any central disturbance to the representation of meaning is characteristic of surface dyslexia. The reverse dissociation has also been documented, and confirms the existence of direct connections between the orthography of whole words and their pronunciation, separate from the ability to understand them. Schwartz, Saffran, and Marin (1980a) have described a dementia patient (W.L.P.) who suffered a major breakdown of semantic knowledge, but who demonstrated extremely accurate reading aloud of words.

The interesting aspect of this case was that irregularly spelled words—including low-frequency items like *tortoise* and *leopard*—were also pronounced correctly, even though the patient could not match the most familiar words (e.g., *chicken*, *sheep*, *cow*) to their pictorial referents, nor on many trials to their category label. Irregularly spelled words like *bowl*—cf. *howl, scowl, growl, fowl,*—*police, liquor,* etc., most of which the patient read correctly, would have been mispronounced if she had only relied on the translation of subword units into sound, because this procedure will deliver the most common value of a segment. The fact that W.L.P. obtained the pronunciation of many irregular words must therefore imply that she retained the ability to translate whole-word orthographic units into their spoken forms without recovering their semantic description, given that the meanings of most words were lost to her. This outcome has been taken as evidence for the existence of a word-specific routine from print to sound that does not involve the semantic mechanism.

The patient reported by Schwartz et al. was capable of reading a wide range of irregular words, indicating near-normal operation of the word-specific route to pronunciation. Another case, documented by Bub et al. (1985), who also had a major comprehension deficit of written and spoken language, could only read familiar irregular words with a high degree of accuracy (e.g., *love*), and produced numerous regularization errors on less familiar items (e.g., *pint*). For this patient, we may conclude that the whole-word mechanism is partially impaired, so that her performance exemplifies surface dyslexia coupled with nonsemantic reading.

Deep Dyslexia

A complex association of multiple symptoms characterizes the highly publicized reading disorder known as "deep dyslexia" (Coltheart, Patterson, and Marshall, 1980). The first and most fundamental finding is that the patient often reads a word by producing a semantically related response to the target (e.g., *table* is read aloud as "chair"). On some occasions, the patient may be aware of the error, but at other times—especially when the word refers to an abstract concept (e.g., *justice*) or the response is a close synonym to the target—the semantic paralexias go undetected. In addition to semantic errors, patients with deep dyslexia are worse at reading abstract words aloud than concrete, high-imagery words. Typically, many of the errors for abstract words are omissions, i.e., the patient fails to produce a response to the written target. Another feature of the syndrome is that reading of nonsense words is completely impossible—the patient either declines to respond or, if pressed, may produce a word that shares some letters with the nonword (e.g., "sift" for *sife*). There are numerous errors to singly presented grammatical function words (e.g., *if, and, when*), which are either omitted or substituted by another word from the same type of vocabulary (*the* may be read as "and"). Derived or inflected words are misread by substituting one affix for another valid but incorrect one (*walking* may be rendered "walked," *helpful* as "helpless"), omitting the affix (*walking* read as "walk") or assigning an extra one to the word (e.g., *helpless* read as "helplessly"). An affix may also be added to the base form, so that *walk* is read as "walking." Finally, patients make visual errors to words, producing responses like "tantrum" for *tandem* and "monument" for *moment*.

There are a number of ways to approach the co-occurrence of impairments that make up this fascinating syndrome. One possibility is that there is no direct functional relationship between them—the patients could form a homogeneous group not by virtue of some underlying property of the reading mechanism, but simply because the damage affected anatomically proximal areas in the brain. However, there may be a functional explanation for the co-occurrence of these abnormalities. Coltheart, Patterson, and Marshall (1987) have recently discussed the possible significance of the pattern observed in deep dyslexia. They note that the conjunction of symptoms hinges crucially on the presence of one error type: if the patient makes semantic errors, then, according to all published cases, the remaining characteristics are always obtained. In the absence of semantic errors, however, one finds patients who cannot read nonsense words (i.e., phonological dyslexia) but show no sensitivity to the other variables affecting the performance of patients with deep dyslexia. There are also patients who fail to produce semantic errors, but whose reading is affected by morphological complexity (Job and Sartori, 1984) or the concrete/abstract dimension (Funnell and Allport 1987). The dissociation of impairments without the apparently binding role of semantic errors led Coltheart et al. to doubt an explanation of the syndrome based simply on damage to contiguous anatomical regions.

But what, then, is the explanation of the co-occurence of semantic errors and the other characteristics of deep dyslexia? We may consider two different attempts at an interpretation, neither of which is entirely satisfactory. The first solution is to argue that the syndrome occurs because of interactions between components of the reading mechanism that emerge after damage to the system. The alternative viewpoint is that deep dyslexia reflects the properties of a right hemisphere mechanism, released after brain damage effectively abolishes reading in the left hemisphere.

The first explanation runs as follows. Patients with deep dyslexia are completely unable to assemble the pronunciation of a written nonsense word, so we may infer that the subword routine from print to sound has been totally abolished. The fact that a semantic variable like concreteness influences reading performance suggests further that the patient must be relying on the direct mapping of whole-word orthography onto meaning to obtain a pronunciation. Thus, many authors contend that for patients with deep dyslexia, neither the subword routine nor the nonsemantic translation of whole words into sound is viable (cf. Morton and Patterson, 1980), leaving the semantic pathway as the only means by which the patient can achieve a response (figure 5.5).

One interpretation of semantic paralexias in the light of the foregoing analysis is that the output of the semantic mechanism activated by a written word may not on its own guarantee the correct pronunciation of the target, even when the routine is operating nor-

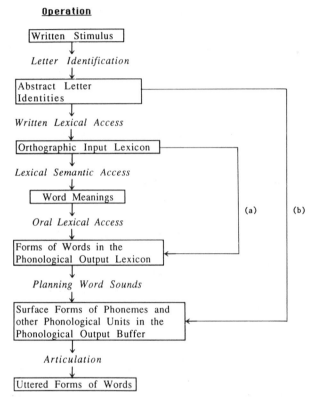

Figure 5.5
The reading model showing the location of the deficits in deep dyslexia.
Two routes are affected: (a) the direct route from lexical orthographic representations to lexical output phonological units, and (b) the route from sublexical orthographic units to sublexical output phonological units.

mally (cf. Marshall and Newcombe, 1973). The idea is that additional information, derived from the procedures that recover phonology
directly from word and subword units, is needed to locate the correct response from a number of alternative options. A word like *gift*,
for example, may address the pronunciation of a conceptually
equivalent word like *present* from the semantic system as well as
its own pronunciation, so that another code—the spoken form
obtained independently of the meaning—must be available to prevent an error. We could argue that the semantic mechanism in isolation is particularly unreliable when the representation of a word
does not contain enough information to uniquely determine the

spoken form. Thus, grammatical function words and bound morphemes (ed, ing, ment) might be particularly vulnerable because they often lack the kind of semantic detail that would unambiguously point to the correct output.

The main weakness of this account is that the normal semantic routine operates without being inherently prone to errors even when there is no reason to assume that it receives additional information from other components of the language mechanism. The naming of visually presented objects presumably takes place by deriving an instance of a concept from its physical structure, which is then used to look up the pronunciation. At least in terms of current theory, there are no extra codes obtained independently of this process, as there are when the normal reader converts a written word to sound, yet we do not often make semantic errors in naming visual objects, unless perhaps we are forced to respond quickly and the objects are relatively uncommon. An alternative hypothesis has therefore been proposed: that the performance of a patient with deep dyslexia is not a natural consequence of reading without phonological back-up, but is in fact the outcome of damage to the semantic mechanism itself (Morton and Patterson, 1980). If we assume that the conceptual description of certain words has been affected, locating their pronunciation from meaning would not be possible. Yet another possibility is that there is a disturbance in activation of output phonological representations from semantically intact representations.

These sources of semantic paralexias may account for different classes of errors—those that the patient recognizes as errors and those that he does not appreciate are erroneous. Semantic substitutions that are identified by the patient as errors (e.g., soldier–"Army, no that's not right") would be considered to be due to a failure in the mechanism that addresses the pronunciation of the word from meaning, so that a related word is inadvertently selected for output after the presented target word has been correctly identified and understood. Unmonitored errors, which usually are responses to abstract words and words that have close synonyms, have been dealt with by falling back on the notions that the semantic route alone cannot normally produce an unambiguous output for many words or that there may be damage to the set of lexical semantic representations. Thus, according to Morton and Patterson (1980): "It is only for some words that the semantic code uniquely identifies one output

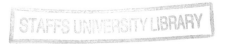

logogen; this may even be true for normal readers. For the patients, who have no other code, abstract words and words with close synonyms will yield semantic paralexias which are unidentified as errors." (p. 114).

We can explain visual errors in terms of the same idea by assuming that a word orthographically close to the target, having an *intact* semantic description, will often become activated to the point where it leads to a substitution error. The fact that visual confusions tend to be responses that are biased away from the production of abstract words (Shallice and Warrington, 1980) lends some support to the claim that words with preserved meaning (i.e., concrete words) are substituted for items lacking an adequate semantic representation.

However, this entire line of explanation is not above criticism. We have already questioned the hypothesis that the normal semantic route is intrinsically error-prone. We have now further assumed two different kinds of semantic-related problems underlying the reading responses in deep dyslexia—a loss of semantic knowledge for certain words, and a disturbance in activation of output phonological representations from semantically intact representations. Coltheart, Patterson, and Marshall (1987) justly voice their discomfort regarding such a proposal: "Must we now postulate several different semantic-routine impairments in deep dyslexia, and if so, why do we not observe patients who have one but not the other: in particular, patients who make semantic errors but do not have difficulty with abstract words" (p. 422).

The second explanation of the co-occurrence of semantic paralexias and the other features of deep dyslexia is that patients with deep dyslexia read with right hemisphere–based mechanisms that produce these kinds of errors (Coltheart, 1980; Saffran et al., 1980a). This argument is based on several findings. One is that the lesions in these patients tend to be large and occupy most of the language zone of the left hemisphere. Obviously, this argument is at most suggestive. A second point is that the right hemisphere of some patients with a division of the corpus callosum (the fibers connecting the two hemispheres) can support considerable language. However, this appears to be a rare phenomenon (Gazzaniga, 1983). It is important to note that if deep dyslexia truly relected the right hemisphere functions of this minority of cases, the syndrome would tell us little about the normal reading process. A third argument is that, in visual half-field studies (in which a visual stimulus is projected to one hemisphere), there is an advantage for recognition of concrete words, compared to abstract words, with left visual field–right-hemisphere projection of stimuli. However, this advantage is rarely found (Patterson and Besner, 1984), and may be confounded by length (Bub and Lewine, 1988a, b; Young and Ellis, 1985). Thus, the right hemisphere account receives little support from empirical studies.

Overall, the effort to link the semantic errors in deep dyslexia to other errors remains unsatisfactory. It appears that the constellation of symptoms seen in this syndrome is likely to reflect a co-occurrence of a number of different impairments in visual word processing (Shallice and Warrington, 1980).

Letter-by-Letter Reading

Certain patients with acquired dyslexia are unable to identify a word without laboriously naming or sounding out each letter. The term "letter-by-letter reading" has been used to describe this syndrome (Patterson and Kay, 1982). Paradoxically, these brain-damaged patients usually have no trouble spelling or writing (though surface agraphia may be observed in some cases; Friedman, 1982), but then experience great difficulty when they are asked a short time later to read the result. Below, we present, by way of an example, the attempts of a French patient, documented nearly a hundred years ago by Dejerine and Pélissier (1914), to decipher the phrase "Le siège d' Andrinople":

Le . . . . yes, that's correct . . . . . L . . . . E . . . . . le . . . . . after that an S . . . E . . . siècle, I have identified, Le siècle, d' . . . . E . . . that's an E, and after that . . . . . what's   that? . . . . d'En . . . . . . d'Endrino . . . . . . d'Andrinople . . . . . . le siècle d'Andrinople . . . . . It can't be that . . . . It must rather be Le siège d'Andrinople

Dejerine (1891, 1892), gave the first description of the reading disorder and interpreted it as a disconnection between the two occipital cortices and the mechanism representing the visual form of words in the left hemisphere. The damage may be cortical or subcortical, but the overall effect must block the transfer of letter codes extracted from sensory features onto word units. The word form system—the permanent description of the word's orthographic pattern—remains intact, however, and can be accessed from the language mechanism to recover the spelling of a word spontaneously or to dictation.

The account offered by Dejerine—later revived by Geschwind and Fusillo (1966)—is based on anatomical evidence, and leaves undefined the notion of a "disconnection" in functional terms. From a processing standpoint, we may conceive of the damage as either a total lack of communication between visual analyzers and the word-form system or as a change in the nature of communication between them. Researchers initially opted for the first of these possibilities.

Dejerine's explanation was abandoned in favor of the view that letter-by-letter reading was the outcome of a more general perceptual disturbance termed *simultanagnosia* (Wolpert, 1924, Kinsbourne and Warrington, 1962a, b). Patients with damage to the occipitotemporal region of the left hemisphere can usually recognize a single percept at brief exposure durations but in many cases are unable to recover the identity of additional elements from a display of two or more items even when the material is presented for a relatively protracted interval (Kinsbourne and Warrington, 1962a,b; Levine and Calvanio, 1978). The claim was made that the breakdown in the simultaneous perception of multiple forms extended to the synthesis of a word from its component letters. Thus, according to Kinsbourne and Warrington (1962b): "Only one letter can be read at a time and the interval before the visual system is ready for perception of the next is so long that reading must be a laborious hardship" (p. 481).

On theoretical grounds, there is reason to doubt this interpretation of letter-by-letter reading. The simultanagnosic patient has difficulty retrieving many perceptual *units* displayed at the same time, be they letters, numbers, or line drawings. Written words appear to have the status of perceptual wholes once they have been recognized perceptually. We might therefore expect simultanagnosia to interfere with the reading of several words presented together, but the deficit might not be expected to impair the recognition of an isolated word. Empirical evidence also provides support for a functional distinction between the two syndromes. Patients described in a group study by Warrington and Rabin (1971) were found to be very impaired on visual span tasks, yet none of them appeared to fit the clinical description of a letter-by-letter reader. More recently, Warrington and Shallice (1980) have documented a case study of a letter-by-letter reader who showed only a moderate reduction in visual span, incommensurate with his profound reading disorder.

Warrington and Shallice conclude that letter-by-letter reading cannot be attributed to visual or perceptual deficits. They offer the following interpretation of the syndrome: The visual word form system normally parses letter strings into familiar units (ranging in size from graphemes to syllables and whole words), and categorizes them perceptually. This automatic synthesis of letters into higher-order units allows for rapid and accurate identification of written words. Damage to the word form system produces letter-by-letter reading— the patient can no longer extract familiar units from a spelling pattern, and is forced to read by explicitly identifying each separate letter in the word. The ability to decipher a word from the name or sound of the letters is mediated by the intact spelling mechanism, which contains a duplicate of the visual word form system.

Warrington and Shallice's analysis is amenable to a direct test. Numerous experiments, beginning with observations made by Cattell in 1886, have shown that normal subjects are able to recognize briefly displayed words more accurately than random letter strings. A procedure devised by Wheeler (1970) and Reicher (1969) has shown clearly that the advantage for words is perceptual in origin. The general method behind these experiments is as follows: A four-letter word or random letter sequence is briefly presented to the subject on each trial, followed immediately by a pattern of random letter segments (a pattern mask) that disrupts further visual processing of the target display after it has terminated. The mask is followed by one of two choices that remain in view until the subject has made a response: one of these is the target item; the other is a foil that differs from the target by one letter only. The subject must say whether the first stimulus was repeated or a second stimulus shown. Reliable performance cannot be based on guesswork in this task, because the two alternatives are equally plausible. Furthermore, the use of a forced-choice procedure with a brief delay between the stimulus and the response minimizes the load on short-term memory (McClelland and Johnston, 1977). Any advantage in the recognition of words (e.g., McClelland, 1976; Johnston, 1978) can reasonably be attributed to the fact that the letters composing them are more accurately encoded than a group of random letters, or even a single letter (cf. McClelland and Johnston, 1977), that fails to activate a familiar orthographic structure.

The word superiority effect, then, is due to the activation of higher-level orthographic units that enhances the recoverability of letter identities, either because the familiar units making up a word are not susceptible to masking in the way that unstructured letter strings are, or because the constituent letters of a word are identified more rapidly than the letters in a random sequence. If Warrington and Shallice are correct, the knowledge mediating the effect, which is stored in the visual word form system, is no longer available to the letter-by-letter reader.

Bub, Black, and Howell (1989) recently evaluated this claim by looking for the absence or presence of a word superiority effect in a patient with the disorder. The patient was a 51-year-old teacher (J.V.) who underwent neurosurgery for removal of a benign left temporo-occipital meningioma. Although clearly reading letter by letter (the time taken to identify a word was massively dependent on word length), J.V. nevertheless showed a pronounced effect of orthographic familiarity on letter recognition when the display was presented briefly under masked viewing conditions and he was asked to discriminate the target from an alternative differing by one letter. His performance was compared with another patient (P.J.) of similar age who also had damage to the posterior regions of the left hemisphere, but whose reading was found to be intact. During a practice session, the exposure duration of the target was adjusted for each patient so that both attained an overall accuracy of roughly 75%. Figure 5.6 indicates the relative abilities of each patient to distinguish letters on trials where the difference between the target and the foil involved positions 1 (e.g., *mark park*), 2 (e.g., *find fund*), 3 (e.g., *ship shop*) or the 4 (e.g., *food foot*) in the array. P.J. demonstrated a U-shaped curve on random letters typical of normal encoding; the string is processed from the outer to the inner elements, so that medial positions are less accurately identified than the letters in external positions (Rumelhart and McClelland, 1982). The curve for word stimuli remains flat and reveals a clear influence of orthographic context on letter recognition. The serial position effect obtained for J.V. on random letter strings indicates that he processes them from left to right; his recognition of the initial two letters is accurate; his performance is at chance when he is required to discriminate either of the last two letters from an alternative choice. The pattern is consistent with the impairment of simultaneous form perception often observed in association with letter-by-letter

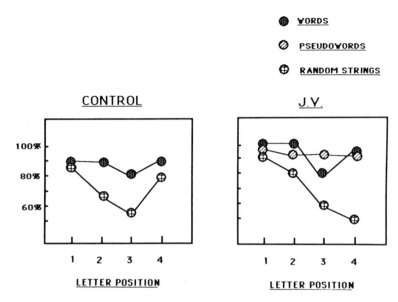

Figure 5.6
Percentage of correct letter identifications in words, pseudowords, and random letter strings made by patient J.V., a letter-by letter reader. (Reproduced with permission from Bub, Black, and Howell, 1989.)

reading. In contrast to the very marked impact of serial position on the recognition of random letter strings, J.V. demonstrates no loss of accuracy over the length of the array when he is presented with familiar words and pseudowords.[6] This indicates that he can make use of orthographic context to facilitate the recovery of letter information, and suggests that his simultanagnosia affects his ability to retain or retrieve multiple letter forms from a short-term memory system *after* they have been activated.

The results obtained by Bub et al. indicate that J.V. is perceptually sensitive to legal orthographic patterns (which include nonsense words as well as words). Though we do not have sufficient grounds to claim that his units of visual processing include whole words, we can, however, reject the strongest version of the explanation for letter-by-letter reading proposed by Warrington and Shallice, namely that the syndrome is due to such a major reduction in the magnitude of the encoding units derived from print that only information about single letters can be processed.

Other evidence suggests that letter-by-letter readers may indeed gain access to a whole word representation, but that the system is not activated strongly enough to permit complete identification of the target. Shallice and Saffran (1986) have described a letter-by-letter reader who could obtain a partial meaning from words presented too briefly for him to decode explictly by naming the letters. Given a forced choice, the patient could reliably determine whether a target word referred to an animate or an inanimate object, for example, even though he was incapable of reporting the word's identity. Coslett and Saffran (1988) reported additional letter-by-letter readers with this residual ability, and proposed that the patients were using a right hemisphere mechanism operating covertly on written language. How general the phenomenon of unconscious reading ability is in the syndrome remains to be established. Perhaps there are a variety of word form deficits, some patients having lost whole word units, others with a disturbance in the activation of word units from letter analyzers. One fact is clear, however; letter-by-letter reading is often a compensatory strategy on the part of the patient that cannot be taken as a direct reflection of the underlying capabilities of the system. A more general lesson to be learned from these cases is that the attempts by a brain-damaged patient to fully recover a word or sentence for an explicit report may give a misleading picture of the deficit, and that to obtain a true understanding of language impairments we need measures that go well beyond the most immediately obvious manifestations of a deficit.

Summary

We have outlined several disturbances that affect the ability to read and understand printed words. These disturbances can be attributed to disruptions of different aspects of the reading process, here described as "routes," in a model of the functional architecture of reading. Though much remains to be learned about these disorders, this approach has clearly indicated that different dyslexic patterns are due to different functional impairments.

AGRAPHIA

Phonological Agraphia

Patients with phonological agraphia are severely impaired in their ability to spell or write nonsense syllables and nonsense words, but are capable of very good performance on legitimate words, even words that are low in frequency and contain unusual spelling patterns (e.g., *leopard*). The extent of this dissociation is striking: Shallice (1981), for example, has documented a patient who could not accurately transcribe more than 26% of single-syllable nonsense words to dictation, though he averaged 90% on a large sample of words varying in concreteness, frequency, and spelling regularity. The patient's difficulty was not merely the result of impaired auditory discrimination, or of any problem in retaining the items in memory for the duration required to assemble their spelling pattern. Shallice tested whether the patient could repeat the dictated nonword *after* each attempt at a response; repetition was clearly very much better than writing the item to dictation, even after a delay of 10 seconds.

The existence of phonological agraphia, now confirmed in several reports (Bub and Kertesz, 1982a; Roeltgen and Heilman, 1984; Baxter and Warrington, 1985; Hatfield, 1985), clearly refutes the suggestion that we can only write words by converting speech segments (e.g., phonemes or syllables) into their corresponding orthographic units. However, the general features of the syndrome do not rule out the possibility that access to the pronunciation of the *whole word* is necessary before its spelling pattern can be obtained. Evidence for the independence of activation of spoken and written word forms comes from patients whose ability to recover the pronunciation of a word is very impaired but who nevertheless can accurately retrieve its orthography.

Dissociations Between Written and Spoken Naming
Certain aphasic patients are able to write down the name of an object that they cannot produce in spoken form. The anomic disturbance in the relevant cases is not simply caused by impairment to lower-level mechanisms responsible for articulation. Bub and Kertesz (1982a), for example, documented a patient (M.H.) whose spontaneous speech, though fluent, was almost totally devoid of content words. Her oral naming of drawings, objects, and written words was extremely poor, and this deficit appeared to involve a complete failure in the ability to access the underlying pronunciation of the target. M.H.'s performance on a variety of tasks requiring the internal manipulation of speech codes (e.g., picture-word rhyme matching) indicated that the sound of the word was simply unavailable.

Despite this profound impairment in spoken language, M.H. displayed a very remarkable capacity to write the names of pictures or objects presented to her. She correctly produced the written names of 19 of 20 objects and 15 of 20 line drawings; by contrast, she could retrieve the spoken names for only 3 of 40 of these items. Further aspects of M.H.'s writing were typical of patients with phonological agraphia. She could not write nonsense words (1/20 correct) or nonsense syllables (0/20 correct) to dictation, but her transcription of words was very accurate over a wide range of frequency values. The errors on nonsense words were clearly not the result of impaired auditory encoding or retention; M.H., like the phonological agraphic patient documented by Shallice (1981), could accurately repeat each nonword before and after attempting a written response. The evidence from this patient and similar patients indicates that the orthography of a word can be available for writing and spelling in the complete absence of its spoken form.[7]

Category-Specific Phonological Agraphia

Patients who are forced, through brain damage, to write without the mediation of speech codes must generate the orthography of the word directly from its meaning. In some cases, this process is not completely intact, and selective difficulty occurs for words belonging to a particular semantic category.

Bub and Kertesz (1982b) documented a patient (J.C.) who wrote concrete words to dictation much more accurately than abstract words, while verbs and grammatical function words (e.g., *the, and, before*) were written very poorly. Several of J.C.'s responses were semantically related to the target : thus, she wrote *funny* for the word *happy, boat* for *yacht, smile* for *laugh*, etc. The authors termed this striking pattern "deep agraphia," to link it with the analogous reading disorder observed in patients with deep dyslexia (Coltheart, Patterson, and Marshall, 1980), but it is perhaps more accurate to think of it as a category-specific phonological agraphia. Unlike these patients, however, J.C. had no trouble reading and comprehending written words, so that her difficulty was specific to the production of an orthographic code. In fact, although J.C. did not seem aware of her errors during the act of writing, she immediately recognized them on completion, because her reading of single words was intact. This suggests considerable independence between the mechanisms for recognizing and producing the visual form of a word.

The nature of category-specific phonological agraphia indicates some disturbance in the process that recovers the spelling of the word after its meaning has been correctly determined. Baxter and Warrington (1985) provide the best evidence for the claim that the impairment can occur subsequent to the point where the word is understood, by asking for definitions of all items that the patient was unable to write or spell correctly. The particular classes of words that were poorly transcribed (verbs, adjectives, and function words caused more errors than nouns) were nonetheless understood without difficulty.

There are two possible explanations for the effect of word type on writing performance in phonological agraphia. We could assume that the functional connections between the meaning of words and their orthographic description are represented in terms of specific categories. If the connections sustain only partial damage, certain classes of words may be more adequately retrieved. Hart, Berndt, and Caramazza (1985) argued for this kind of interpretation in their analysis of a patient with a selective naming disorder for fruits and vegetables. The patient had trouble generating the precise label for items from these categories but he attained a high level of accuracy when asked to name objects from a wide variety of other categories (e.g., animals, vehicles, and food products not including fruit and vegetables). Further tests indicated that the anomia could not be due to a loss of semantic knowledge for the impaired items, leading the authors to conclude that "the lexical/semantic system is organized categorically and specifically at the level of the input and output processes to and from the system" (p. 440). (See chapter 3 for further discussion of category-specific processing deficits.)

An alternative proposal is that category-specific agraphia involves changes to the actual structure of the word-form system (cf. Baxter and Warrington, 1985). A processing component that deals with whole words as orthographic units may contain information about their grammatical class for correct insertion into sentence frames. It should be emphasized, however, that this higher-level knowledge could pertain only to the role of a word as a syntactic unit. Other conceptual attributes that represent the meaning of the word (e.g., whether it refers to a fruit or vegetable) form part of semantic memory and exist independently of the orthographic lexicon. Thus, we may expect the word-form system to fractionate in ways that distinguish nouns from verbs and adjectives from function words, but any effects of word class that cannot be linked to the processing of syntax would most probably originate outside this component.

Visual Aspects of Phonological Agraphia

Some patients with phonological agraphia have commented that they feel as if they are writing by looking at the word registered on an "internal screen" (e.g., Shallice, 1981). In one very unusual patient with right parietal damage, the syndrome was accompanied by errors at the beginning of the word (Baxter and Warrington, 1983), which the authors attributed to unilateral neglect of space. This patient could spell with equal accuracy both forward and backward, and the position of the errors remained the same regardless of the response direction. Hatfield (1985) has described an agraphic patient whose writing suggested a visual approach: B.B. often wrote the letters composing a word in a nonlinear order, sometimes beginning with the last or intermediate letter before attempting to reconstruct the rest of the word. Hatfield suggested that, "If a patient was forced to rely on some kind of visual representation it would seem less surprising that he or she would proceed in this way. . . . A visual form need not imply a left-to-right succession but could be a simultaneous event with or without prominence of certain (nonsequential) features" (pp. 17–18). A similar observation on the nonlinear retrieval of letters in agraphia has been made by Morton (1980b).

The claim that spelling in phonological agraphia may demand an ability to visualize the words raises questions about the relevance of the syndrome for our understanding of the normal writing mechanism. Conceivably, the retrieval of whole-word orthography without the mediation of sound can only occur in exceptional persons who are skilled at forming detailed visual images. This type of explanation has been offered by Levine, Calvanio, and Popovics (1982), who document a patient showing extremely good written language skills and a complete loss of spoken language that included both word pronunciation and the recovery or manipulation of internal speech codes. The authors go so far as to suggest that the patient's talent for visual imagery along with extensive practice in speed reading caused a functional reorganization in the brain that "resulted in his unique pattern of disability instead of a more ordinary aphasia" (p. 407).

But there are reasons for doubting the assumption that imagery provides the functional basis for written word production (or comprehension) in the examples we have discussed. The orthographic knowledge of whole words, though based on a visual representation, is highly abstract in nature, and should not be thought of as a sensory description of letter elements (Clarke and Morton, 1983). A mental image of the word may be generated from this higher-level information but it is unclear why the image would be required as a necessary intermediate step for correct performance.

The evidence, then, provides little support for the direct contribution of imagery to writing in phonological agraphia. The subjective impression of certain patients, that they are using an "inner screen" to retrieve the visual form of a word, cannot be given much credence without more objective evidence that this is how they activate written word forms. The observation that letter retrieval is not always sequential in certain cases is of interest, but this approach to spelling may be more a reflection of a disturbance in accessing the orthography of the word than a manifestation of imagery. As for the suggestion that only exceptional persons may be capable of writing without the mediation of sound, Shallice (1981) argues that the errors occurring in phonological agraphia are identical to the "slips of the pen" observed in normal writers (Ellis, 1979b). This correspondence can be attributed to the "use of a common mechanism in the two situations, namely, excessive reliance on the . . . [whole word] . . . route in one case because of necessity and the other for speed" (p. 424).

Writing Without the Visual Word Form: Surface (or Lexical) Dysgraphia

Phonological agraphia is an agraphic syndrome that reveals the existence of an orthographic procedure allowing direct access to the visual form of entire words. This cannot be the only procedure available to normal writers, of course, who, unlike patients with phonological agraphia, can also use more analytic units to represent the spelling of any spoken form, even an unfamiliar one. The nature of phonological agraphia suggests that this component may function independently of the word-specific routine, since legitimate words can be written even when the ability to write nonsense words has been compromised. The assumption of independence predicts the occurrence of another major writing disorder, involving the reverse of the dissociation observed in phonological agraphia. If whole word orthographic knowledge has been damaged (or if this knowledge cannot be retrieved), the patient will be forced to use sublexical spelling-to-sound correspondences to assemble the spelling of the word. When the orthography of the language permits several legitimate ways of capturing the same pronunciation, we should expect that numerous responses to irregularly spelled words will be produced that are phonologically valid transcriptions of the target but which are not the conventional form of the word. There have been a number of published cases that provide clear examples of this spelling disorder, termed *surface agraphia* or *lexical agraphia*.

Beauvois and Derouesné (1981) have documented a patient, R.G., who experienced spelling difficulty after surgery for a left parieto-occipital angioma. He could accurately write nonsense words to dictation, demonstrating adequate knowledge of the correspondences between sound and print, but he often made errors when asked to write orthographically ambiguous words or irregular words. The degree of ambiguity was indicated by the number of silent letters in a word or by the relative frequency of the orthographic value for a given speech segment (e.g., the vowel in *care* can be signaled by the digraph EA, as in PEAR and WEAR, but this correspondence is not used very commonly). The patient's accuracy deteriorated systematically as the orthographic ambiguity of the target increased, though the effect was less pronounced for familiar words, which were often transcribed correctly. The influence of word frequency on performance is characteristic of surface agraphia, and suggests that the vulnerability of whole word orthographic units depends on their history of prior activation (Bub et al. 1985).

In a more recent case report, Hatfield and Patterson (1983) began to explore the size of the units used by a surface agraphic patient in converting phonological representations to orthographic representations. They examined the ability of a patient with surface agraphia (T.P.) to spell homophonic words (dictated in a sentence to convey their meaning) relative to words with a spelling pattern that is completely predictable from the pronunciation alone. The patient's numerous errors on these items (e.g., *bean* rendered as "been") and her very accurate performance on predictable words (e.g., *lunch, thing, spent*), indicated the use of a procedure that translates phonemic segments into orthographic code when the specific form of the word had not been accessed. Further analysis of the mistakes produced by T.P. to a variety of dictated words confirmed the observation that her responses often captured valid correspondences between sound and spelling (e.g., *nephew* spelled as NEFFUE). A substantial number of the errors, however, could not be classified in this manner (15%), and in fact appeared to violate the principles of correspondence. For example, the patient wrote *bake* as BAK and *pan* as PANE, which reveals an inadequate grasp of vowel lengthening in the context of a final E. Hatfield and Patterson argue that many of these anomalous responses can still be interpreted as *correct* transcriptions if we assume the patient is not consistent in her choice of orthographic units and if she is insensitive to the constraints between segments. Thus, for example, the spoken target BAKE could yield the letter sequence BA as instantiated in *baby*, *basin*, etc. and the patient would then appropriately terminate her response with the letter K.

To justify their interpretation, the authors point out that each sound segment may be treated as an independent unit of translation for writing or spelling via a speech-based code. The mapping of print into sound (i.e., reading aloud), by contrast, must include a processing stage where phonemic segments are blended together to form a single utterance, and this requires sensitivity to a variety of contextual influences. They also note that the patient's lack of consistency in her choice of an orthographic correspondence for a given speech segment is entirely compatible with the multiple graphemic options available for numerous phonemes in English.

The tendency to employ a range of correspondences rather than to follow invariable mapping principles has been observed in other cases of surface agraphia. The patient R.G. documented by Beauvois and Dérouesné spelled *rameau* as RAMO, *copeau* as COPOT, and *faisceau* as FAISSAU. O, OT, and AU are all legitimate French spellings of the sound /o/. Goodman and Caramazza (1986) have recently analyzed the number of different graphemic values that a surface agraphic patient assigned to each phoneme by comparing them with norms of English orthography compiled by Hanna and colleagues (1966). These tables list the relative frequency of every correspondence for a given phoneme in the appropriate syllable position. The results indicated that the probability of selecting a particular graphemic value depended on the relative frequency of its occurrence, leading the authors to conclude that the mechanism for converting phonemes into spelling units has mapping options with activation levels determined by their frequency of use in the language.

We have described two aspects of surface agraphia that have emerged from studies of individual patients : (1) lack of consistency in the selection of an orthographic correspondence for a phonemic segment and (2) apparent failure to always employ correct principles of translation between sound and spelling. It should be emphasized that individual patients can exhibit considerable heterogeneity with respect to these characteristics, a fact which must be accounted for by any theory of the disorder. Campbell (1983), for example, notes that a patient, E.E., (first described by Coltheart, 1982), produced spellings that were highly consistent from one week to the next. The patient R.G. (Beauvois and Derouesné, 1981) made very few mistakes that were due to the application of invalid correspondences; this type of error accounted for only 9% of his responses.

We noted in our discussion of the sublexical spelling mechanism that phonological spelling can be based on orthographic segments of varying size. Damage to the processing mechanism will tend to reduce the size of the unit available for transcoding (Shallice et al., 1983), and the degree of shrinkage will presumably depend on the extent of functional damage in each case. Many patients with surface agraphia are clearly relying on very small units to assemble the orthography of a spoken word. Newcombe and Marshall (1985) have described a particularly extreme version of this disorder, where the phoneme-grapheme correspondences were consistently limited to a single letter for each phoneme. Thus, the patient (whose spelling was normal prior to a closed head injury) wrote *motor* as MOTA, *tone* as TON and *goes* as GOZ. The authors conclude that the functional disturbance in this patient affected both whole word knowledge and the phonological routine, which could no longer assign multiletter graphemes to a phoneme. The performance of other surface agraphic patients indicates a similar dual deficit, although the constraint on their spelling appears to be less severe.

When responses are assembled from minimal orthographic segments, we can expect frequent violation of mapping principles that require sensitivity to contextual influences (cf. Hatfield and Patterson, 1983). Larger units of translation, however, will not produce such errors (cf. Beauvois and Derouesné, 1981). In addition, the size of the unit may determine the overall consistency with which a mapping option appears: very small segments (e.g., an individual

letter for a phoneme) can only yield a limited number of correspondences for each vowel or consonant, and spelling performance
should be highly consistent. If the units available to the patient
extend to multiple letters (e.g., graphemes or syllables), a greater
variety of mapping options become available to the patient, which
may be chosen on a probabilistic basis (Goodman and Caramazza,
1986). Finally, still larger units (e.g., entire word endings) may re-
introduce constraints on the possible values that could mediate a
response. For example, the word *priest* could never be written
PREEST if the terminal segment EEST is considered as the relevant
unit, because this particular orthographic ending does not occur in
English.

The degree of impairment to the whole word writing routine may
also be partial (as is the case for the whole word reading routine, see
the discussion of the surface dyslexic patient, M.P., above). Support
for such a partial impairment of this route comes from results presented by Goodman and Caramazza (1986), who examined the way
their patient spelled homophones disambiguated by the appropriate
sentence context. They reasoned that, in the absence of a mapping
from the input phonological to the output orthographic word form
systems, the correct spelling of a homophone must depend entirely
on its meaning. If the particular orthographic address of a word were
not available, the patient would be forced to use phoneme-grapheme
correspondences to assemble a response, and the errors would tend
to be phonologically valid nonsense words (e.g., KORSE for *course*)
rather than the alternative homophonic word (*coarse*). Different predictions can be made if the spoken word is directly mapped onto
both orthographic representations in the visual word form system.
When each member of a homophone pair is a relatively familiar
item, the patient would be expected to produce many responses
involving homophone substitutions (e.g., *wore* instead of *war*),
because the two forms have an equally strong likelihood of being
activated from auditory input. A similar situation would arise when
one of the alternative homophones has a lower frequency of occurrence; the more frequent orthographic version of the auditory word
will be contacted, yielding many errors. The authors found that
the relevant misspellings were mostly homophone substitutions,
unless both members of a response pair were low in frequency.
For these items, access to whole word orthography could not take
place, and the patient often produced nonsense words that were

plausible translations of the auditory target. The authors concluded that the activation of written word forms from whole word phonology is frequency sensitive.

Asemantic Writing

Evidence for the proposal that the contents of the visual word form system can be addressed from spoken input without first looking up the conceptual representation (i.e., meaning) of the word has recently been presented by Patterson (1986). She described a patient (G.E.) who could not write spontaneously but whose writing to dictation was relatively accurate. Further investigation of G.E.'s performance disclosed that he could not have been relying on subword units to perform the task, because his ability to spell nonsense words was clearly impaired. Tests of the patient's comprehension also revealed a significant discrepancy between his understanding of a spoken word (which was impaired) and the accuracy of his spelling to dictation. The accurate transcription of words in the *absence* of (a) preserved comprehension and (b) phoneme-grapheme translation suggests that there is a direct route from whole word input phonology to whole-word output orthography in which word meanings are not activated.

The Role of Phonological Codes in Writing Sentences

We indicated above that some theorists maintain that the phonological forms of words are stored in a buffer in writing sentences. According to this theory, these forms activate the written forms of words via the direct whole word phonology→ whole word orthography route in writing sentences. As yet, evidence from brain-damaged patients has failed to confirm or disconfirm the hypothesis that speech codes are needed to fluently produce a written sentence. Bub and Kertesz (1982a) observed that the patient M.H., described above, whose written performance at the level of single words occurred entirely without the mediation of phonology, was very impaired in her ability to write sentences. The nature of the errors indicated poor control of grammatical morphemes (e.g., function words like *the, but,* and word affixes like *ing, ment, er*) as well as complete omission of verbs. For example, M.H.'s written description of a picture illustrating a boy closing a window was: "A boy is close the window." By contrast, her spoken response, tested approximately 1 hour later, revealed correct use of grammar along with the expected failure to produce the necessary content words ("It looks as if he is putting down the . . . "). Although the constraints on M.H.'s performance in the written and spoken modalities are strikingly discrepant, we should be cautious in our interpretation of the results. They indicate only that M.H. has sustained damage to some processing component involved in the construction of written sentences, and that this component is not required to generate the structure of a spoken sentence. It may be the case that the functional lesion responsible for the disorder is indeed confined to the phonological mechanism, but we need relevant evidence that bears directly on this question.

We must also note that E.B., a patient who demonstrated a breakdown in phonology that appeared very similar to the one affecting M.H., had no major difficulty writing sentences. According to Levine et al. (1982), E.B. wrote slowly, but: "His syntax was sophisticated, and his writing included frequent compound sentences, complex sentences and participial phrases" (p. 405). Unless we are willing to accept the suggestion that E.B.'s performance was based on the development of highly atypical skills (which, the reader may recall, is the interpretation the authors put on this case), the ability of this patient to write sentences indicates that speech codes are not essential for producing written language.

Independence of Reading and Writing

The general model of the writing mechanism includes a number of higher-level processing components. The visual word form system holds the permanent orthographic description of the word, its meaning is located in semantic memory, and a rule-governed procedure exists for mapping phonological information onto graphemic segments. To what extent are these different functional components restricted to the writing mechanism? Does the reading mechanism make use of the same components, or must we assume that another set of orthographic and phonological representations are available for encoding (as opposed to production) of written words?

There is no doubt that the reading performance of patients with phonological or surface agraphia can be strikingly different from their writing performance. The patient J.C. (Bub and Kertesz, 1982b) was unable to write nonsense words to dictation, but read these items aloud without difficulty. R.G., studied by Beauvois and Dérouesné (1979), produced numerous misspellings when attempting to write orthographically irregular or ambiguous words. In marked contrast, his reading problem appeared to be the complete reverse of the spelling disorder—he accurately read the majority of legitimate words, but could not assemble the pronunciation of a written nonsense word. Astonishingly, this patient often failed to read his own transcription of dictated words; if the resulting pattern (obtained by converting phonemes into spelling units) was found to be an orthographic nonword, R.G. was incapable of a valid response!

The dissociation they observed led Beauvois and Derouesné to infer that "the orthographic knowledge necessary for word recognition in reading is different from the orthographic knowledge necessary for correct spelling in writing" (p. 32). Similar arguments have been made for a distinction between the word form system mediating reception and production of auditory language (Morton, 1979a, b; 1980a, b; Shallice, McLeod, and Lewis, 1985; see chapter 4). The proposed organization of these functionally separate input and output components is depicted in figure 5.7.

The assumption of dual word form systems in each modality, though accepted by many researchers, has also been the subject of controversy. Allport and Funnell (1981) have pointed out that a dissociation of the kind reported by Beauvois and Dérouesné is in fact theoretically neutral with respect to the question. It may be the case that R.G.'s spelling disorder involves damage to a visual word form system required only for written output. However, the results are equally compatible with the hypothesis that written language is processed via a single orthographic mechanism, with functionally distinct channels allowing access to whole-word representation for reading, and retrieval of this information for writing. A diagram of this proposal is depicted in figure 5.8.

Examining dissociated performance (e.g., surface agraphia with phonological dyslexia) to decide between the two rival claims requires clear proof that impairment found on one set of tasks (writing) is the result of damage to a visual word form system and not to an output channel. In many cases, it may be difficult to provide such evidence because we still lack definite criteria for distinguishing the loss of a particular mental representation (e.g., orthographic knowledge) from an access or retrieval problem. (See chapter 3 for dis-

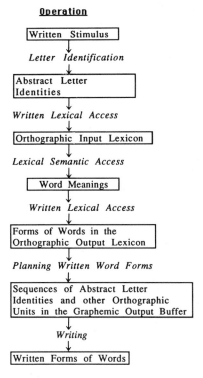

Figure 5.7
A model of the reading and writing process that includes a separate input and output orthographic lexicon.

cussion of attempts to make this distinction with respect to the semantic system.)

Further information relevant to the question of a duplicated word form system can be sought by considering instances where the disturbance in reading and writing is qualitatively the same. Thus, we look at patients who demonstrate associated deficits rather than dissociations in performance. Coltheart and Byng (1983) have analyzed a developmental case of surface agraphia and dyslexia (S.L.) in order to determine whether the reading and writing errors originated from a common mechanism. They focused on the numerous confusions made by S.L. when he was asked to produce or comprehend a written homophone. If these errors reflect damage to the contents of a unitary word form system, the particular items that are misspelled in writing should be the same items that are confused with their homophonic counterparts in reading.

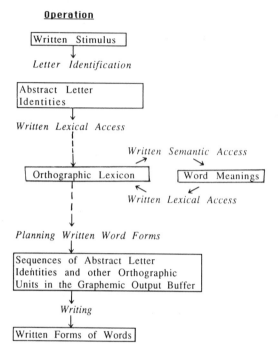

Figure 5.8
A model of the reading and writing process that includes a single orthographic lexicon.

The results gave no indication of the predicted consistency. S.L.
correctly spelled many homophonic words that he misunderstood
when they were presented to him in written form. Conversely,
words that he successfully recognized were not spelled better than
words yielding homophone confusions in writing. Finally, items
that were misspelled did not yield more reading errors than the
alternative correctly spelled member of a homophone pair.

The authors then considered whether S.L.'s dyslexia and agraphia
may have been the outcome of a disturbance in gaining reliable access to orthographic knowledge. This possibility would explain the
lack of any significant correlation between his reading and spelling
mistakes without forcing us to reject the assumption of a unitary
word form system. They reasoned that impaired access to a word
should result in fluctuations of word activation over time, so that
even on very similar tasks, the item-by-item comparison of performance will not reveal consistency. Analysis of S.L.'s ability to com-

prehend a visual word, though, did produce reliable overlap between items. For example, a homophonic word was spelled aloud to him and he was asked to supply a definition of its meaning. If S.L. correctly understood the item, he also demonstrated comprehension of it on a previous reading test. By contrast, spelled words that were confused with their homophonic alternatives, also caused many errors in the reading task.

Coltheart and Byng favor the conclusion that reading and writing are mediated by separate word form systems, and they account for S.L.'s impairment in terms of two functional lesions, one affecting the contents of the output system, the other disrupting the pathway from the input system to semantic memory. We may question these results, given the discrepancy between the techniques used to compare the encoding and retrieval of orthographic knowledge. The activation of whole-word orthography from print was measured by asking S.L. to determine the meaning of a written homophone. In this task, the familiarity of the word would be expected to dictate the choice of response; an item like SOLE, for example, may be misunderstood as SOUL, because the frequency of the target is very low. S.L.'s ability to produce the orthography of a word was assessed more directly—he was required to spell it after he grasped the meaning. Here, we do not expect familiarity to be the only variable affecting his performance. Instead, the frequency of the particular spelling pattern in the word could also be relevant. Thus, SOLE has a very common pattern and may be spelled correctly, while the pattern SOUL is much less common and will produce an error. The difference in the nature of the reading and writing tasks may therefore explain the failure to obtain a correlation between them.

More recently, Bub, Black, and Behrmann (1986) have carried out an item-by-item analysis of the transcoding errors made by a patient (M.P.) with a documented impairment of the whole-word routine, whom we described earlier in our discussion of surface alexia. M.P. is a surface dyslexic patient, who derives the pronunciation of many written items by relying on her intact ability to translate sublexical spelling patterns into sound (Bub et al., 1985). As discussed above, this causes her to misread orthographically irregular words. The same constraints affect her spelling of dictated words; though phonologically plausible, the responses often indicate a failure to retrieve the correct visual form. The question of interest is whether the particular items misread by M.P. are also the items she misspells. Since her disorder is only partial, M.P. accurately transcodes a considerable number of irregular words; for these items, we again wished to know whether a significant overlap in performance could be found.

The results indicated a very clear association between reading and writing: over 75% of M.P.'s responses were either both correct or both incorrect, consistent with the hypothesis that a single functional locus was responsible for the errors in both tasks. The damaged processing component may well be the visual word form system, though an alternative locus is also possible. M.P.'s ability to retrieve the orthography of a word in writing to dictation cannot depend on the activation of its meaning, because M.P. has a major comprehension deficit that precludes the use of the semantic component. If the representation needed for spelling a word is obtained from the output system that mediates pronunciation (cf. Patterson, 1986), we can explain the results without giving up the assumption that reading and writing are based on separate orthographic mechanisms. M.P. has a severe naming disorder, involving a disturbance in the retrieval of phonological codes. She may have lost the phonological entries of certain words. She would then be unable to produce the visual form of those items when they are dictated to her, nor could she achieve the reverse process of translating their orthography into a word-specific pronunciation (see figure 5.9).

Clearly, the issue of a dual vs. unitary word form system has not yet been resolved. We have discussed the available work on the subject to illustrate a number of different methodological approaches that have been utilized in the search for an answer. The dissociation of reading from writing implies that reception and production of written words are functionally separate at some level, but this fact alone does not prove that the word form system is doubly represented. The analysis of cases where reading and writing are both similarly impaired could provide a test of the hypothesis, but the disturbance must be shown to affect the patient's knowledge of whole word orthography, and the proportion of errors must be low enough to permit a valid comparison between tasks.

Peripheral Mechanisms

The abstract graphemic representation of familiar and unfamiliar words is ultimately converted by the writing mechanism into a

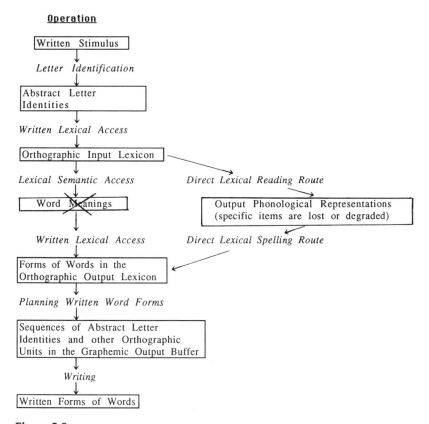

Figure 5.9
A model of the writing process incorporating both an input and an output orthographic lexicon, illustrating a possible deficit in M.P. that accounts for the consistency of her reading and spelling errors over lexical items.

sequence of rapid movements that generate letters on the page. The peripheral components mediating the output requirements of the system are not well understood at present, though we have some knowledge of their general organization.

The Graphemic Buffer
The higher-level codes available for written production range from whole-word units to more analytic spelling patterns, whereas the components behind motor output deal with the programming of individual letters (Ellis, 1982). According to Caramazza, Miceli, Villa and Romani (1987), a specialized working memory device is needed

to maintain the graphemic code in a buffer zone while the spatial identity of each letter is chosen at the next processing stage.

To obtain neuropsychological evidence for a graphemic buffer, the authors document a patient (L.B.) whose writing disorder originated in a functional component that was sufficiently peripheral to be: (1) the destination of all possible input channels, and (2) used whenever an orthographic sequence was translated into a response. Caramazza et al. report that L.B. made the same kind of errors in writing, oral spelling, and typing, a result which justifies the conclusion that the disturbance arose *before* the planning and execution of a particular motor program. They also found that mistakes occurred when the patient was asked to write spontaneously, transcribe dictated words, produce the written name of an object, and even when delayed copying was tested. This result, along with the fact that nonsense words and words gave an identical pattern of errors, implies that the relevant processing stage is located *beyond* the point where orthographic information has either been retrieved from the word form system or assembled from the correspondences between phonemes and spelling units.

The authors proceed by making a number of intuitively plausible assumptions: First, they note that the role of the buffer is to temporarily store an orthographic representation. The effect of damage to the buffer should presumably be a deterioration in the specificity of its contents, which may involve substitution, deletion, addition, and transposition of graphemic units. The kind of spelling errors made by L.B. were largely consistent with the expected pattern.

An additional claim by the authors is that the hypothesized degeneration of traces within the buffer would probably be more extreme for longer than for shorter items. They point out that deletion of letters increased as a function of stimulus length while the number of transpositions showed the opposite tendency. The occurrence of deletions can be attributed to the fact that the "graphemic representation is so deformed as to be unusable for guiding the selection of specific letter forms" (Caramazza et al. 1986, p. 27). Transposition errors, however, may only be possible when "the graphemic representation is sufficently spared to contain information about the specific graphemes even if their respective order is not retained" (page 27).

Finally, the authors turn to an empirical result obtained from a study of normal writing errors. Wing and Baddeley (1980) have observed that "slips of the pen" are more common in the middle portion of a word than at the beginning or final positions. They suggested that active letter units interfere with neighboring items in the output buffer; letters with fewer neighbors (i.e., at the beginning or end of the word) suffer less interference and are usually produced correctly. Caramazza et al. (1986b) found the same inverted U-shaped distribution of spelling errors with respect to word length when they examined the performance of L.B., and they view his deficit as being a more extreme version of the normal constraints on the recovery of memory traces from the graphemic buffer.

An important point is that L.B. was consistently better at spelling words than nonsense words. This outcome conflicts with the interpretation of the buffer as a device that passively maintains the description of any graphemic sequence without reference to whole-word levels of representation. Other instances of damage to peripheral output mechanisms have been reported showing a similar effect of word familiarity on production (Caramazza et al., 1986a; Bub et al., 1987). Caramazza et al. tentatively propose that the greater number of spelling errors for nonwords may reflect an additional impairment to the system. However, it is not clear what this additional impairment might be. The concept of a response buffer operating in isolation from the rest of the system may be too simple-minded if whole-word codes are distinguished from other spelling units at this level. It would seem that output processes function dynamically, monitored by more central components that help to preserve the structure of legitimate words. (See discussion of similar issues regarding spoken word production in chapter 4.)

The Allographic Procedure

Written production takes place by generating the spatial form of each letter in the correct order. Ellis (1982) refers to these letter descriptions as allographs and considers them to be relatively abstract in nature; allographic codes would specify the shape of a letter without determining the overall dimensions or the muscle system (hand, foot, etc.) executing the reponse. According to Ellis (1979b), certain writing slips typical of normal spellers may be due to a temporary malfunction in allographic processing. For example, the omission of a letter occurring twice in the word (LISTEING for *listening*) has only been observed when the members of the pair are identical allographic variants of the same letter. A mistake like this would not arise when upper- and lower-case versions of the letter occur in the same word.

A possible explanation of these inadvertent slips is that the output mechanism cannot simultaneously activate two tokens of the same allograph during the planning of a response. A recurring allograph may introduce a temporary block in the motor program until the first instance of the letter has been successfully produced. If the output chain resumes before enough time has elapsed to reactivate the allograph, it will be omitted from the second position in the word. Errors that involve the omission of letters next to the repeated item may be the result of the same limitation on the processing of allographs. All words containing two or more instances of a letter must be divided into segments, because each duplicated allograph cannot be set up for a written response until the first one has been completed. A word like *dependence* might be parsed as /DEP/END/ ENC/E at the graphemic level in preparation for allographic conversion. If the read-out mechanism does not always keep track of its location in the output sequence, a segment may be skipped during the production of a word.

Other writing errors linked to the functioning of the allographic mechanism include letter substitution and reversal. Ellis (1979b, 1982) comments that these mistakes, found in normal writers, usually involve allographically similar forms (N and M, P and B, etc.) and suggests they arise through misselection of a graphic motor pattern with a spatially close alternative.

A few agraphic patients have been documented whose impairment is plainly confined to the retrieval of elements in the allographic code. In these patients, adequate knowledge of the word's orthography can be demonstrated, because oral spelling is carried out extremely well. When tested, other methods of forming a printed word that do not require a written response (typing or use of block letters) may also yield a high degree of accuracy. Writing, however, is characterized by numerous errors of omission, substitution, reversals, and insertions (Rosati and De Bastiani, 1979; Kinsbourne and Rosenfeld, 1974; Bub et al., 1987; Rothi and Heilman, 1981). The agraphia is not merely a disturbance in the production of a graphic motor pattern, because the patients can write single letters to dictation, and their writing of words, though flawed, is clearly legible.

While the general quality of the performance does implicate the allographic component, there are no detailed analyses of the different errors, conducted within a theoretical framework, to enable us to have a more precise understanding of the disorder. It may be the case that certain patients, whose writing errors consist mainly of letter substitutions, have trouble in the mapping process from the allographic store to the appropriate motor pattern. More complex errors (e.g., omissions and insertions) may reflect an impaired ability to monitor the retrieval of ordered segments planned in the graphemic buffer.

Graphic Motor Output

The motor schema for a letter appears to distinguish between the movements denoting the shape of a letter and the parameters that govern scale factors like magnitude and orientation (Van Galen and Teulings, 1983). Cases of apractic agraphia reveal a loss of the motor programs necessary for producing letters. Written characters are poorly formed and may be indecipherable (e.g., Margolin and Binder, 1984; Coslett et al., 1986), though even severely affected patients maintain the distinction between cursive and printed letters, and between upper and lower case (Margolin, 1984). Evidence indicates that the disturbance need not be associated with limb apraxia; Coslett et al. (1986) described a patient with apractic agraphia who showed no difficulty in performing other skilled movements. The authors concluded that the graphemic code is separately represented from the engrams mediating the execution of other complex motor acts. Baxter and Warrington (1986) have reported a patient with apractic agraphia who nevertheless retained his ability to copy letters and drawings. They infer that the disturbance could not have been at the final stage of motor output, and propose a slightly higher level of representation, where graphic motor patterns are stored.

Finally, certain patients with right hemisphere damage have no difficulty constructing written letters or words, but they exceed the correct number of strokes on letters needing recursive movements (e.g., M, U, E). Ellis (1982) suggested that the motor program must be continuously updated by sensory and proprioceptive feedback, to keep track of the movements being produced. Right parietal lobe damage may interfere with the feedback mechanism, causing re-·duplication of strokes.

SUMMARY

Writing is achieved by a number of distinct processing components that translate sound and meaning into orthographic units. This information leads to the compilation of a motor program and the execution of a response. Agraphic disorders can be interpreted by localizing the damage to one or more of the components specified within a proposed functional architecture. The analysis of brain-damaged performance may in turn provide relevant evidence for a theory of the mental processes that mediate our ability to write and spell.

Research supports the claim that the orthography of entire words can be activated directly from their meaning. Two additional routines obtain a spelling pattern from the spoken representation of the target, either by mapping whole-word phonology into whole-word orthography (if the item is familiar), or by translating phonemic segments into graphemic units. We have described results showing that each of these procedures can be independently affected by brain damage.

Future work should clarify a number of unresolved issues. We remain uncertain about the role of speech codes in writing continuous text. Although the data are inconsistent, the marked discrepancy between spoken and written construction of sentences, noted in some patients, is intriguing and requires further investigation. The size of the units governing the translation of sound into spelling has not been fully determined, nor are we certain about the possible effects of brain damage on the use of segments of different sizes. The question of dual word form systems, separately mediating the recognition and production of written words, has not yet been answered. A valid approach to this problem requires experimental techniques that would demonstrate a central impairment to word-level representation in one modality, followed by a comparative analysis of performance in the alternative modality. We also are just learning about the peripheral components dealing with the organization and execution of a handwritten response; progress in this area may profit from recent theoretical developments in the study of a related motor skill like typing, and from more sophisticated, computer-based techniques for measuring the flow of movement across the page as it unfolds in real time.

NOTES

1. We shall have little to say about the additional mechanisms that are involved in the processing of written sentences, for several reasons. First and foremost, there is virtually no work that deals specifically with reading or writing deficits at the sentence level in brain-damaged patients. A second reason for our emphasis on the reading and writing of single words is that they constitute the input into sentence processing. Any disturbance at the word level will inevitably be a limiting factor in the patient's ability to read or write sentences. There are patients whose sentence production or comprehension is abnormal in the auditory-oral modality despite good single word processing. No comparable patients have been described in the written modality who do not also have disturbances in auditory-oral sentence processing. Of course, such acquired, written-modality-specific, sentence- and discourse-level problems may well exist. These isolated problems may be more common in developmental disorders. Many young adult patients with developmental disorders affecting written language processing (collectively termed "developmental dyslexia") complain of problems in reading and writing texts. However, these are not well described, and the integrity of single written word processing is not well attested in these cases.

Another reason for our focus on single words is that they are the basic units of orthographic representation. Orthographies represent words, not sentences. Finally, on a positive note, considerable progress has been made during the last 15 years on the functional components of the reading mechanism that recognize and produce the orthography of isolated words and disorders of these processes.

2. The 19th century founders of neurological aphasiology held briefs on this issue. Wernicke (1908), for example, was quite explicit that "we accept the existence of memory images for letters only, and not for entire words" (see Eggert's translation of Wernicke's monographs, p. 243). Wernicke's claim in this statement was that the *visual* (orthographic) form of words did not have a permanent representation in the brain. Reading occurred by converting sequences of letters into a pronunciation which then gave access to meaning. Writing was mediated by the reverse process of activating the spoken form of a word and translating it into the appropriate sequence of letters.

Other researchers of that time disagreed with Wernicke, and favored the idea of a specialized mechanism containing the visual form of whole words that could mediate written production even when the equivalent spoken form was not immediately available. Charcot (1883) described a patient who appeared to rely on the internal visual image of a word to recover its pronunciation. Wernicke (1908), in discussing this observation, commented: "I do not believe that such cases represent the general rule and therefore consider them exceptions" (p. 244).

Dejerine (1891, 1892) used the concept of a visual word form to account for the selective impairment of reading (with intact writing and spelling) in certain patients. His explanation of this particular dissociation was that the center containing the permanent description of visual words had become disconnected from the perceptual mechanism but was still available for written production. Interestingly enough, Dejerine did not believe that writing (and reading) took place from this center without first activating the spoken form of the word. The "proof" in support of this claim, according to Dejerine, is that "when we read even silently, we hear the words resounding in our ear at the same time as we are conscious of the movements necessary for pronouncing them" (p. 111).

3. A second theory, advocated by Hansen and Rodgers (1968), holds that the letter groups relevent for phonologically mediated reading are related to syllables. A third theory, developed by Marcel (1980), holds that any orthographic unit may yield a phonological value. There are many difficulties in putting both the second and third models into operation, mostly centering around how a reader can identify orthographic units such as syllables and intermediate units. Though the idea that orthographic units as large as a syllable, or intermediate between syllables and graphemes, such as the sequence of letters *ear* in the word *search*, might be relevant to reading by a phonologically mediated route, we shall not discuss these aspects of phonologically mediated reading here. We postpone discussion of them at this point primarily because, if there is a phonologically mediated route, it almost certainly makes use of basic regular grapheme-to-phoneme correspondences as well as any other larger orthographic-to-phonological correspondences.

4. Seidenberg and his colleagues caution against accepting the conclusion that GPCs play no role in normal word recognition on the basis of the results obtained in lexical decision tasks. They point out that a lexical decision task requires a *decision* as to whether a stimulus is a word or a nonword, and, therefore, that it can be performed in various ways depending upon the nature of the stimuli used in a particular experiment. For instance, a lexical decision task in which the nonwords were all pictures could be performed without recognizing any of the words, simply because subjects would realize that anything that is not a picture must be a word. Conversely, if most of the real words in a lexical decision task are exception words or irregular words, the use of a GPC strategy for recognizing words might be minimized. Therefore, there is likely to be a great deal of task specificity in the results of a lexical decision task because part of the task requires setting some criterion for deciding what is and is not a word. Part of setting or applying this criterion could involve the use of strategies that determine to what extent word recognition is to be accomplished through a direct, whole word route and to what extent it might be accomplished by a phonologically mediated route.

5. Note that such a patient must have a problem accessing the spoken form of a word from both its written form and its meaning. The relationship of this disturbance to anomia will thus bear on the types of semantic information that are accessed from pictures and from written words and how these

types of information gain access to spoken word forms. See chapters 3 and 4 for discussion of these issues.

6. Pseudowords (e.g., *fabe*), as well as words, produced an advantage compared to random letter strings for J.V., as is true of normal readers. Any effect of real words beyond that found for legal letter strings is typically quite small in forced-choice tasks and shows considerable interindividual variability (Manelis, 1974).

7. As a point of interest, M.H. eventually learned to use the spelling of a word to evoke its pronunciation. For example, presented with the picture of a mountain, her response was: "That's a M-O-U-N-T-A-I-N, mountain." This adaptive strategy, which we observed when her oral reading of single words began to improve, apparently took place by generating the visual form of a word and translating it into sound. This strategy is very reminiscent of Charcot's (1883) early interpretation of the same approach to naming in a patient.

6 Recognizing and Producing Morphologically Complex Words

To this point in this book, we have been considering the internal phonological structure, orthographic form, and meanings of simple, underived words. We now turn our attention to words that have what is called internal morphological structure. They consist of words formed from a root plus one or more affixes, and compound words. We begin by considering the structure of these words, then turn to how they are recognized and produced, and finally describe disturbances affecting word formation processes.

WORD FORMATION IN ENGLISH

English words may be formed from other English words (Aronoff, 1976). In English, there are basically two processes that create new words: morphological constructions and compounding. Morphological constructions mostly use affixes; compounding forms words from other words without usually using affixes.

Morphological word formation can be divided into two mechanisms: inflectional morphological processes and derivational morphological processes. Though there is no hard-and-fast definition of these two types of morphological word formation processes, there are several differences between the two.

One way to conceive of inflectional morphology is that inflections are morphological forms that are related to the syntactic structure of a sentence (see chapters 7 and 8 for discussion of syntactic structures). Typical examples of inflectional morphological forms are affixes that are determined by agreement features, such as the third person singular present tense marker -s. English is relatively poor in its inflectional agreement affixation processes, and in other inflectional processes. Languages such as French and German have more complete and complex agreement systems that affect adjective-noun agreement, verb inflections, and the case markers on nouns.

For the most part, inflectional morphological processes do not change the category (noun, verb, adjective) of the roots to which they are attached. By this criterion, certain semantic affixes (past tense marking, plural marking, etc.) are inflectional affixes. In addition, prefixes, which do not change the category of a stem, would be considered to be inflectional affixes by this definition.

Derivational affixes, in contrast, are those that create new categories of words from existing words. Therefore, most derivational affixation changes the category of a root (e.g., *destroy* → *destruction*; *happy* → *happiness*), though some do not (e.g., *orphan* → *orphanage*). Derivational affixes fall into two classes in English. We have already seen (in chapter 2) that the patterns of stress assignment on English words are a consequence of both a Latinate (Romance) stress assignment rule and an Anglo-Saxon stress assignment rule. These two major contributors to modern English—Romance and Anglo-Saxon—also contribute different affixes to the inventory of derivational affixes in English. Latinate suffixes (also called "level I" suffixes) attach to Latinate roots; Anglo-Saxon suffixes (also called "level II" suffixes) attach more freely to many simple, underived words, as well as to derived words with Latinate suffixes. Latinate suffixes differ from Anglo-Saxon suffixes in other respects as well. They attach before Anglo-Saxon suffixes and in many cases they affect the phonological structure of the words to which they are attached. Anglo-Saxon derivational suffixes attach after Latinate suffixes have been attached, and do not influence the sound patterns of the roots to which they are attached.

A few examples will illustrate this system (see Kiparsky, 1982, and Anderson, 1982, for additional discussion). Consider the affix -*ive*, which changes verbs into adjectives. It applies to Latinate stems, to produce words such as *receptive, deceptive, perceptive,* etc. In each of these cases, it changes some of the phonological features of the stem (the final vowel and consonant). The Anglo-Saxon derivational affix -*ness* can now apply to the form derived by Latinate affixation, yielding *receptiveness, deceptiveness, perceptiveness,* etc. The opposite order affixation is not possible in English: we have no words such as *homelessity* in which the Anglo-Saxon affix -*less* has been added to the root *home* to form the adjective *homeless* and then the adjective turned into a noun through further application of the Latinate derivational affix, -*ity*.

Inflectional suffixes apply after all the derivational suffixes have applied to form a word. Thus we have examples such as *horrifies*, in which a noun, *horror*, has been changed to a verb by a Latinate affix, to yield *horrify*, and then the third person singular present tense ending is added. Similarly, if we consider that "semantic" affixes are inflectional, we have examples such as *considerations*, in which the verb *consider* has been turned into a noun by the affix *tion*, and then pluralized by the inflectional affix, *-s*. We do not, however, have forms such as *considersation* in which the third person singular inflectional affix *-s* is added to a verb, *consider*, and the result turned into a noun. Note that the absence of forms such as *considers-ation* is not likely to be due to its semantic impossibility: *considers-ation* could mean something that a single individual is presently considering; it simply does not exist as a derived word of English because it violates the rules which form words from roots and affixes.

In addition to "regular" inflections, such as the third person singular present marker *-s* or the progressive affix *-ing*, some inflectional forms affect the form of the words to which they are added. Thus, alongside of the "regular" past tense forms that make use of the suffix *-ed*, English also has special past tense formation rules for subsets of verbs. For instance, irregular verbs whose stems end in *-ng* fall into several classes: *ring - rang; hang - hung; bring-brought*, etc. In addition, there are completely irregular inflectional forms, such as *woman - women; go - went*, etc. These subregularities and exceptions do not apply to words that are derived from other words, even if the derived words have exactly the same phonological forms as the stems which produce nonstandard inflected forms. Thus, for instance, suppose we form the verb *ring* from the noun *ring*, to indicate that something surrounds something else. Then we would say (1):

(1)   The army ringed the town.

not (2):

(2)   The army rang the town.

The fact that subregularities and irregularities in morphological forms are not productive—that is, that they do not apply freely to form new words but only apply to a specified set of vocabulary items—raises questions about whether they are processed the same way as more productive regular morphological forms.

We have already noted that inflectional affixation has semantic consequences. Agreement features such as the third person singular present tense marker -s convey the semantic features inherent in the agreement. In the case of the third person present tense marker -s, this information is that an action is being accomplished (or is habitually accomplished) by an individual (or a set of individuals considered as whole) who is neither the speaker nor the listener. In many languages, these inflectional processes are sufficiently explicit and distinctive to stand alone as indications of these semantic values. For instance, in Italian, there is no need for subject pronouns in sentences, as the information expressed by these pronouns is explicitly marked by the agreement features on the verb. Other semantic features, such as past tense markers and plural markers in English, and affixes indicating continuous action in the verbal system of French, etc., also explicitly convey particular semantic features.

Derivational morphology also has effects upon semantics. For instance, the thematic roles assigned by a verb (information about who is doing what to whom; see chapters 7 and 8) are reassigned to different nouns when certain adjective-formation suffixes are added. Consider, for instance, the verb *hug*. It assigns the thematic role theme to its object and the thematic role of agent to its subject, as in (3):

(3)   The boy hugged the child.

In (3), the child receives the hug and the boy does the hugging. The adjective derived by the suffix *-able* keeps these thematic roles but reassigns them. A noun modified by the adjective *huggable* is understood as the theme of the action of *hugging*, as in (4):

(4)   The boy is huggable.

In one formal system for representing this change in how thematic roles are assigned by the verb-adjective pair *hug/huggable*, Williams (1981) represents theme as the "internal" argument of the verb *hug*, which is turned into the "external" argument of the adjective *huggable*. This is one way of expressing the changes in semantic values associated with the formation of an adjective from a verb using the suffix *-able*.

Many derivational processes also relate the meanings of derived words and their roots or stems in ways that do not involve the nature of thematic role assignments. In these cases, though there is a general relationship between the meaning of the derived word and its stem, this relationship can be quite varied. For instance, the words in the pair *discuss - discussion* are related in a way that those in the pair *congregate - congregation* are not: "congregations congregate, but discussion arises when *discussants* discuss" (Henderson, 1985, pp. 38–39; see also Jackendoff, 1975, p. 651).

The other major word-formation process in English is word compounding. Compounding is a fairly productive process in English, responsible for forms such as *blackboard, boathouse, greenhouse, housefly*, etc. These forms, originally derived by compound formation of their constituent words, may become "lexicalized," that is, they may be sufficiently frequent so as to form single lexical items in most people's vocabulary, perhaps indistinguishable from simple words as far as their being listed in a "mental dictionary" goes. On the other hand, words such as *chair-cushion, record-cleaner, bottle-breaker*, etc., are not lexicalized, but are nonetheless possible words of English, which could be constructed by a speaker in an appropriate context. Such words illustrate the productivity of the word-compounding process in English.

As all other aspects of linguistic structure, word compounding, though very productive, is not totally unconstrained. In English, for instance, so-called major category items enter productively into word formation processes. The major categories are nouns, verbs, and adjectives; prepositions, determiners, pronouns, auxillary verbs, most classes of adverbs, and the like are so-called minor categories. Thus, we can form the compounds described above and many others using major category items, but there are only a few examples of compounds using minor category words (such as *run-off, check-out*). The productivity of the compounding process is a feature of English that distinguishes it from languages such as French, where virtually no compounding exists, and German, where a much greater range of compounding processes is frequently used.

Compounding also affects meaning. In newly coined compound words, the meaning of the compound word is related to the meanings of its constituent parts (i.e., they retain some degree of what is called "semantic transparency"). Compounding establishes a relation between the two lexical items in the compound such that, in some sense, the first item tends to modify or restrict the meaning of the second. Thus, the compound *horsefly* refers to a fly that is found on horses, not a horse that flies or a horse that has flies on it; similar relationships hold between the two items of the compounds in all of the examples cited above. Lexicalized compounds tend to lose the close relationship between words in the compound: a blackboard need not be black.

Compounding has syntactic consequences as well. With very few exceptions, the final item in the compound acts as the "head" of a compound by giving its category to the entire compound: *blackboard* is a noun, not an adjective, because *board* is a noun, and is the head of the compound, not the adjective *black*. There is a syntactic similarity between the process of compounding and the process of derivational word formation, in that the final derivational suffix in a series of derivational suffixes determines the category of the derived word. Thus, for instance, *considerate* is an adjective, because *-ate* is an adjective-forming suffix, while *consideration* is a noun, because *-ion* is a noun-forming suffix. Word formation is "right-headed" in English, in the sense that it is the final item of a complex word that determines the syntactic category of the entire derived word (excluding inflectional suffixes). This "direction of headedness" is different for lexical items (derived and compound words) and for phrases (see chapter 7).

PROCESSING MORPHOLOGICAL FORM

Two questions arise regarding the processing of the morphological structure of words. The first is whether and how morphological structure influences the recognition and production of morphologically complex words. The second issue is how the information carried in affixation is utilized in constructing higher-order syntactic and semantic structures.

Clearly, to understand a word like *happiness*, we must realize that it is different from the word *happy*, but we must also appreciate that its meaning is related to that of *happy*. How do we understand words that are derived from others? Is a word like *happiness* decomposed during the recognition process into its stem and affix (so-called affix stripping), each of which is separately recognized, with the meaning of the complex word assembled in some way from the meanings of its parts? Or are words like *happiness* represented in a mental dictionary in the same way as simple words with no internal syntactic structure, and recognized and understood in the same way as these simple words? Similar questions arise regarding speech production: Are the two parts of a complex word accessed separately and combined in the word production process or are complex words listed as units that are accessed as entire wholes by word production system? If morphological decomposition occurs in either comprehension or production or both, is the process of decomposition the same for all affixes—prefixes as well as suffixes, suffixes which change the phonological form of the words to which they are attached as well as phonologically neutral suffixes, and irregular morphological forms as well as regular ones? We shall discuss research bearing on these questions here.

The second issue is how the information carried in affixation is utilized in constructing higher-order syntactic and semantic structures. The grammatical category of a derived lexical item (determined by its rightmost derivational affix), the agreement and semantic features such as tense and aspect marked by inflectional morphemes, and other syntactic and semantic consequences of morphological forms, may be part of the input into aspects of the process of constructing higher-order (supralexical) structures and meanings. We shall leave the question of the role of morphological forms in sentence processing to chapters 7 and 8.

Though we have mentioned compound forms, there is very little work on how normal subjects process these forms and no work at all on the question of how processing compound forms breaks down after neurological disease. We therefore will not discuss this aspect of the word formation process; hopefully, research into this question will develop in the future.

Recognition of Morphologically Complex Words

Most studies of processing morphologically complex words deal with how these words are recognized (not understood), and most of these studies have been carried out in the written modality. It may well be that the conclusions that have been drawn from these studies are applicable only to written language processing, but I discuss them here as a guide to what might be true of spoken language as well. Two basic opposing positions have been developed regarding the recognition of morphologically complex words. The first, which has been called the "decomposition" model, is that the various morphemes that make up a morphologically complex word are processed individually.[1] The second major point of view regarding recognition of morphologically complex words is that they are recognized as entire units. There is also a third view that holds that morphologically complex words are recognized by both a decomposition and a whole-word recognition mechanism. Evidence regarding these models comes from various sources: the time it takes to recognize stems and pseudostems; the time it takes to recognize affixed and pseudoaffixed words; the effects of morphology on priming; and the effects of morpheme frequency in recognition tasks. These experimental approaches have been applied separately to prefixes, and to inflectional and derivational suffixes. The experimental evidence is controversial (see Taft, 1985, and Henderson, 1985b, for detailed reviews with largely opposing viewpoints; see also Monsell, 1985, 1987, and Seidenberg, 1989, for reviews of this literature). I first present the data that support the morphological decomposition theory, and then present some of the criticisms of this interpretation of these data. The data most strongly support the case for morphological decomposition for accessing regularly inflected forms. Irregular inflected forms and derived words are more complex.

We begin with a discussion of processing prefixed words. Rubin, Becker, and Freeman (1979) reported that pseudoprefixed words (e.g., *relish*) took longer to recognize than truly prefixed words (e.g., *revive*) in a lexical decision task (a task in which words and nonword letter strings are displayed and the subject must indicate as quickly as possible whether a stimulus is or is not a word; see chapters 3 and 5). This suggests that pseudoprefixed words are decomposed into possible stems and prefixes, and these stems and prefixes combined leading to a morphologically nonexistent form (*re-lish*). Only after this process is finished is the entire stimulus identified as a simple word. In the case of truly prefixed words, the attempt to put together the identified parts succeeds, allowing for a faster response. Though Rubin et al. (1979) argued that this result depended on very particular experimental conditions in the lexical decision task (they believed it required the presence of pseudoprefixed nonwords in the nonword set), Henderson et al. (1984) found a similar effect in a weak form in an experiment in which this factor was minimized. Taft (1981) found a similar effect in a reading-aloud task in which there were no nonwords at all (though here the effect could be due to the reading-aloud part of the task, not the recognition aspect). Taft and Forster (1975) also found that if a stimulus was both a freestanding real word and a stem (e.g., *vent*, which is both a real word and a part of words like *prevent* and *invent*), and if the frequency of the prefixed word was higher than that of the freestanding word (i.e., *prevent* and *invent* are more frequent than *vent*), then lexical decision reactions were longer for these stimuli than for simple freestanding words matched for frequency (i.e., *vent* takes longer to recognize than a simple word like *coin*). Again, the conclusion the authors drew was that the form *vent* was recognized as a stem first (because its frequency as a stem was higher than that as freestanding word) and considered for rejection because, as a stem, it is not an acceptable word. Though the fact that items like *vent* are really words eventually led the subjects to the correct response, this process of considering *vent* as a stem occupied time and slowed down response latencies. All these results are consistent with the decomposition model for prefixed words. However, the objection has been raised that most of the prefixed words used in these experiments consist of stems that are not real words (e.g., *vive*) and that words that add prefixes to these stems (e.g., *revive*) are not really morphologically complex at all but only particular types of simple words. Thus, though these results show that words that contain internal stems that are not themselves words differ from other words, this may not generalize to truly prefixed words.

Similar effects show up in processing nonwords. Taft and Forster (1975) reported that it took longer to reject bound stems (e.g., *vive*, from *revive*) than parts of pseudoprefixed words (e.g., *lish* from *relish*). This result was also found when bound stems with inappropriate prefixes (e.g., *devive*) were compared to pseudostems with inappropriate prefixes (e.g., *delish*). They argued that this pattern indicated that the bound stems were stored as part of an inventory of lexical forms, and were only rejected when the subject found that they could not stand alone as words or be combined with a particular prefix. Taft (1976, 1979) also reported that it took subjects longer to indicate that pseudoprefixed nonwords (e.g., *revilk*) were not words than unanalyzable nonwords (e.g., *lomalk*). Caramazza, Laudanna, and Romani (1988) reported that nonwords that consist of either a real stem and a pseudoaffix or a pseudostem and a real affix were harder to reject than nonwords that had no real morphological components (see below). These results suggest that the pseudoprefixed items were decomposed into nonsense stems and possible prefixes, and that the rejection of a nonword was slowed if nonword status depended on a prefix not being combinable with a nonsense stem to form a real word.

Studies of words with suffixes have investigated both inflectional suffixes and derivational suffixes. We first turn to evidence regarding derivational suffixes, beginning with word recognition tasks. Taft (1976), Manelis and Tharp (1977), and Henderson et al. (1984) found that pseudoderived words (e.g., *bounty*) were no more difficult to recognize than nonderived words (e.g., *morsel*) or truly derived words (e.g., *roomy*) in a lexical decision task. Taft (1976) found no difference in rejecting nonword stems of derived words (e.g., *groce* from *grocer*) and the nonwords that resulted from presenting the first syllables of underived words (e.g., *trink* from *trinket*), and no difference in rejecting derived nonwords (e.g., *boithy*) and nonderived nonwords (e.g., *foutha*). Snodgrass and Jarvella (1972) found that rejection times were no longer for derived nonwords (e.g., *diltness*) than their nonword stems (e.g., *dilt*). Smith and Sterling (1982) found that subjects had equal trouble with a letter cancellation task (crossing out all the "e"s in a word) for targets in both true derivational suffixes (e.g., *-er* in *driver*) and derivational pseudosuffixes (e.g., *-er* in *river*). All these results suggest that derived words with suffixes are processed as entire units. Some of these results may have resulted from incidental properties of the materials used in these experiments and there are some discrepant data (see Taft, 1985, for discussion). For instance, Smith and Sterling found that the letter cancellation task was much easier when the subject had to cancel out letters in similar positions in simple, nonpseudoaffixed words (such as *money*), which suggests that both derived and pseudoaffixed words differ in their processing from simple words that cannot be mistaken for derived words. Overall, however, the evidence from these studies suggests that derived words are processed as entire units.

Inflectional suffixes behave differently in similar experiments. Pseudoinflected words (e.g., *kindred*) were more difficult to recognize in a lexical decision task than noninflected words (e.g. *shuffle*) (Taft, 1976, 1979). Inflected nonwords (e.g., *molks*) were harder to reject than noninflected nonwords (e.g., *porld*) (Taft, 1976, 1979). Reisner (1972) found longer reaction times to reject inflected nonwords (e.g., *drilked*) than derived nonwords (e.g., *dralkor*). Gibson and Guinet (1971) reported fewer errors in identifying the last letters of words and nonwords with inflectional endings than in identifying the last letters of uninflected words and nonwords. Letter cancellation was worse in inflectional suffixes than in the same letter strings when they were not inflectional suffixes (*-ed* in *hunted* vs. *-ed* in *hundred*) (Smith and Sterling, 1982). Drewnowsky and Healy (1980) found that the "n" was found less reliably in the suffix *-ing* than it was in the suffixes *-en*, *-ion*, and *-ment*. This was taken as an indication that the frequency of a suffix influenced detection of its constituent letters. It may have occurred because *-ing* can be an inflectional ending while *-en*, *-ion*, and *-ment* are derivational; if so, it suggests that inflectional and derivational endings are treated differently.

Laudanna et al. (1989) reported a series of experiments in Italian that provide additional support for the decomposition model for regularly inflected words. They had subjects perform a "double lexical decision task," in which the task is to say whether both of two stimuli are words. They presented four types of word pairs: (1) different inflected versions of a single root, (e.g., *volt-are* (to turn) and *volt-avo* (I was turning); (2) words whose stems are homographic but different lexical items, e.g., *port-are* (to carry) and *port-e* (door); (3) orthographically similar inflected words, e.g., *contare* (to count) and *corta* (short); and (4) unrelated word pairs, e.g., *causa* (cause) and *ponte* (bridge). In this task, reaction times for different inflected versions of the same root (type 1) were faster than for any other pair of stimuli. Homographic stems (type 2) were significantly slower than orthographically related pairs of words (type 3) and unrelated words (type 4). Orthographically similar words (type 3) did not differ from unrelated words (type 4). The fact that reaction times for different inflected versions of the same root (type 1) were faster than for any other pair of stimuli supports the view that recognizing one word helps in recognizing a morphologically related word. The fact that orthographically similar words (type 3) did not differ from unrelated words (type 4) indicates that mere visual similarity between two words does not help in this way. Finally, the fact that unrelated words with homographic stems (type 2) were significantly slower than orthographically related pairs of words (type 3) and unrelated words (type 4) is consistent with the view that recognizing one stem inhibits the recognition of an unrelated homographic stem. All these results are thus in keeping with a decomposition model of lexical access for inflected words.

All these results are consistent with inflectional endings being stripped off, stems and these suffixes each being recognized, and the entire word being recognized by a combination of these parts. Findings that contradict this conclusion do exist (e.g., Manelis and Tharp, 1977, experiment 2) but may be explained by other aspects of the experiments (see Taft, 1979a, 1985, for discussion).

Another approach to investigating recognition of morphologically complex words is to analyze frequency effects in these words. As we saw in chapters 3 and 5, word frequency exerts a significant effect on reaction times in lexical decision and reading-aloud experiments. But what determines a word's frequency? The frequency of the presented form in isolation (its "surface" frequency), or the frequency of the presented form plus its derivationally and/or inflectionally related forms (its "stem" frequency). Taft (1979b), Reisner (1972), and O'Connor (1975) showed that the combined frequency of a presented form and its inflectionally related forms determined reaction times for inflected words in a lexical decision task. Words like *sized* (coming from a high-frequency word, *size*) were recognized faster than words like *raked* (coming from a low-frequency word, *rake*), even though *sized* and *raked* are of equal frequency. Reisner (1972) found a similar effect for low-frequency derived words. Bradley (1979) found a similar effect for derived words in which the derivational suffix did not change the phonological form of the stem (level II derivational morphology, such as *-er*, *-ness*, and *-ment*), but not for derived words in which the affix changed the phonological form of the stem (level I derivational morphology, such as *-ion*). These results suggest that both inflected and certain derived words—those with infrequent and/or regular level II suffixes—are recognized by a decomposition mechanism.

A third experimental approach to the problem of recognition of morphologically complex words is to see if the stem of one form primes a related form. (See chapter 3 for a discussion of priming.) If so, researchers argue, processing of the second form must be affected by its morphologically defined components, consistent with the decomposition model. Several results indicate that suffixed words prime their stems and other suffixed words. Stanners et al. (1979) reported that regularly inflected words (e.g., *lifting*) primed their stems (e.g., *lift*) as much as the stems themselves did. They found the same for prefixed words. Murrell and Morton (1974) reported a similar result: previously memorized words facilitated recognition of related stems (e.g., memorizing *sees* helped in the recognition of *seen*) but memorizing visually similar words had no such effect (e.g., memorizing *seed* did not help in the recognition of *seen*). These results are consistent with a decomposition model for regularly inflected words. (See also Laudanna et al., 1989, experiment 3.)

The data on derived and irregularly inflected words are less clear. Stanners et al. found an effect in priming for derivationally related words (*selective-select*), but it was less strong than that for regularly inflected words. They also found intermediate strength effects for irregularly inflected words (*hung-hang*). Fowler, Napps, and Feldman (1985), however, using a variant of the same technique, found no difference in priming effects for the same word repeated twice, inflectionally related words, and derivationally related words (in the Fowler et al. experiment, the number of words intervening between the prime and the target was increased to 40 or more items, instead of 8 to 10 in the experiment of Stanner et al.). Kempley and Morton (1982) had subjects rate spoken words for imageability and then identify words in noise after an interval of between 10 and 40 minutes. Prior exposure to a word did not help in recognizing related irregularly inflected words (e.g., hearing *stink* did not help in the recognition of *stank*). These results make the evidence for a decomposition theory of lexical access less clear in the case of derived and irregularly inflected words than regularly inflected words, and also suggest that there may be important differences between the way these items are processed in the written and auditory modalities.

Burani and Caramazza (1987) and their colleagues have tried to reconcile the decomposition and whole-word models in a hybrid model of complex word recognition, called the "augmented accessed morphology" model. This model postulates a separate access process for both the components of complex words and for the entire word itself. The theory thus maintains that lexical access for morphologically complex words may take place through a whole-word recognition procedure or through a decomposition mechanism. Both procedures are used for words that the subject knows; only the decomposition procedure is available for new words. The authors assume that activation of a word via the whole-word recognition mechanism is faster than via the decomposition procedure (which requires finding the components of the word and putting them together).

The motivation for this hybrid model comes from several sources. We indicated above that there is an effect of stem frequency (the summed frequency of all the inflectionally related forms of a word) upon lexical decision response times, even when stimuli are matched for surface frequency (the frequency of the presented form). This was taken as evidence for the decomposition model of lexical access for complex words. However, there is also an effect of surface frequency on reaction times in these experiments. Taft (1979b) found that inflected words that were matched for their stem frequencies but that differed in their surface frequencies differed in their reaction times. For instance, the combined frequency of all forms of *follow* is equal to that of all forms of *number*, but *followed* alone is more common than *numbered* alone. In a lexical decision task, *followed* was recognized more quickly than *numbered*. Similar effects were reported by Burani and Caramazza (1987) for very productive, phonologically regular derived words in Italian. These findings suggest that surface forms are accessed directly, in addition to any decomposition-based access process. There are also effects in rejecting nonwords that have similar implications. Reaction times are progressively faster and errors progressively less frequent for three classes of nonwords: (1) those that consist of real stems and affixes (e.g., *walkest*); (2) those that contain either a pseudostem (e.g., *walkost*) or a pseudoaffix (e.g., *wilkest*); and (3) those that have no real morphological component (e.g., *wilkost*) (Taft and Forster, 1975, 1976; Henderson et al., 1984; Caramazza et al., 1988). This pattern would follow from the existence of several recognition mechanisms sensitive to the lexical status of both a whole word and its morphological consitituents.

We have presented many results that support the idea that recognition of some morphologically complex words involves recognizing the stem and affix of the word separately. However, these results do not prove that this is the case. All the results we have reported rely on tasks in which the effects of morphological form could have occurred *after* a word has been recognized—lexical decision, letter detection, reading aloud (Henderson, 1985b). For instance, in a lexical decision task, a subject may recognize a morphologically complex word without splitting off the stem and affix, but still have the decision as to whether or not what he or she saw was a word be influenced by the presence of the stem and the affix (see Seidenberg, 1989, for discussion). The same is true of letter detection and reading-aloud tasks: the effects of morphological structure could be postlexical. Thus, caution is required before concluding that prelexical decomposition occurs, even in the cases where the evidence for it is strongest. However, morphological structure does appear to affect performance in a wide variety of tasks, many of which do not require verbal production of a morphologically complex word. Thus we may tentatively conclude that morphological decomposition takes place for certain classes of words somewhere in input-side lexical processing, though where it occurs in the course of lexical access—as part of the "contact representation" before stimuli activate lexical items, or in the "activation," "selection," or accessing" stages of this process (see chapter 2)—remains unclear.

In summary, there appears to be a mechanism that identifies the components of morphologically complex words. It is possible that this mechanism is part of the lexical access process. It does not appear that this decomposition process applies to all morphologically complex words: at least some derived words and irregular inflections appear to be processed by a whole-word recognition process. The whole word processing mechanism may operate together with the decomposition process in recognizing and processing regularly inflected words. The written modality may differ from the auditory modality with respect to the role of morphological decomposition in lexical access for complex words. The experimental evidence supporting decomposition—even in the case of inflected words with regular suffixes and prefixed words—remains controversial because of the many technical problems involved in controlling nonmorphological variables in these experiments (see Henderson, 1985b) and because of the problems in attributing effects in the experimental tasks that have been used to pre- and post-lexical-recognition stages of processing. It is even possible that at least some of the effects that have been attributed to morphemes are in fact due to morphemelike units that are used by the perceptual system in the initial coding of a stimulus (see Taft, 1979, and Seidenberg, 1989, for discussion of this issue). Despite these possibilities, there is good evidence that listeners are sensitive to the presence of morphological units that make up many complex words at some point in input-side processing of these words.

Production of Morphologically Complex Words

We have just seen that there is evidence that some morphologically complex words are broken up into constituent morphemes at a stage of language processing prior to oral or written word production. Are morphologically complex words subject to similar decompositional processes when being produced? If so, at what level of speech planning and speech production does this decomposition occur? Does a speaker think of the semantic features associated with a stem (e.g., a domestic animal that has fur, chews on bones, and is a good friend to man) and those associated with an affix (e.g., that there are two such animals he wishes to talk about), access the stem (*dog*) and the plural affix (*-s*) separately, and combine them to form the word he needs? Does he think of the concepts separately but combine them to access a single inflected word (*dogs*) that is already listed in the output lexicon? Or does he think of the concept of TWO DOGS as a whole? Are these processes different for derived and inflected words, for regular and irregular forms, and in writing and in speech? There are no definitive answers to these questions, but we shall review several studies that bear on some of these questions.

We have seen in chapter 4 that one theory of speech production maintains that complex words are accessed from concepts as wholes. Levelt's (1989) model of word sound production hypothesizes that the first phonological representation of a word is what he calls the morphological-metrical form of the word. This representation specifies the number of morphemes in a word, and the metrical pattern of the word (its syllable and stress make-up). In this model, morphologically complex words are listed in the output lexicon, and accessed from concepts as wholes.

The opposite model—that affixes are accessed independently of their stems and combined with stems at a later point of processing—also has its advocates. This model is supported by the considerable amount of data that indicate that affixes are processed differently from stems in sentence production. We shall review this evidence in more detail in chapter 8, but we give a preview of it here. One argument is based on the existence of a type of speech error called a "stranding" error, as in *"he is schooling to go,"* for *"he is going to school."* In a stranding error, the suffix (*-ing*) has been "stranded" in its original position and the verb stem to which it was originally attached has been moved elsewhere in the sentence (Garrett, 1976, 1980). The elements that are "stranded"—that is, those that are left in their syntactic positions—are affixes; it is the content words that are moved. Garrett argues that, for an error to occur, the vocabulary elements that are involved in the error must be processed simultaneously during a certain stage of the sentence production process. Using this principle to analyze these data, Garrett posits the existence of a "positional level" of structure in the sentence planning process at which the syntactic form of a sentence is produced, and the phonological forms of words are inserted into their appropriate positions in the syntactic structure of the sentence. The stranding errors, in which function words and bound morphemes are stranded while the content words and stems are moved, arise during the creation of the positional level, when content words are misordered. The fact that bound morphemes remain in place while stems move suggested to Garrett that the syntactic structures accessed during the creation of the positional level of representation already contain bound morphemes and function words in their final position. Garrett thus postulates a specific relationship between affixes and their stems in sentence planning: the two are accessed separately and combined only during the process of planning the syntactic structure of a sentence.

Garrett's hypothesis, that the phonological forms of affixes are in some way accessed during the process of constructing the syntactic forms of sentence, may well be too strong. Levelt's analysis— according to which morphologically complex words are accessed as units—may apply to some classes of words, such as those with derivational morphology. Stemberger and MacWhinney (1986) have provided evidence that high-frequency inflected words are accessed as entire units in the output lexicon. However, given the evidence that the components of complex words are processed separately during sentence production, there must be some point at which the phonological forms of at least some affixes are processed separately from their stems.

There is some experimental evidence from single word production tasks that bears on the issue of where in the production process the components of complex words are treated separately. Unfortunately, this evidence is far from definitive, and even contradictory. Steinberg and Krohn (1975) presented subjects with printed words and had them attach an inappropriate suffix to these items and then utter the resulting nonword (e.g., presented with *maze*, the subject had to add the suffix -*ity* to form *mazity*). Subjects rarely changed the vowel in the root (as in *sane*—*sanity*). Had they done this, it would have provided evidence of their producing the derived form by a general morphophonological rule; since they did not, the result provides no evidence for the use of this rule. Since this rule would be expected to be available if subjects generally produced derived forms by adding a suffix to a root, this result provides (weak) evidence against the use of such a rule, and therefore against a decompositional model of production of isolated derived forms.

A different picture emerges from an experiment conducted by MacKay (1978). He required subjects to produce derived forms that varied in their phonological relationship to their roots. For instance, the phonological relationship between the word *decision* and *decide* is more complex than that between *conclusion* and *conclude*, because it includes a vowel change as well as a consonantal change. Production times were longer for the more complexly related pairs, consistent with the view that the production of these words involved accessing the base and changing it in a way required by the addition of the suffix. However, since this task required the subject to produce a derived form from a root, it does not prove that stems and affixes are accessed separately and combined when complex words are accessed from semantic representations. This result therefore only provides evidence that there is a stage of word production at which affixes and stems can be combined, not that this stage is the one at which words are accessed from semantics.

Overall, there are few data regarding the production of morphologically complex words. Though the speech error data and experimental results such as those of MacKay indicate that at least some morphologically complex words have their stems and affixes processed separately in speech production, whether they are always processed separately or whether complex words are accessed as wholes and only later decomposed into constituent parts (perhaps when syntactic structures are constructed; see chapter 8), remains unclear.

DISTURBANCES OF PROCESSING MORPHOLOGICALLY COMPLEX WORDS

Many aphasic subjects have trouble with the production of morphological forms. Some of the best known disturbances affecting sentence production are the classic aphasic symptoms of agrammatism and paragrammatism, in which morphological affixes are omitted and changed. I deal with these disturbances in the discussion of sentence production in chapter 8. In this chapter, I discuss disturbances of processing morphological aspects of words in written and auditory word recognition and comprehension, and in single word production.

Disturbances of Input-Side Processing of Morphologically Complex Words

Perhaps the first modern studies that suggested a disturbance of processing morphological forms in single word tasks were those of the oral reading of single words by patients with deep dyslexia (Coltheart, Patterson, and Marshall, 1980; Patterson, 1980). As we saw in chapter 5, these patients make semantic reading errors (e.g., *dad→ father*), visual errors (*earn→ learn; proof→ roof*), and other errors (function word substitutions and omissions; omissions in reading nonwords aloud). They also make numerous morphological errors (e.g., *write→ wrote; fish→ fishing; directing→ direction*). Patterson (1980) provided the most detailed account of these derivational paralexic errors in the early literature on deep dyslexia, reporting on two cases (D.E. and P.W.). She found that 58% of these errors on derived words involved suffix deletions, 38% involved substitutions, and there was a tiny percentage (4%) of other errors involving morphological forms. Additions of suffixes to simple words were also common. Suffixes varied in their likelihood to be produced: *-ing, -er, -ly,* and *-y* were likely to be produced, while *-est* and *-ed* were hardly ever read aloud.

Patterson suggested that these errors indicated that these patients had some disturbance of morphological processing—either in word recognition, comprehension, or in word production. She undertook a series of tests to see where in the processing system these errors arose. She first tested these patients in a lexical decision task. In one test, the contrast was between truly affixed words (e.g., *feared, roomy*) and incorrectly affixed words (e.g., *fearest, roomly*); in a second test, it was between truly affixed words (e.g., *hardest*) and affixed nonwords (e.g., *neakest*); and in a third test, it was between the stem of real words the patient had missed in the first two tests (e.g., if the patient missed *feared*, the word *fear* was presented) and the base of any nonword that had been classified as a word in the second test (e.g., if the patient had said that *firching* was a real word, he was given the stimulus *firch*). Both patients performed well above chance on all these tests. However, both showed signs that input-side morphological processing was not normal.

This evidence revolves around the patients' better performances on isolated base forms of words than on complex forms. D.E. correctly rejected the base nonwords in the third test (e.g., he rejected *firch*, even though he had said that *firching* was a real word), and P.W. correctly recognized the base words for 19 of 22 derived words he had missed earlier. Both patients were better on the test with just base forms (test 3) than the test with affixed nonword base forms (test 2), and better on test 2 than on the test with real word base forms and simply illegal stem-affix combinations (test 1). Suffixes had opposite effects on words and nonwords: D.E. was more likely to accept a nonword base as a real word if it had a suffix (e.g., *firching* vs. *firch*), but less likely to accept a real word as real if it was suffixed (e.g., *feared* vs. *fear*). This indicates that the results are not just due to the patients' treating all stimuli with suffixes as either words or nonwords.

Patterson argued that this pattern of performance was in keeping with the decompositional theory of lexical access derived words. The biggest problem the patients had was in knowing whether a real affix could combine with a particular real stem. This would be easily explained if affixes and stems were recognized separately and later combined to form entire complex words; the step of recombination could go wrong in these patients. This conclusion was reinforced by a fourth lexical decision test based on Taft and Forster (1975) (see above), in which the patients were asked to judge nonword stems from real prefixed words (e.g., *juvenate* from *rejuvenate*) and parts of pseudoprefixed words (e.g., *pertoire* from *repertoire*). The two patients performed worse in rejecting the bound stems than the parts of morphologically simple words (as did normal subjects). This could be explained if the patients identified stems independently of affixes.

Patterson performed several additional tests and made other observations that bolstered the conclusion that these patients had input-side disturbances affecting morphological processing. She found that the patients had considerable trouble matching a written word to one of three spoken words (a spoken version of the written word itself, of a morphologically related word, and of a visually similar word). The patients could not pick the correct morphological form of a visually presented word to fit a context (e.g., could not say if the written form *ruler* or *rule* fits into the sentence: *Prince Charles will one day ____ the country*), although they could do this if the morphologically related words were spoken aloud. The patients frequently could not read derived words they correctly identified as real words, and they read many more stems (e.g., *soft*) correctly than affixed words with the same stems (e.g., *softly*). Patterson also commented on the fact that most errors made in reading aloud simple abstract words (e.g., *truth*) were omissions of letters, while most errors made in reading aloud abstract complex words (e.g., *honesty*) were morphological errors. These results also indicated that these patients had particular difficulty with the processing of written derived words, though, of course, the errors made in reading aloud may have reflected disturbances on the output side of processing.

Patterson (1982) also was one of the first researchers to discuss the occurrence of morphological errors in phonological dyslexia. In chapter 5, we indicated that phonological dyslexic patient can read real words quite well but cannot read nonwords well at all. Patterson presented one patient with phonological dyslexia (A.M.) whose rate of producing morphological errors (e.g., *book → books*; *recent → recently*; *disposal → dispose*) was ten times higher than his rate of producing any other type of error in reading real words. He was tested on several of the tests used with the patients with deep dyslexia that we have just reviewed. Though A.M. performed well above chance in a lexical decision task with correctly derived words (e.g., *costly*) and incorrectly derived words (e.g., *passly*), this performance was not as good as his performance in a similar task with simple, noncomplex words. He scored 79% correct in matching a printed word with one of three spoken morphologically related words (e.g., matching the written version of *angry* with one of the spoken words *anger*, *angry*, *angrily*). He made four errors (more than normal control subjects did) in selecting the correct written derived form in a sentence. All these results suggested that A.M. had a problem with input-side processing of written morphologically complex words.

On the basis of the co-occurrence of this (presumed) deficit in processing derived words and A.M.'s problem in reading by the phonological route (i.e., converting parts of words to their corresponding sounds), Patterson suggested that the normal process of oral reading of morphological affixes—and even understanding them—might involve the spelling-sound correspondence mechanism. The idea that the normal process of recognizing and understanding morphological affixes requires the spelling-sound correspondence mechanism is quite a radical suggestion, since it would mean that affixes are not recognized as wholes during the process of recognizing written complex words (see chapter 5 for arguments against the view that the recognition of most simple written words necessarily requires the sublexical spelling-sound correspondence routine). Patterson (1982) argued for this point of view on several grounds. First, she pointed out that, at the point of her writing, all patients who had disturbances of the spelling-sound conversion system (deep and phonological dyslexia) had troubles affecting morphological forms. Second, she pointed out that, in languages like Japanese in which there are both ideographic forms and phonologically more transparent forms (see chapter 5), affixes are written in the phonologically more transparent form. Finally, she pointed out that most errors in rapid reading occur in morphological affixes and function words (Morton, 1964; Drewnowsky and Healy, 1977, 1980). Based on results of Kolers (1966), she argued that rapid reading involves the semantic reading route. The fact that errors are more common on affixes in rapid reading is consistent with the view that affixes are read by the less well-developed and less preferred spelling-sound correspondence route in rapid reading.[2]

Morphological processing in another case of phonological dyslexia in an Italian patient (Leonardo) was reported by Job and Sartori (1984). The authors called any error that involved either an affix or a stem alone a "decomposition error." Leonardo made many such errors in reading. He read 23 of 33 infinitive forms, 15 of 33 verbs with irregular inflections, and only 5 of 33 verbs with regular inflections. He read only 20% of prefixed words correctly, and 53% of pseudoprefixed words. All these findings suggested a problem with affixed forms. The nature of this problem was investigated in an experiment in which Leonardo was required to read various types of nonwords. Since Leonado could not read nonwords (he was a phonological dyslexic patient), he performed poorly on this task. However, he read prefixes and suffixes better than nonword stems in nonwords that were formed by combining real affixes with nonsense stems. His better performance on the affixes than on the stems in these words suggests that he decomposed the stimulus into a stem and an affix and processed each separately. His problem with real morphologically complex words could have been due to a disturbance affecting the recombination process.

Leonardo demonstrated that he could understand the meanings of some prefixes and suffixes in a test in which he was required to match a written affix (e.g., *-issimo* [*very*]) with one of three spoken words: *niente* (*nothing*); *molto* (*very*); and *buono* (*good*). He performed above chance in lexical decision tasks with derived word targets and nonword foils that consisted of either illegal combinations of stems and affixes, changes of one letter in the affixes in correctly formed derived words, and changes of one letter in the stems in correctly formed derived words. He continued to be able to do the lexical decision task when derived words on which he had previously made a decomposition error were used as targets. However, his lexical decision performance was better for simple words than for affixed words, and for pseudoprefixed words than for truly prefixed words. There was a close relationship between correctly classifying derived nonwords and reading those words: nonwords classed as words were read much better than nonwords classed correctly as nonwords.

The authors concluded that, if a word is decomposable, it is more likely to be mistaken for a nonword in a lexical decision task and to be misread or not read in a reading-aloud task. Like A.M., Leonardo's performances were interpreted as indicating that he had a problem involving the decomposition/recombination aspects of lexical access for written words. Though Job and Sartori did not claim that this problem had any relationship to Leonardo's problems with using the reading route based on spelling-sound correspondences, the co-occurrence of phonological alexia with this problem is consistent with Patterson's hypothesis that affixes are read by a mechanism that utilizes sublexical spelling-sound correspondences.

Patterson's hypothesis is rendered unlikely, however, by a patient with phonological dyslexia reported by Funnell (1983), W.B. W.B. showed the disturbance in using the spelling-sound correspondence–based reading route characteristic of phonological dyslexia, but made almost no morphological paralexias. This indicates that the two problems are separable, and are likely to be due to two independent deficits in patients where they co-occur, such as A.M. and Leonardo.[3]

The studies by Patterson and Job and Sartori have been subjected to a detailed analysis and critique by Badecker and Caramazza (1987). These authors raise the concern that what the authors take to be morphological errors may in fact be visual errors or semantic errors. After all, morphologically related words are also semantically related, and morphologically related words are often visually similar. These patients, who made morphological errors, also made some semantic and visual errors. Perhaps all the morphological paralexias were really due to semantic or visual problems or a combination of the two, not to problems with decomposition of visually presented complex words.

Badecker and Caramazza specifically suggest the following possibility. Suppose a presented pseudoprefixed word (e.g., *religion*) activates a set of visually related words. Many of these will be derived from its pseudostem (e.g., *legion, lion*, etc.). These will not be semantically related to the presented word. On the other hand, if a morphologically complex word—especially one with a regular morphophonological relation to its stem—activates a set of visually related words, many will also be derived from its stem (e.g., *repayment* activates *payment, pay, repay*) and these words *will* be semantically related to the presented word. These words are morphologically related to the presented word. If the subject has a problem with both the visual and the semantic aspects of processing visually presented words, more of these morphologically related words may be produced when he reads affixed words than when he reads pseudoaffixed words. Thus, it is difficult to prove that errors such as those found in the patients we have been describing are due to morphological decomposition disturbances rather than to a complex interaction between disturbances of visual word processing and semantic processing.

Badecker and Caramazza presented a patient their own, F.M., in whom they tried to address some of these concerns. F.M. made more errors in reading truly affixed words (e.g., *reader*) than pseudoaffixed words (e.g., *corner*) or simple, nonderived words that contained other words (so-called embedded word stimuli, such as *rustle*, which contains *rust*, or *bland*, which contains *land*), suggesting that he had a disturbance in morphological processing. He also read words with the agentive *-er* suffix (e.g., *driver*) better than frequency- and length-matched words with the comparative *-er* suffix (e.g., *taller*). This difference also is consistent with F.M. having a disturbance that affects certain morphological forms (comparative formation) more than others (agent formation). However, Badecker and Caramazza were concerned that both these findings might not be due to disturbances of morphological processes. In the case of the reading of affixed, pseudoaffixed, and embedded words, though the stimuli in these different categories were matched for surface frequency, it was possible that this pattern of errors arose because the true stems were more frequent than the pseudostems. That is, the pattern may have simply reflected frequency factors that affect visual processing, not the morphological structure of the presented words. In the case of F.M.'s better production of agentive than comparative -er forms, this may have been due to his greater ability to read nouns than adjectives.

Badecker and Caramazza tried to rule out these possibilities by constructing a smaller list of simple words from the sets of pseudoaffixed and embedded word stimuli. In this smaller list, all items were such that the embedded word or pseudostem was of higher frequency than the presented item, the embedded word or pseudostem was a noun and the presented form an adjective or verb, and the embedded word or pseudostem was more concrete than the presented form. Thus the list was set up so that F.M. was likely to read the pseudostems or embedded words rather than the presented forms. F.M.'s performance on this list was compared with his reading of agentive and comparative forms ending in -er. Despite the fact that the control stimuli would be expected to induce many errors, F.M. made more errors on the truly suffixed words (agentive and comparative -er words) than on these selected control stimuli. In particular, more *morphological* errors were made on the comparative and agentive items than on these selected items. Badecker and Caramazza concluded that at least some errors were really due to a morphological processing disturbance in this patient.[4]

Disturbances in recognizing morphologically complex words have also been described for recognizing auditorily presented words, at least in context (Tyler and Cobb, 1987; Tyler et al., 1990; Lukatela, Crain, and Shankweiler, 1988). Tyler and Cobb (1987) presented a study of a patient with agrammatic speech (see chapter 8). D.E. was shown to have normal auditory word recognition abilities, using a variety of tasks. His responses to words presented in the gating paradigm (see chapter 2) and in an auditory lexical decision test were normal. He could monitor for specific words in normal prose passages and scrambled word passages normally. However, he differed from normals in monitoring for words in semantically nonsensical but syntactically well-formed passages (e.g., *Apparently, at the distance of the wind some ants pushed around the church and forced a new item*).[5]

D.E.'s ability to recognize morphologically complex words in sentences was tested using the monitoring technique. D.E. was asked to monitor for specified words in sentences. These targets were immediately preceded by "test words" that had either derivational or inflectional suffixes, or by nonwords. The real, morphologically complex, "test words" were either syntactically correct or not. For instance, D.E. would have to monitor for the words *cook* and *pain* in the following situations:

(5) Derivation.
    Context: Sarah could not understand why John used so much butter.
    Continuation (target: *cook*).

a) Correct: He was the most wasteful cook she had ever seen.

b) Incorrect: He was the most wastage cook she had ever seen.

c) Nonword: He was the most wastely cook she had ever seen.

(6) Inflection.
    Context: I have to be careful when eating ice cream.
    Continuation (target: *pain*).

a) Correct: It often causes pain in my loose filling.

b) Incorrect: It often causing pain in my loose filling.

c) Non-word: It often causely pain in my loose filling.

A group of matched control subjects were faster in detecting the targets in the correct condition than in the incorrect and nonword conditions for both derived and inflected words. This pattern indicates that normal subjects are sensitive to grammatical and lexical well-formedness and are slowed in recognizing a word that occurs after an inappropriate item. D.E. was also faster overall in detecting the targets in the correct condition than in the incorrect and nonword conditions. However, D.E. only showed this pattern for derivational affixes. For inflectional affixes, D.E. was as fast in recognizing the target in the incorrect condition as in the correct condition, and in both of these was faster than in the nonword condition. This pattern indicates that D.E. was sensitive to the well-formedness of words and the syntactic well-formedness of sentences when derived words were misused, but not when inflections were misused. Tyler and Cobb concluded that D.E. had trouble with on-line processing of inflectionally affixed words but not derivationally affixed words.

The trouble that D.E. had might have affected lexical representations themselves or, more likely in Tyler and Cobb's view, his ability to access syntactic and semantic features of inflectional affixes. These possibilities were explored in more detail in a second patient, B.N., investigated by Tyler et al. (1990). B.N. performed poorly on the word-monitoring task that had been used with D.E. Unlike D.E., B.N. showed abnormal monitoring for words following both inflectional and derivational affix anomalies, and he also showed no sensitivity to violations of verb voice (active vs. passive) and tense in a similar monitoring task. He also was unable to make grammaticality judgments about these sentences—that is, to say if a sentence that contained an anomaly due to a morphological mistake was a well-formed sentence or not (see chapter 7 for discussion of the use of grammaticality judgment tasks in assessing sentence comprehension). However, B.N. showed normal effects in a monitoring task in which the relationship between a noninflected verb and its object was varied (see chapter 7 for a description of this task), and in a wide variety of tasks involving processing morphologically complex words in isolation (gating, lexical decision). Tyler and her colleagues concluded that B.N. was able to recognize morphologically complex words, but suffered from a disturbance of the ability to use syntactic and semantic information derived from morphological suffixes to construct aspects of sentence form and meaning.

Disturbances of Output-Side Processing of Morphologically Complex Words

As we indicated above, the classic disturbances affecting the production of morphological forms are agrammatism and paragrammatism, which arise in producing sentences, and which are described in chapter 8. In this chapter, we discuss disturbances affecting morphological processing in single word production tasks.

One of the most detailed case studies of a patient with a disturbance in producing morphological forms is that of Miceli and

Caramazza (1988), who presented an Italian patient, F.S., with agrammatic speech. F.S.'s problem with morphological forms did not just arise in sentence production, however. His pattern of repeating single words also strongly suggested a primary morphological processing impairment in single word oral production.[6]

F.S. was tested on a variety of single word processing tasks. He performed well above chance in a word discrimination task, in which he had to say whether two words that were either identical or that differed in one distinctive feature of one phoneme were the same or different. He also did well in a lexical decision task in which the targets were morphologically complex words and the foils were illegal combinations of roots and affixes. He made both phonemic and morphological paraphasias in repeating single words. Given his level of performance on the word discrimination and lexical decision tasks and the fact that he made similar errors in spontaneous speech, his errors in single word repetition are likely to have arisen in the process of producing the forms of words (see chapter 4).

F.S. repeated 919 of 1832 words incorrectly in an initial test of repetition (50% error rate). Seventy-one percent of errors to words that allow morphological affixes (nouns, adjectives, verbs) were morphological paraphasias. Ninety-seven percent of these errors consisted of the correct repetition of the word stem and a substitution of an affix for the one on the presented word. Miceli and Caramazza showed that, though there were different error rates for repeating long and short words and high- and low-frequency words, the proportion of morphological errors remained constant despite variation in word frequency, length, and grammatical category (noun, verb, adjective). This pattern suggests that F.S. decomposed derived words into roots and affixes and had particular trouble repeating affixes.

Though F.S. made phonological paraphasias, his morphological errors appear to be different from his phonological errors. This was demonstrated by examining his repetition of adjectives. In Italian, adjectives are marked for number and gender. The masculine singular form of an adjective is the form that is usually cited when people refer to the word (it is known as its "citation" form). F.S. had a strong tendency to substitute the masculine singular form of a suffix on an adjective for whatever suffix was presented. This was true regardless of the phonological form of the masculine singular suffix. For instance, F.S. substituted the phoneme /o/ for the phonemes /a/,

/e/, and /i/ when given words from a set of adjectives in which /o/, /a/, /i/, and /e/ mark the masculine singular, feminine singular, masculine plural, and feminine plural, respectively [e.g., *caro* (masc.-sing.), *cara* (fem.sing.), *cari* (masc.pl.), *care* (fem.pl.)]. However, he had an overwhelming tendency to produce the masculine singular ending /e/ for adjectives that only have two forms, /e/ and /i/, e.g., *forte* (masc.sing. and fem.sing.) and *forti* (masc.pl. and fem.pl.). Thus, the morphological status of an adjectival ending, not its phonological form, determined which ending would be produced.

Not all affixes were equally affected in F.S. He had almost no trouble repeating prefixes, and much less difficulty with derivational affixes than inflectional affixes. The authors argue that he had a selective deficit in the oral production of inflectional affixes, which arose in part in the process of specifying the form of individual lexical items.

A second patient, S.J.D., with a disturbance in oral output-side processing of morphological form was described by Badecker and Caramazza (1987). In a series of carefully controlled single word reading studies, the authors showed that S.J.D.'s errors were unaffected by the variables of concreteness, frequency, and orthographic regularity, but were affected by grammatical category (verbs were more affected than nouns or adjectives) and length measured in terms of number of syllables. She was tested on the materials described above for F.M., and made more errors in reading truly derived and inflected words (e.g., *useful*, *listed*) than simple words with embedded words (e.g., *yearn*, *pierce*). She made more errors on regularly inflected verbs (e.g., *packed*) than on irregularly inflected verbs (e.g., *knew*), and more errors on all suffixed verbs than on simple verbs (e.g., *gather*). Finally, she was tested on her ability to read suffixed and nonsuffixed homophones (e.g., *frays* vs. *phrase*), and was better on the nonsuffixed forms. Morphological paralexias were the predominant type of error. All these findings are consistent with her having a disturbance of morphological processing.

In this case, like the cases of phonological and deep dyslexia described above, the patient's errors were studied in a set of reading-aloud tasks. However, unlike the patients described above, S.J.D. performed flawlessly on a task that required recognition and comprehension of written morphologically complex words but did not require her to produce the printed word orally. She had to say which of two printed words referred to a person, and was able to do this for word pairs in which this possibility resided in the affix (e.g., *electricity* vs. *electrician*). In addition, she frequently made comments indicating that she understood a word she misread. For instance, seeing the word *written*, she said, *"writer, writed, not today, but before."* These performances indicated that her problem did not lie in recognizing and comprehending the written forms of complex words, but in producing their oral forms.

S.J.D. produced both morphological paralexias and phonological errors in reading single words, and the authors took pains to establish that her morphological errors were not simply phonological ones that happened to be affixes. There are several pieces of evidence that indicate that the two sorts of errors are different. First, errors on affixes that produced nonwords were almost all other affixes, not simply nonsensical phonological forms (78 of 79 errors). Second, 42% of her errors in affixed words in the homophone test were morphological, but none of her errors on the nonaffixed words in that list were morphological. Third, S.J.D. produced errors that appeared to be due to both morphological and phonological disturbances. For instance, she read *sequence* as [kwensel]. This error may have resulted from her first intending to say *sequential* (a morphological error) and then making a phonemic error in producing that form. These aspects of performance indicate that two error-generating processes were at work in S.J.D., both affecting her ability to produce the oral forms of words.

Finally, the authors were interested in the question of whether S.J.D.'s morphological errors reflected the substitution of an entire word for another, or of one affix for another. This bears on the question of whether the decomposition model is correct for the production of spoken words. There are several reasons that Badecker and Caramazza give in favor of the decomposition analysis. The most important is that S.J.D. produced a reasonably high number of nonwords that consisted of a nonexistent or illegal combination of the presented stem and an affix (e.g., *newing* from *newer*; *discussionly* from *discussing*). These could not have resulted from the substitution of an entire word for another, because the item produced does not exist (and, in some cases, such as the examples above, cannot exist). This, therefore, suggests that the speech output system makes use of affixes and stems separately in producing words.

Patients have also been described who have disturbances in the written production of morphological forms. One such case, described by Badecker, Hillis, and Caramazza (1990), is the patient D.H. whose spoken language was fluent and grammatical with only occasional word-finding problems. His auditory comprehension and oral reading were also unimpaired. His problems consisted of a selective agraphia. On the basis of his written and oral spelling to dictation, and written naming and delayed copying performances, Hillis and Caramazza (1989) concluded that D.H. was unable to hold items in a buffer store that maintains the graphemes in a word while they are being produced in sequence either in writing or in oral spelling (the grapheme output buffer; see chapter 5). The principal evidence for this analysis was that D.H. made errors that the authors associated with a disturbance of the graphemic output buffer (omissions, substitutions, insertions, and transpositions of letters) in all these tasks at about the same rate for words and nonwords. Consistent with the idea that the representations in the grapheme output buffer decay over time, these errors were more frequent toward the ends of words than at the beginnings of words.[7]

Badecker and his colleagues investigated the effects of this disturbance on the production of morphologically complex words. D.H. made the same types of errors on morphologically complex words as on simple words (omissions, substitutions, insertions, and transpositions of letters), but the distribution of errors differed in the two sets. As with simple words, there was a larger number of errors as D.H. progressed through the stem of a morphologically complex word, but the error rate dropped to a very low level at the beginning of the suffix of a word and began to climb again throughout the suffix. Using the materials we have described above, the authors compared the distribution of errors in truly suffixed words with that of errors in simple words containing other words, and that of errors in compound words with that in simple words. In both cases, the distribution of errors differed statistically, with a drop-off in the frequency of errors at the beginning of the suffix of a truly suffixed word or the second word in a compound word, but not at the end of an embedded word in a simple monomorphemic word. This pattern indicates that complex words behaved as if they were composed of stems and affixes, consistent with the view that they are decomposed in the written output processing system.

Two additional points are of interest regarding D.H. The first is that level I suffixes—suffixes that affect the form of the words to which they are attached—and level II suffixes—those that keep the form of the words to which they are attached the same—differed. Words with level I suffixes acted like simple words, suggesting that they are listed and processed as wholes. This is consistent with several results found in normal experimental work (see above). Second, the same error patterns were observed for both written output and oral spelling, indicating that the decomposition of complex words (with level II affixes) into stems and affixes occurred before the final motor output mechanism was operative.

SUMMARY

Linguistic studies indicate that words may have internal morphological structure, and that there are different types of word formation processes (compounding, derivation, and inflection; different levels of affixation). Psychological studies, though not definitive or uncontroversial, suggest that parts of morphologically complex words are handled by different components of the language processing system at some stages of input- and output-side processing. The case studies we have reviewed indicate that patients can have selective impairments of morphological processing. These impairments can affect either input- or output-side processing, in either the auditory-oral or written modalities.

Not every error that affects morphological form reflects a disturbance of morphological processing. Semantic and visual errors can masquerade as morphological errors. If the clinician wants to be sure that morphological errors are truly due to disturbances of morphological processing mechanisms, he or she must test the patient with materials that vary the factor of morphological structure, but which are controlled for other factors that affect performance: length, surface and stem frequency, the lexical status of the stems and pseudostems, etc. Despite these diagnostic challenges, made worse by the fact that morphological processing impairments often co-occur with other disturbances that affect single word processing, morphological processing impairments can be distinguished from other disturbances. They are potentially important as contributers to disturbances of sentence processing, and should be looked for as part of the investigation of a language disorder.

NOTES

1. There are two variants of this basic theory. The first, known as the "decomposition first" model, is that, when the perceptual system is presented with a morphologically complex word, it strips off the various morphological elements, recognizes the root and affixes, and recognizes the word by putting the root together with the morphological elements. If the perceptual system has stripped off a part of a word that is not really an affix (a "pseudoaffix," such as the *er* in *father*), the root will not be found, and the perceptual system will then search for the entire presented item. The second version of this model, the "decomposition second" variant, maintains that complex words (e.g., *lender*) are searched for as a whole in the lexicon but are not found, because they are not listed as wholes, but only their roots and affixes being listed. When a stimulus is not found, it is then decomposed into possible root-affix combinations, which are then searched for and then combined.

Both these variants of the decomposition model have to specify how the recognition system "knows" that a stem and an affix can be combined. In some versions of the decomposition first model, this is accomplished by having the combined form be listed in a second list of words (Taft and Forster, 1975). One might then ask why that list is not consulted first or in parallel with the initial decompostion process. In fact, this possibility has been explored, in terms of a slightly different model, by Caramazza and his colleagues (see text below).

2. She also based her argument on results in lexical decision tasks by Bradley, Garrett, and Zurif (1980), but these results involve function words, not suffixes, and they have not been replicated. These results are discussed in chapter 8.

3. W.B.'s performance posed another problem. He was not able to read inappropriately suffixed words and isolated suffixes, which suggested that these items were not recognized by the whole word reading route. Job and Sartori (1984) suggest that these aspects of W.B.'s problem may be due to a lowered ability to recognize written suffixes compared to written stems, and support this analysis by pointing to different patterns of errors in reading affixes in illegal affix-word combinations (50% suffix substitution) and in reading simple nonwords (mostly omissions).

4. Additional evidence for such a deficit came from F.M.'s performance in reading irregular morphological forms.

5. For more discussion of this patient's monitoring functions, see chapter 7.

6. The relationship between F.S.'s deficits in his single word and sentence production is discussed in chapter 8.

7. It may be that this left-to-right effect was due to a spatial attention disturbance affecting the right side of space, rather than to decay of letter information in the grapheme output buffer. However, this possibility is not directly relevant to the issues regarding the effects of morphological structure on written production that we are concerned with here.

7 Sentence Comprehension

Words in isolation convey a limited set of semantic features. With some limited exceptions, English words convey semantic values pertaining to individual items, actions, and properties. In addition to these semantic features, language conveys relationships between the items designated by individual words. Information about thematic roles—which person or object is accomplishing an action, which is being acted upon, where actions are taking place, etc.—depends upon the relationship of words to each other within a sentence. Similarly, sentences convey information about which adjectives are associated with which nouns (attribution of modification), which pronouns refer to particular nouns (co-reference), which items are qualified by negative and other numerical elements (scope of quantification), and other semantic features not inherent in single words themselves. These aspects of meaning make up the propositional content of a sentence, an essential aspect of the information conveyed by language. Propositions are the basis for drawing inferences and structuring discourse, and are thus essential to the communicative functions served by language.

SENTENCE MEANING AND ITS RELATIONSHIP TO SYNTACTIC STRUCTURES

The information conveyed by sentences depends upon the relationship of the meanings of the words in a sentence to each other, dictated by the structure of a sentence. Syntactic structures provide the means whereby the meanings of individual words can be combined with one another to add to the information conveyed by language.

Syntactic structures are hierarchically organized sets of syntactic categories. Individual lexical items are marked for syntactic category (e.g., *cat* is a noun [N]; *read* is a verb; *of* is a preposition [P]).

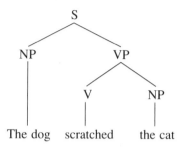

Figure 7.1
Syntactic structure of sentence 1.

These categories combine to create nonlexical nodes (or phrasal categories), such as noun phrase [NP], verb phrase [VP], sentence [S], etc. The way words are inserted into these higher-order phrasal categories determines a number of different aspects of sentence meaning. Consider, for instance, the very simple sentence (1):

(1)   The dog scratched the cat.

In (1), we know that the dog did the scratching and the cat was scratched. This is not because the world is set up so that only dogs can scratch and only cats can be scratched; it is because of the way the words in the sentence are placed in a syntactic structure. The syntactic structure of (1) is shown in figure 7.1. The noun *dog* is part of the NP *the dog* that is attached to the sentence node, S. I will refer to categories as nodes, and say that any node that is connected to another node by an upward-directed line is "dominated" by that "higher" node, and that one node is "immediately dominated" by another if no other nodes intervene along such a line. In this case, the NP, *the dog*, is immediately dominated by the node S. We shall say that the NP that is immediately dominated by S is the "subject" of the sentence. The notion of subject is thus a syntactic notion, defined by the position of words in syntactic structures. We shall call subject a "grammatical role," and say that *the dog* plays the grammatical role of subject in (1). The way this notion is related to the fact that the dog accomplishes the action of scratching (i.e., that *the dog* is the "agent" of *scratch*) is via the way thematic roles are assigned by the verb. Part of the meaning of a verb is its "argument structure"—how it assigns actors, recipients of actions, and other thematic roles. The subject of a verb is the "external argument" of the verb, and the verb *scratch* assigns the thematic role of agent to

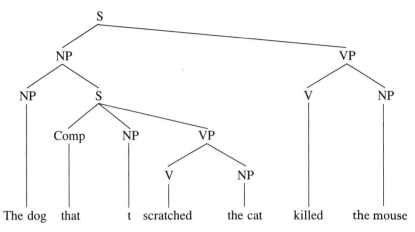

Figure 7.2
Syntactic structure of sentence 2.

its external argument. In a similar way, *the cat* is the "object" of the verb, the object of the verb is (one of) the "internal" arguments of the verb, and *scratch* assigns the thematic role of theme to its internal argument. This is how sentence (1) comes to mean that the dog is doing the scratching and the cat was scratched.

Things can get considerably more complicated than this. Consider sentence (2):

(2) The dog that scratched the cat killed the mouse.

In (2) there is a sequence of words—*the cat killed the mouse*—which would be a well-formed sentence if it were presented by itself, but which is not understood as a proposition in (2). The reason that this sequence is not understood as a sentence—that is, that sentence (2) does not indicate that the cat actually killed the mouse—is that the structure of (2) does not group together *the cat* with *killed the mouse*. A sequence of words that is grouped together syntactically is known as a syntactic "constituent." A sequence of words is a constituent in a sentence if (and only if) it is dominated by a single syntactic node that does not also dominate other words. Thus, *the cat* is a constituent of (2)—it is the NP that is the object of the verb *scratched*—and *killed the mouse* is a constituent of (2)—it is the VP of the main clause of the sentence, but *the cat killed the mouse* is not a syntactic constituent of sentence (2). The syntactic constituents of sentence (2) are shown in figure 7.2.

Figures 7.1 and 7.2 not only demonstrate the way syntactic categories like N, V, NP, VP, etc. are organized hierarchically. These figures also indicate that the hierarchical structures that make up the syntactic structure of a sentence have a certain direction of branching. In English, when a higher-level node is divided, the category that gives its name to the higher-order node is usually on the left-hand branch. In both figures 7.1 and 7.2, when the VP node branches into a V and an NP, the V is on the left. In figure 7.2, when the subject NP branches into another NP and an S, the NP is on the left. We say that a node that gives its character to the node that immediately dominates it is the head of its phrase. In English, heads of phrases are on the leftmost branches of hierarchical structures. The result is a language with a certain order of words—a "word order" known as "subject-verb-object," or S-V-O. Two points about the direction of headedness are of interest. First, the direction of headedness for word formation processes and for sentence structures may differ in a language. English is a case in point. In chapter 6, we noted that a word like *decision* receives its syntactic category from its *right*most derivational affix—the opposite of how a phrasal node receives its category. Second, the direction of headedness in phrases differs across languages. In Japanese, for instance, heads of phrasal categories go on the right-hand branches, leading to a subject-object-verb (S-O-V) word order.

In English, syntactic grammatical roles such as subject are largely indicated through word order. In other languages, other markers are used to convey these grammatical roles. Especially common devices in Indo-European languages such as German, French, and Italian are case markers and agreement features. In German, for instance, the subject of a sentence is marked by a particular morphological suffix that expresses nominative case and the object by another suffix that conveys accusative case; in Italian, the subject agrees with the verb in person and number, and these features are indicated through suffixes on both the subject noun and the verb. Thus languages have at their disposal a variety of formal means of expressing grammatical roles. Interestingly, these formal devices tend to express features of *syntactic* structures such as *grammatical roles*, not features of sentential *semantic* structure such as *thematic roles*. In German, for instance, as in English, the subject of the sentence may be the theme of an action (when a verb like *hit* is used in the passive voice, for instance), and when this happens, the subject is still given nominative, not accusative case. In Italian, a sentence subject in this situation still determines the form of the morphological affixes attached to the verb. Formal markings such as word order, declensional morphology, inflectional agreement, etc. tend to encode syntactic structure, not semantic structure.

The modern study of the nature of syntactic structures and the way they contribute to sentence meaning began with the pioneering work of Noam Chomsky (1955, 1957, 1965, 1970, 1981, 1985). It was Chomsky who changed the study of syntax from an effort to enumerate the patterns that make for well-formed sentences in a language to the study of the relationship between syntactic structures and aspects of meaning. The relationship between subjects and objects and thematic roles that lies at the basis of the meanings of sentences (1) and (2)—though appreciated for many years before Chomsky's work—was integrated into general theories of syntactic representations and their relationship to meaning for the first time in his research.

At the heart of Chomsky's work and subsequent research in modern linguistics lies the effort to represent the syntactic structure of sentences in such a way as to capture regularities in sentence structure. For instance, the fact that subjects and objects of sentences receive the thematic roles assigned to the external and internal arguments of verbs is a regularity of the relationship between sentence structure and sentence meaning. Representing syntactic structure so as to define the notions of subject and object allows us to express this regularity. The existence of the notion of a "subject of a sentence" explains the fact that *the dog* in (1) and *the dog that scratched the cat* in (2) are the agents of their clauses. Both *the dog* and *the dog that scratched the cat* are NPs in subject position, and this fact determines their thematic role. The fact that they differ in their internal structure (*the dog that scratched the cat* contains a relative clause and *the dog* does not) does not affect the fact that they are both subjects.

Modern linguistics attempts to extend the ability of representations to account for regularities in sentence structure and in the relationship of structure to meaning to a wide range of structures. The most interesting (and controversial) analyses are those where the simplest generalizations do not appear to hold; that is, where syntactic structures become more complex. For instance, Chomsky has emphasized the fact that thematic roles are the same in sentences of different types, in actives such as (1) and in passives such as (3):

(3)   The cat was scratched by the dog.

In (3), the simple generalization that the subject receives the thematic role assigned to the external argument of the verb is violated. *The cat* is the subject of the sentence, but it is is the theme of *scratched*; that is, it plays the thematic role assigned to the internal argument of the verb *scratch*.

Chomsky has developed models of syntactic structures that explain this fact. These models postulate a so-called underlying syntactic structure where thematic roles are assigned directly. This structure was known as "Deep Structure" in earlier models and is called "D-structure" in more recent work. The D-structures of (1) and (3) are shown in figure 7.3. In Chomsky's theory, sentences (1) and (3) share aspects of D-structure; namely, the fact that *the cat* is the object of *scratch* in the D-structure of both sentences. This fact guarantees that *the cat* will be the internal argument of *scratch* and play the role of theme. The role of agent is assigned to *the dog* because it is the *subject* of scratch in (1), as discussed above, and because it is in a *by* phrase in (3). This theory thus accounts for the identity of one of the thematic roles in actives and passives on the basis of the fact that these two sentence types share one crucial aspect of their D-structures—the same NP (*the cat*) is in object position in both D-structures. In this respect, the theory behaves exactly as it did in explaining how *the dog* in (1) and *the dog that scratched the cat* in (2) are the agents of their clauses—identical grammatical roles lead to the identical processes of thematic role assignment. Chomsky's theory of the passive creates a new question, however: How does *the cat* get to be the subject of the sentence in (3) and why is it not assigned the role of agent by virtue of its being the subject of the sentence? Chomsky answers these questions by postulating that *the cat* is moved by a syntactic rule from its position in D-structure to its final position in what is now called "S-structure," shown in figure 7.4. (S-structure is similar to what was formerly called "surface structure.") A simple way of thinking of Chomsky's theory is to say that that it postulates that thematic roles are determined by the grammatical roles of lexically specified NPs in D-structure, not S-structure.[1]

Sentence 1

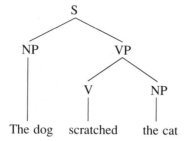

Sentence 2

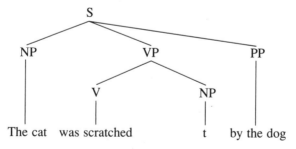

Figure 7.3
D-structures of sentences 1 and 3.

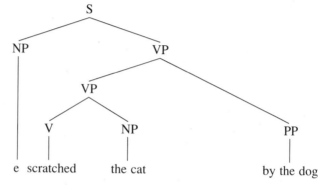

Figure 7.4
S-structure of sentence 3.

$$S \quad \text{-----} \rightarrow NP + VP$$

$$NP \text{-----} \rightarrow Determiner + N \ (+S)$$

$$VP \text{-----} \rightarrow V \ (+NP) \ (+PP) \ (+S)$$

Figure 7.5
Some sample phrase structure rules. The category on the left of the arrow is replaced by those on the right. Categories in parentheses are optional.

Of course, there must be a motivation for this complication of syntactic structure—the idea that each sentence has several levels of structure, one (or possibly more than one) quite different from that found on the surface. The justification for postulating D-structure and S-structure is complex and cannot be reviewed properly here. However, the rationale behind it can be sketched. In Chomsky's theory, the S-structure of a sentence is due to two different sorts of rules. The first set of rules creates the D-structure; the second set creates the S-structure from the D-structure. Rules of the first sort are known as "phrase structure rules." Phrase structure rules (illustrated in figure 7.5) rewrite syntactic categories as other syntactic categories. Phrase structure rules are responsible for two important properties of sentences: (1) their hierarchical syntactic structure, and (2) the fact that they are potentially infinite in length. This second property is due to the fact that the rules in figure 7.5 can be used over and over again. The second set of rules are so-called movement or transformational rules. These rules move categories in D-structure to their positions in S-structure.[2]

Despite many changes in Chomsky's thinking over more than 30 years of developing his theory, the basic idea that there are two processes involved in creating syntactic structures has remained an important part of his theories. One set of rules is related to the creation of underlying structures, and is responsible for the potentially infinite number of syntactic structures of a language. These rules create structures in which the thematic roles of a sentence are easily related to the position of NPs in the syntax. The second set of rules (or processes) are responsible for relating underlying structures to overt structures. These rules move NPs and other constituents around in ways that complicate these simple relationships between thematic roles and grammatical positions. We can see how the effort to describe the syntactic structures of sentences such as (1)–(3) has led to quite an elaborate set of rules and structures, all designed to describe the structure of sentences and to capture (and thus explain) the regularities in the relationship between sentence form and sentence meaning.

In early versions of Chomsky's theory, the second type of rule we just mentioned—rules that rearrange the order of words set by the phrase structure rules—consisted of a large set of rules, each devoted to creating a particular structure. Thus, there were rules for forming the passive, for creating questions, for inserting words like *There are* at the beginning of a sentence, etc. In the latest version of the theory, all these rules have been replaced by one simple rule that basically allows any constituent to be moved anywhere at all! Obviously, this state of affairs is unsatisfactory. It would lead to a situation in which almost any sequence of words was a possible sentence in any language. Therefore, an important part of the modern theory of syntax is a set of constraints on the application of the general rule that moves constituents. The general form of these constraints is thought to apply to all languages, and to reflect an innate, specifically human, mental capacity to structure sequences of words into sentences. For instance, movement rules apply only to constituents, and not to sequences of words or syntactic categories that are not constituents. Moreover, a given application of the movement rule cannot result in a constituent being moved arbitrarily far away from its original syntactic position. Within this general framework of possible constraints on movement of constituents, specific constraints apply in individual languages, contributing to the syntactic differences among languages.

The development of theories of syntactic structure that attempted to describe and explain the systematic relationships between syntactic structures and the meanings of sentences naturally led linguists to explore a variety of aspects of meaning that arise at the level of the sentence. Aside from the assignment of thematic roles, one phenomenon that has been extensively studied is co-reference—the relationship of referentially dependent items such as pronouns (e.g., *him*) and reflexives (e.g., *himself*) to referring NPs. A noun like *boy* can refer to a class of items in the real world by virtue of its intrinsic meaning (see chapter 3 for a discussion of what the meaning of a nominal item like *boy* might be and how it might be represented and processed). A word like *him* or *himself* cannot refer to a class of items in the real world in quite the same way.[3] Words like *him* or *himself* can only refer to an entity in the real world by being connected to another word in a sentence or a discourse. The position of a word like *him* or *himself* in a syntactic structure constrains or even determines the word to which *him* or *himself* refers.

How syntactic structure affects the interpretation of reflexives and pronouns is illustrated in sentences (4) and (5) (the subscripts in these sentences indicate identity and distinctness of reference):

(4a)   Susan said that a friend$_i$ of Mary's washed herself$_i$.

b)   Susan said that a friend$_j$ of Mary's washed her$_i$.

(5a)   Susan said that Mary's$_i$ portrait of herself$_i$ pleased Helen.

b)   Susan said that Mary's$_j$ portrait of her$_i$ pleased Helen.

In (4a), *herself* refers to *friend* and cannot refer to *Susan* or *Mary*. In (4b), *her* cannot refer to *friend* but can refer to either *Susan* or *Mary*. Similarly, *herself* refers to *Mary* in (5a), not *Susan* or *Helen*, and *her* cannot refer to *Mary* in (5b) but may refer to *Susan* or *Helen*.

Pronouns (e.g., *her, him*), reflexives (e.g., *herself, himself*), and other words that refer to other NPs are said to be "co-indexed" with those NPs, and the NPs with which they are co-indexed are said to be their "antecedents." Sentences (4) and (5) document an interesting fact about English—one that is true of all languages. This is the fact that if a NP is in a syntactic position where it can be the antecedent of a reflexive, then it cannot be the antecedent of a pronoun that occupies the same syntactic position as the reflexive.

Sentences (4) and (5) also show that there are heavy constraints on which NP can function as the antecedent of a reflexive and be unable to be the antecedent of a pronoun. First, this NP must be within a particular syntactic domain. In the case of sentences (4a) and (4b), this domain is the clause within which the reflexive or pronoun occurs; in sentences (5a) and (5b), it is the complex NP within which the referentially dependent item occurs. This constraint limits how far away an NP may be from a reflexive and still function as the antecedent of that reflexive (or, for pronouns, this constraint limits how far away an NP may be from a pronoun and still be affected by the constraint that eliminates certain NPs as possible antecedents of the pronoun). Second, an NP that must be the antecedent of a particular reflexive (or that cannot be the antecedent of a given pronoun) must stand in a particular structural relationship to the reflexive or pronoun. In (4a) and (4b), the head of the subject NP stands in

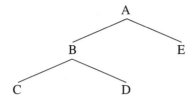

C-command relations:

C   c-commands D
D   c-commands C
B   c-commands E
E   c-commands B, C, and D

C and D do not c-command E, because they are dominated by the branching node B which does not dominate E

Figure 7.6
Diagram illustrating the notion of c-command.

that relationship; in (5a) and (5b), the NP that occupies the determiner position in the complex NP stands in that relationship. The relationship—known as "c-command"—that permits co-indexation of reflexives and rules out co-indexation of pronouns to an NP is defined in terms of the hierarchically organized syntactic structure in which the reflexive or pronoun is found (Chomsky, 1981; Reinhardt, 1983). One node c-commands a second if and only if the first branching node above the first dominates the second. This relationship is illustrated in figure 7.6, and how it is relevant to sentences 4 and 5 is illustrated in figure 7.7. The reader who has been following the details of these syntactic structures will appreciate that the structural relationship of c-command, which is relevant to determining the antecedents of pronouns and reflexives, differs from the structural relationships of "subject" and "object," which are relevant to thematic roles.

The assignment of thematic roles and the assignment of co-reference come together in Chomsky's theory in the determination of the meaning of sentences with what are known as "phonologically null, logically co-referential" elements or "empty categories" (or "empty NPs")—referentially dependent items that are not phonologically specified. Passive sentences such as (3) have such empty NPs, illustrated by the symbol t in figure 7.4, as do sentences with

Sentence 4

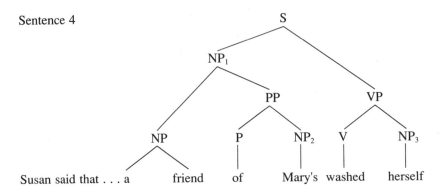

NP₁ c-commands **NP₃** because it is dominated by **S** which dominates **NP₃**
NP₂ does not c-command **NP₃** because it is dominated by **NP₁** which branches
and does not dominate **NP₃**

Sentence 5

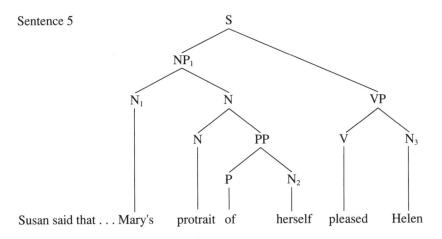

N₁ c-commands **N₂** because it is dominated by **NP₁** which dominates **N₂**
N₃ does not c-command **N₂** because it is dominated by **VP** which branches and
does not dominate **N₃**

Figure 7.7
C-command relationship in the sentences in the text. (Reproduced with
permission from Chomsky, 1981, p. 154.)

relative clauses, such as (2). So do sentences with question words, such as (6) and (7):

(6) Who$_i$ did John introduce $\mathbf{t}_i$ to Mary?

(7) Who$_i$ did John introduce Bill to $\mathbf{t}_i$?

Who is the theme of *introduce* in (6) and the goal of *introduce* in (7). This exactly parallels the roles of *Bill* and *Mary* in (8).

(8) John introduced Bill to Mary.

Furthermore, the grammatical roles occupied by *Bill* and *Mary* in (8)—the direct and indirect object positions—are empty in (6) and (7): an NP is "missing" after *introduce* in these positions in (6) and (7). In Chomsky's theory, all these sentences—(6)–(8)—have the same D-structure, generated by phrase structure rules, and sentences (6) and (7) are derived by movement of the interrogative *who* into sentence-initial position when a question is to be created. According to this theory, the application of the movement rule leaves a **trace (t)** in the original position originally occupied by *who*. The trace is an "empty NP." It receives a thematic role [theme in (6), goal in (7)], on the basis of its position in a phrase marker, just as the overt NPs *Bill* and *Mary* do in (8). This trace is co-indexed with *who*, and its thematic role is transmitted to its antecedent, *who*. These sentences begin to illustrate the complex interactions that Chomsky's theory postulates between the assignment of thematic roles and the process of co-indexation, all of which combine to determine aspects of sentence meaning in sentences like (6) and (7).

Having introduced the concepts of co-indexation and empty categories like **trace**, we can consider some of the constraints on movement of syntactic constituents that we mentioned earlier, that constrain the application of the movement transformation that creates S-structure from D-structure. One example of these constraints is the fact that in English an NP cannot be moved beyond two S or NP boundaries. Consider the sequence in (9a):

*(9a) The boat that you believed the claim John painted is red.

The sequence of words in (9a) is not a well-formed sentence even though it is quite clear what it would mean if it were a sentence. The reason it is not well-formed is that the relative pronoun *that* is related to a **trace** across two S boundaries and an NP boundary, as indicated in (9b). This is not allowed by the grammar of English.

*(9b)   The boat [$_{\bar{s}}$ that$_i$ [$_s$ you believed [$_{NP}$ the claim [$_s$ John painted t$_i$]]]] is red

Contrast (9a) with (10a):

(10a)   The boat that you believed John painted is red.

The sequence of words in (10a) is a well-formed sentence, because the relative pronoun *that* is related to its **trace** across two S boundaries, as indicated in (10b). This is allowed by the grammar of English.

(10b)   The boat [$_{\bar{s}}$ that$_i$ [$_s$ you believed [$_s$ John painted t$_i$]]] is red.

It is generally the case that a language sets a limit on how far an NP can move, just as it sets a limit on the possible distance between a reflexive and its antecedent. This limit differs from language to language, but it is always expressed in terms of a certain number of major higher-level nodes such as NP and S. The study of the constraints on movement of constituents in natural languages is one of the most active (and technically complex) areas of linguistic research (see Radford, 1988, for an introductory presentation, and Chomsky, 1985, for a technical discussion).

Let us return to the issue of referentially dependent nominal categories. According to Chomsky's theory, there are several different types of referentially dependent empty categories in natural languages. The **trace** in (2), (6), and (7) is a "wh-trace" because the trace is related to "wh-word" (*who*). The **trace** in the passive sentence (3) is an "NP-trace," because it is related to a common noun. Chomsky also postulates the existence of an **NP-trace** in sentences such as (11), which the reader can verify also involve the transmission of a thematic role from one syntactic position to another NP (*John* is not the agent of *seems* but is the agent of *shaving*). The **NP-traces** in (3) and (11) function similarly to a **wh-trace** in the sense that they receive the thematic role assigned by the verb, are co-indexed with another word in the sentence, and transmit their thematic roles to that word.

(11)   John$_i$ seems to Bill t$_i$ to be shaving.

According to Chomsky, sentences (12)–(14) contain a different empty NP, indicated as **PRO**. In (12), **PRO** is co-indexed with *John* and in (13) with *Peter*. In (14), **PRO** refers to anyone; that is, its reference is free. Unlike the antecedent of a **trace**, which lexical NP is the antecedent of **PRO** depends upon the main verb of the sentence.

(12)   John$_i$ promised Peter **PRO$_i$** to shave.

(13)   John persuaded Peter$_i$ **PRO$_i$** to shave.

(14)   It is hard **PRO** to shave.

The empty NPs **PRO** and **trace** are similar to reflexives and pronouns in that all these NPs share the property of receiving their reference by being related to a lexical NP (i.e., they are both "referentially dependent" NPs), and they are similar to each other because neither is phonologically realized (i.e., both are "phonologically empty" NPs). However, in Chomsky's theory, **PRO** and **trace** are two quite different types of phonologically empty referentially dependent NPs. **PRO** does not transmit a thematic role, while **trace** does. In addition, **PRO** may refer outside the sentence it is in, while **trace** must refer to an NP within its sentence. In this latter respect, **PRO** and **trace** are similar to pronouns and reflexives, respectively. Like **PRO**, a pronoun (e.g., *him*) may refer to other nouns in the sentence it is in or may refer to an entity outside the sentence. The only restriction on pronouns or **PRO** is that there are certain NPs which they may *not* refer to. Like **trace**, reflexives (e.g., *himself*) must refer to a particular NP in their sentence.

Chomsky's theory is just one of several that seek to capture the structural relationships between words that determine or constrain sentential semantic features such as thematic roles and co-indexation of referentially dependent items. There are many differences among these different theories (see Sells, 1985, for a presentation of three major approaches). For instance, Bresnan (1982) has developed a theory of syntactic structures in which sentences such as (11)–(14) do not have an empty NP in their syntactic representation. Bresnan's theory easily captures one regularity in these sentences: the fact that the relationship between the subject of the embedded infinitive and the nouns in the main clause is determined by the verb of the main clause. In Chomsky's theory, this regularity is not expressed as directly as in Bresnan's theory. On the other hand, Chomsky's theory captures a similarity between sentence (11) and passive sentences such as (3) (whose structure was shown in figures 7.3 and 7.4); namely, in both sentence (11) and passive sentences, the noun that plays a thematic role around a particular verb [the embedded infinitive in (11) and the main verb in a passive clause] is not located in the syntactic position to which that thematic role is usually assigned. Chomsky's theory expresses this regularity through its use of the empty category **NP-trace** and the idea that a thematic role can be transmitted from an **NP-trace** to an NP that has been moved from one syntactic position to another. There is no simple way to capture this similarity between sentences like (11) and passive sentences in Bresnan's theory of syntactic structure.

Linguists do not know which of the several contemporary theories of syntactic structure is correct. In all likelihood, all will need to be revised to be empirically adequate. But this does not imply that the study of syntactic structures is so full of uncertainties and controversies that psychologists and aphasiologists cannot use theories of syntactic structures to guide research into language processing and language disorders. All syntactic theories have several features in common. First, they all agree that there are lawful ways in which words can combine to form larger structures responsible for conveying sentence-level semantic features such as thematic roles and co-indexation. Second, they agree that syntactic structures consist of hierarchically organized sets of syntactic nodes coupled with relationships defined over these hierarchical structures (e.g., subject, object, c-command, etc.). Third, they all recognize that different relationships defined over these structures are relevant to different aspects of semantics; for instance, the relationships of subject and object are relevant to the determination of thematic roles, while c-command is relevant to the determination of certain aspects of co-indexation, etc. Fourth, most linguistic theories group together language elements that are not intuitively related, such as Chomsky's suggestion that the subject of *to shave* in (12) and pronouns belong to the same class of referentially dependent categories. Finally, most linguistic theories maintain that syntactic structures, the relationships between nodes defined over these structures, and the mapping of these structures and relationships to semantic values differ from the representations in other linguistic domains, such as phonology, lexical semantics, discourse, and so on. This suggests (but obviously does not prove) that syntactic structures are a special domain of mental representations, likely to be associated with their own processors. These commonalities among existing theories of syntactic structures are the basis for aspects of the work on the nature of sentence comprehension and its disorders that we shall discuss shortly.

ALTERNATIVE ACCOUNTS OF SENTENCE STRUCTURE

I have emphasized the role that syntactic structures play in determining aspects of sentence meaning. However, it is possible to understand some of the aspects of sentence meaning without reference to these complex structures. For instance, consider sentence (15):

(15)   The bone was eaten by the dog.

We do not have to structure this sentence and understand the effect of the passive form on the assignment of thematic roles to understand (15). In sentence (15), it is possible to know that the dog did the eating and that what it ate was a bone, simply by knowing that dogs, being animate, can eat bones, and bones, being inanimate, cannot eat dogs. In other words, we can arrive at an understanding of the thematic roles in (15) by a "lexico-pragmatic" route.

Or, consider sentence (16):

(16)   The dog chased the cat.

A lexico-pragmatic route will not work to assign the thematic roles in (16), because both cats and dogs can chase one another. However, we may not have to structure the sentence in a complex way to extract the thematic roles. We may rely on the fact that, in English, the NP that precedes the verb is usually the agent of the verb and the NP that follows the verb is usually its theme. In other words, we may use short cuts ("heuristics") based on simple syntactic analyses—such as which word immediately precedes a verb or which word comes first in a sentence—to relate words to thematic roles, rather than use the entire syntactic tree to assign these semantic features. Of course, these heuristics will not work for all sentences. They will not work for sentences such as (2), which we discussed above, for instance. However, they may suffice for some sentences.

Some researchers have elaborated upon the notion that nonsyntactic mechanisms, such as a lexico-pragmatic route to sentential semantic meanings, and simplified syntactic analyses, such as an assignment of thematic roles based on the order of major lexical items, are the basis for sentence comprehension (Bates et al., 1982; Bates and MacWhinney, 1989). According to these researchers, the types of nonsyntactic and simplified syntactic factors that influence sentence processing are not restricted to the two examples we have just mentioned. Rather, there are many such factors. For instance, these researchers point out that the first noun in a sentence tends to play the discourse role of topic, and that topics tend to be agents of a sentence. Therefore, there is a tendency for the first noun in a sentence to be the agent of that sentence. Similarly, there is a tendency for animate nouns to be agents. According to some researchers who emphasize these tendencies, these tendencies are all there is by way of sentence structure. That is, these researchers argue that there are no such things as the syntactic structures we have been describing. Instead, they say, sentential semantic information such as which item mentioned in the sentence plays which thematic role is encoded in a wide set of structural and lexical semantic features, each of which enters into a large-scale calculation of the probability that a given sentential semantic feature is assigned to a given lexical item. Formal mathematical models of this approach to the representation of sentence form and meaning are being developed within the PDP framework we have described in connection with word processing before (see chapters 2, 4, and 5 for some discussion of these models). We shall review this work in our discussion of sentence processing.

At this point in the development of linguistics, these probabilistic-type models pose no serious challenge to the need for the more complex syntactic structures we have been describing.[4] The sentences that have been explored within this framework are all very simple sentences, and there is no clear way (yet!) to extend these models to more complex sentence types. This situation may change in the future, but for now these models are not serious contenders for syntactic representations: they are unable to represent the range of form-meaning pairings found at the level of sentences in natural languages.

Formal, computer-implemented PDP models and related psycholinguistic models may, however, have a lot to offer to our theories of sentence processing. Given that it is possible to extract sentence meaning in some circumstances through a lexico-pragmatic or heuristic route, or through both, and that there are tendencies for nouns in certain positions or that have certain intrinsic semantic features to be assigned certain sentential semantic functions, it is an empirical question whether and when comprehension involves the construction of syntactic form. This question leads naturally to our next topic: psycholinguistic studies of sentence comprehension.

PROCESSES INVOLVED IN SENTENCE COMPREHENSION

In many previous chapters, we developed models of language processing according to which a language-related task could be accomplished in a variety of ways, each involving the computation of different linguistic representations. For instance, in chapter 4, we presented a model of spoken word repetition according to which words could be repeated semantically, lexically, or nonlexically. Though it is somewhat unorthodox to do so, it is possible to look at sentence comprehension the same way. Following the discussion above, we can investigate the possibility that there are several "routes" to sentence meaning. Three of these would be: a syntactic route that computes a full syntactic representation for a sentence and uses this representation to assign aspects of meaning; a heuristic route that uses a reduced syntactic structure for this purpose; and a lexico-inferential route that infers aspects of sentence meaning from word meanings and knowledge of real world events. The types of structures constructed by these three routes are illustrated in figure 7.8.

I begin my consideration of the psycholinguistic processes involved in sentence comprehension by reviewing research that deals with the construction and interpretation of syntactic form. I then discuss other routes to meaning, dealing with both the heuristic and lexico-pragmatic route and with theories that amalgamate several different routes into a single comprehension process.

The Syntactic Route to Sentence Comprehension

Several lines of evidence suggest that there is a specialized processing mechanism dedicated to the construction of syntactic form. Such a mechanism is called a "parser." We begin with some general considerations about what a parser might be like, and then review evidence that bears on its existence and the nature of its operations.[5]

Many researchers have begun their thinking about the mechanisms that assign syntactic structures to sentences with the observation that the rules that generate the syntactic structures of a language can produce an unlimited number of different structures. This fact has prompted researchers to develop parsers that are capable of assigning syntactic structure to any possible sentence, not simply to a small list of commonly occurring syntactic structures.

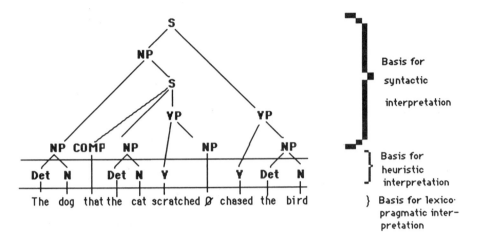

Figure 7.8
Different bases for sentence comprehension, each possibly associated with a different "route" to sentence comprehension.

In these parsers, the syntactic structure of a sentence is not recognized as a whole. Rather, it is built up by the application of a number of rules that assign structure to its parts.

One way to create a parser that accomplishes this incremental assignment of syntactic structure involves the use of so-called pattern-action rules (see chapter 4 for some discussion of the use of these types of rules in word production). A pattern-action rule takes as its input a syntactic category, such as Determiner, Noun, or Noun Phrase, and creates a syntactic structure as its output. For instance, the "pattern" *Determiner* can trigger the creation of the larger category *Noun Phrase*; the category *Noun Phrase* can trigger the category *Sentence*. The pattern-action rules specified in any particular parser must bear a close relationship to a particular theory of syntax, because their output must be a structure specified in that theory. Thus, there now are parsers that are related to Chomsky's theory (Marcus, 1980; Berwick and Weinberg, 1984) and to other theories (Bresnan, 1982).[6]

How does a parser operate? I shall present one model—that developed by Frazier (1987a). Key aspects of Frazier's model are based on the existence of preferences in interpretation and so-called garden path effects in understanding locally ambiguous syntactic structures. Locally ambiguous syntactic structures are sequences of words that could be assigned more than one syntactic structure when they are initally encountered in the speech stream. In most situations, there are preferences in the interpretation of locally ambiguous syntactic structures; that is, one of the possible interpretations of these ambiguous stretches is considered more likely to be the correct analysis than another. Frazier has attempted to use these preferences as indications of how the parser works. In some sentences, these locally ambiguous syntactic structures are never disambiguated by subsequent material (i.e., the entire sentence remains syntactically ambiguous), but in many sentences, locally ambiguous syntactic structures are ultimately analyzed one way and not another when more of the speech stream is heard (i.e., the local syntactic ambiguity is resolved). When a preference for one of several possible interpretations of a locally ambiguous syntactic structure is consistent with a later resolution of the local syntactic ambiguity, all goes well. The listener may never realize that he heard a sentence that was temporarily ambiguous. But when a preference for one of several possible interpretations of a locally ambiguous syntactic structure turns out to be inconsistent with the subsequent resolution of the local syntactic ambiguity, the listener must reconsider his initial syntactic analysis. At such times, the listener has been temporarily misled as to the syntactic structure that he should be assigning to a part of the sentence. When these misinterpretations of part of a sentence attain consciousness, they go by the name of "garden path" effects. Frazier has also attempted to use garden path effects as indications of how the parser works.

Perhaps the best-known garden path effect, illustrated in (17), was first brought to psychologists' attention by Bever (1970):

(17)   The horse raced past the barn fell.

Subjects analyze (17) as containing a main clause, *the horse raced past the barn*, and then do not find a grammatical role for the last word. In fact, the "correct" (i.e., grammatical) structure of (17) is the same as that of (18):

(18)   The horse racing past the barn fell.

Sentence (17) is related to (19), with the relative pronoun *that* and auxiliary *had been* deleted:

(19)   The horse that had been raced past the barn fell.

Why is sentence (17) so difficult to structure? Most theorists agree that this is due to the fact that *raced* can be both a main verb and a participle, and that the human sentence comprehension system has a tendency to take it to be a main verb in this sentence context. Pursuing this idea somewhat further, we may ask what it is about this context that leads us to take *raced* as a main verb. Bever (1970) originally suggested that what was crucial about (17) was the sequence of categories N-V in sentence-initial position. He suggested that listeners match sequences of this form to the grammatical roles of subject-verb, using a heuristic.

Frazier (1987a) agreed with the basic point that the difficulty in structuring (17) is due to the existence of syntactic operations that automatically misanalyze the first words in the sentence. However, she argued that these operations are not due to the application of heuristics, but reflect basic aspects of how the parser operates. She argued that the parser incorporates each new word in a sentence into a syntactic structure, following principles that minimize the work that it must do. Two of these principles are known as "minimal attachment" and "late closure." Minimal attachment specifies that the parser does not postulate any potentially unnecessary nodes. Late closure specifies that new items are attached to the phrase or clause being processed, if grammatically possible. Minimal attachment leads to the structure (A) in figure 7.9 for (17), rather than the ultimately correct structure (B).

How exactly does minimal attachment work? When the parser encounters the words *the horse* in (17), it creates an NP, which it attaches to the S node that dominates the entire sentence. When it then hears the word *raced*, it creates a verb phrase VP. The easiest way to connect the VP to the structure that it has already created is to attach the VP to the S node, as shown in figure 7.9(A). The alternative analysis shown in figure 17.9(B) requires that the previously created NP node be revised to allow the new VP node to be attached to a new S node that is dominated by the revised NP node. Frazier argued that the parser does not make such changes in structures it has already created unless it is forced to by later developments within a sentence, as actually happens in (17). Late closure works the same way: it essentially says that the parser will continue to work on the node that it is presently working on, unless something forces it to jump to another part of the structure it has already created.

(A)

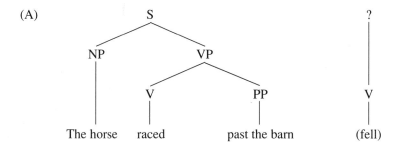

(B)

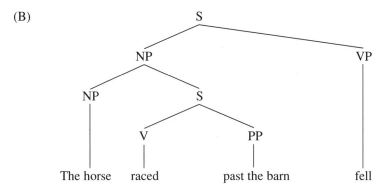

Figure 7.9
Garden path (A) and correct (B) structures in sentence (17).

Minimal attachment and late closure are general principles that lead to systematic preferences regarding the higher-order syntactic structures assigned to sequences of words. One or the other, or both, create a whole host of preferences and garden path situations. A partial list, given by Frazier (1987a), includes:

(20) John hit the girl with a book (the preferred reading attaches *with a book* to *hit*, not to *the girl*).

(21) Ernie kissed Marcie and her sister laughed (a temporary misanalysis yields the interpretation that Ernie kissed Marcie and her sister).

(22) Since Jay always jogs a mile seems like a short distance to him (a temporary misanalysis yields the interpretation that Jay always jogs a mile).

(23) Joyce said that Tom left yesterday (the preferred reading attaches *yesterday* to *left*, not to *said*).

(A)

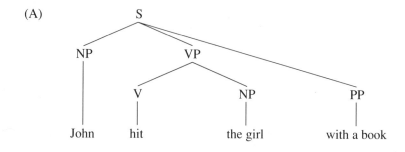

(B)

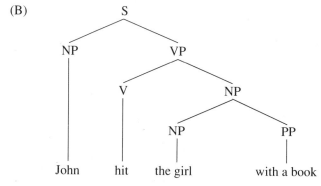

Figure 7.10
Garden path (A) and correct (B) structures in sentence (20).

To see Frazier's point about the generality of principles such as minimal attachment, compare sentences (20) and (17). Figure 7.10 illustrates the two structures that underline the two possible interpretations of sentence (20). The relevant aspect of this structure is the syntactic configuration into which the prepositional phrase (the node PP) is inserted. In figure 7.10(A) the prepositional phrase *for Susan* is attached directly to the VP, whereas in figure 7.10(B) it is attached to an NP that is itself attached to the VP. It is clear that, although the nodes differ significantly from those found in figure 7.9, the choices for the parser are very similar in the two sentences. One possibility is to attach a phrase to the existing phrase marker without revising it, and the other choice is to revise a phrase marker to create a more complex set of nodes to which the incoming phrase can be attached. In both cases, the basic operation of the parser is the same: it attaches an incoming phrase to the existing phrase marker with as few intervening nodes as possible, consistent with the principle of minimal attachment.

Minimal attachment and late closure are "natural" principles, in the sense that they make first-pass parsing simpler. They preclude the creation of potentially unneeded nodes and keep attachments local, at least initially, thereby presumably reducing both the number of structures created by the parser and the number of times the parser must move from place to place in the syntactic tree it is creating. Thus, both principles reduce the workload of the parser.

We have thus far been dealing with parsing operations that attach lexical category nodes to higher nodes, subject to constraints such as minimal attachment and late closure. Some researchers have suggested that the parser consists of several different types of processes, of which these structure-building operations are but one. Weinberg (1987) has argued that structure-building operations are separate from operations that connect referentially dependent items to their antecedents. I shall briefly review the processing of empty referential dependencies. Sentences with these elements are called "filler-gap" constructions in the psycholinguistic literature because a word appearing early in a sentence is related to an empty syntactic position occurring later in the sentence. The filler-gap constructions that have been most thoroughly explored involve "wh-words," as in (24) and (25):

(24)   What did John buy ____ ?

(25)   The little girl who the teacher liked ____ sat on the grass.

In both (24) and (25), the phonologically empty position following the verb is "filled" by the wh-word that occurs at the beginning of the verb's clause. How is this "filling" accomplished?

Two aspects of the process of handling these long-distance dependencies must be to identify both potential fillers and gaps, and then to relate the correct ones to each other. For sentences like (24) and (25), the filler-gap relationship can be relatively easily described: the filler (the wh-word) is not assigned a thematic role by virtue of its position in a phrase marker, and a single gap exists at a spot where a thematic role must be assigned to complete the argument structure of the verb. It is straightforward to assign this filler to this gap. Moreover, in (24) and (25), there is an overt indication that the sentence contains a filler—the wh-word. Thus, it is possible for the parser to actively search for a gap once the wh-word is encountered in (24) and (25), and some research suggests that such a search in fact occurs (Frazier and Clifton, 1989). For all these reasons, sentences such as (24) and (25) are ones in which the filler-gap relationships are relatively easy to identify.

Not all constructions with filler-gap relationships are so simple, however. Consider examples (26)–(28):

(26)   What did John buy (___) the paint with ___ ?

(27)   What did John buy (___) the paint ___ $_1$ to decorate ___ $_2$?

(28)   What did John buy ___ $_1$ ___ $_2$ to paint the porch with ___ $_3$?

In (26), the gap does not occur until after the preposition *with*, but the fact that the verb *buy* is transitive coupled with the fact that the parser has already identified a filler leads to a preliminary assignment of the filler to the role of object of *buy* (Stowe, 1986, 1989; Tanenhaus, Stowe, and Carlson, 1985a). In other words, sentence (26) creates a local garden path because of the possibility of there being a filler-gap relationship that turns out not to exist in the actual sentence (a so-called pseudogap). Sentence (27) contains two gaps—one that functions as the subject of the infinitive *to paint* (that is filled by *John*), and one that functions as the object of *decorate* (that is filled by *what*)—and a "pseudogap" as in (26). Sentence (28) is yet more complex. It contains three gaps—the two in (27) plus a real gap after *buy* that is filled with the filler *what*.

In circumstances with more than one filler and/or more than one gap, there seem to be several principles that apply to constrain the parser's assignment of fillers to gaps. Fodor (1978), Crain and Fodor (1985), Frazier et al. (1983), and Engdahl (1983) have all provided evidence that, in sentences with two gaps, the parser assigns the more recent of two possible fillers to the first gap, and the more distant to the second. This creates a nested filler-gap structure, illustrated in (29) and (30) (taken from Fodor, 1978):

(29)   Who$_j$ did you$_i$ want ___ $_i$ to make a potholder for ___ $_j$?

(30)   What$_j$ are boxes$_i$ easy to store ___ $_i$ in ___ $_j$?

There is evidence for a number of distinct processing operations within the related set of procedures that deal with filler-gap relationships. Frazier and Clifton (1989) have suggested that the most-recent-filler strategy does not apply in cases where lexical "control" information determines filler-gap relationships, as in (31). Though research on these topics is too limited to assert any general theory with confidence, it may be that differences among types of empty referentially dependent NPs that are expressed in linguistic theory (see above) may map onto different procedures for relating fillers and gaps. One possible generalization is that co-indexation procedures differ for the different empty NPs **PRO** and **WH-trace**.

(31)   John promised Mary ____ to read the book on vacation.

The operations involved in filling gaps occur very quickly. As best as can be measured at the moment, they are as rapid as structure-building operations. For instance, Tanenhaus and his colleagues (Tanenhaus, Stowe, and Carlson, 1985; Garnsey, Tanenhaus, and Chapman, 1987) reported as rapid detection of the anomaly at the point marked by an asterisk (*) in (32) as in (33):

(32)   Which snake did the little girl force to hop * over the fence?

(33)   The little girl forced the snake to hop * over the fence.

To detect the anomaly in these two sentences, the listener must recognize that *the snake* (or *which snake*) is the agent of *to hop* and that snakes cannot hop. If we ascribe to a parser that has operations that correspond to the structures described in Chomsky's theory, determining that *the snake* is the agent of *to hop* in (33) proceeds as follows: *the snake* is the object of *force* and is co-indexed with the empty NP, **PRO**, that is the subject of *to hop*. **PRO** is assigned the external theta role of *to hop*. In this way, the listener comes to assign *the snake* as the agent of *to hop*. In (32), however, determining that *the snake* is the subject of *to hop* is much more complicated. The listener must find the agent of *to hop* by co-indexing the empty category, **PRO**, that is the subject of *to hop* with a second empty catgeory, **Wh-trace**, that is the object of *force*, and then co-indexing this **Wh-trace** with the phrase containing a wh-word, *which snake*. Whether or not this is actually how the agent of *to hop* is found in sentence (32), it is clear that finding the agent of *to hop* is much harder in sentence (32) than in sentence (33), simply because *which snake* is farther from *to hop* in (32) than *the snake* is in (33). Nonetheless, by the time the parser encounters the words *to hop*, the agent of the verb is already established and the judgment that the sentence is anomalous can be made as rapidly in the one sentence as in the other.

Frazier (1987a) makes the point that there are several similarities between the way the parser handles long-distance dependencies and the way it handles structure-building operations. In both cases, the parser operates quickly. It does not wait for all the relevant linguistic input to be available, but makes decisions about structure quite early. In both cases, relatively simple structures are postulated— minimal attachment and late closure result in the simplest possible attachments and the least moving around of constructed phrase markers; the most-recent-filler strategy requires a minimum of look-back in cases of long-distance co-indexation.

These studies of sentence comprehension suggest that there is a component of the language-processing system that constructs syntactic phrase markers and uses these phrase markers to constrain and determine aspects of sentence meaning. This component of the language-processing system may consist of a set of different types of operations, each related to constructing different aspects of syntactic structure. The parser appears to operate as quickly as the other language processors we have described in chapters 2 through 6. This may at first seem a bit surprising, given the fact that syntactic structures are determined by sequences of words, whereas the language processors we have been discussing so far are all devoted to processing single words. However, it appears that this is the case, and this suggests that many language processors operate simultaneously ("in parallel") during normal language comprehension.

Nonsyntactic Routes to Sentence Comprehension

It appears that listeners use both lexico-pragmatic and heuristic routes to sentence meaning as well as the syntactic comprehension mechanisms we have been discussing. Evidence that this is the case comes from results such as those reported by Slobin (1966). In Slobin's experiments, subjects were required to indicate whether a sentence and a picture conveyed the same thematic roles. Sentences were of four types: active irreversible, active reversible, passive irreversible, and passive reversible [types (34)–(37)].

(34)   The man ate the cake (active irreversible).

(35)   The man pushed the woman (active reversible).

(36)   The cake was eaten by the man (passive irreversible).

(37)   The woman was pushed by the man (passive reversible).

Subjects were faster at matching the active sentences to the pictures than the passive sentences, and faster at matching the passive irreversible than the passive reversible sentences to the pictures. However, matching active irreversible sentences to pictures was no faster than matching active reversible sentences.

One way to interpret these results is as follows. The fact that active sentences were more easily matched than passive sentences is an indication that comprehension can proceed by the application of a heuristic based on word order (that N-V-N sequences are to be mapped onto agent-verb-theme interpretations). The fact that reversibility affected the matching of any sentences indicates that a lexico-pragmatic route to meaning is operative. However, the fact that reversibility affected the matching of only passive and not active sentences indicates that the lexico-pragmatic route to meaning is too slow to affect the comprehension of sentences that can be understood by the appplication of a heuristic. There are other possible interpretations of these results, but it is hard to understand this pattern without postulating that lexico-pragmatic factors can affect comprehension and do so differently in sentences with different syntactic structures.

As we indicated above, several researchers have pursued this line of investigation in considerable detail. Bates and MacWhinney (1989) review a series of studies of sentence comprehension in several languages, the results of which have provided a basis for the development of a theory of sentence processing. These experiments were designed to investigate the relative importance of different types of "cues" regarding the assignment of thematic roles in a variety of languages. The cues that were used included syntactic cues (e.g., word order, subject-verb agreement, declensional markings), semantic cues (e.g., animacy of NPs), and discourse-level cues (e.g., prosodic contours). Stimuli were presented to subjects, who were asked to identify the perpetrator of the action (agent or instrument) of each spoken utterance. In many cases, the different "cues" as to which noun was the agent of the sentence were in conflict. Stimuli included sentences that are completely well formed, such as (38), but also semantically odd sentences, such as (39), and even syntactically ill-formed sentences such as (40).

(38)   The boy pushes the sweaters.

(39)   The sweaters push the boy.

(40)   Pushes the boys the sweater.

In these stimuli, word order, subject-verb agreement, and animacy are varied. In sentence (38), all these variables converge on the assignment of agency to *the boy*. In (39), the first two factors make it more likely that *the sweaters* are the Instrument, while the animacy factor again suggests that agency should be attributed to *the boy*. In (40), word order is less clearly a factor, since the V-N-N sequence is not a well-formed sentence in English (though the fact that *the boys* follows *pushes* is consistent with its being the theme). In (40), subject-verb agreement places *the sweater* as the instrument, while animacy leads to the assignment of agency to *the boy*.

Bates and MacWhinney (1989) report that "cue validity" determines how subjects assign agency and instrumentality in these stimuli. Cue validity refers to the *availability* of a particular cue, the *reliability* of that cue when it is available, and the *conflict validity* of the cue—the number of times that cue dominates over other cues when two or more cues are in conflict. A cue is available if it is present and detectable in the signal. Cue availability is defined as "the ratio of cases in which the cue is available over the total number of cases in a task domain" (Bates and MacWhinney, 1989, p. 41), and can be estimated from an analysis of texts and transcripts. For instance, subject-verb agreement is not highly available in English, because there are so few markers of subject-verb agreement in English, but it is very available in Italian, where such markers abound. Certain cues may be present but hard to discriminate because of their phonetic make-up; such cues rank lower in availability than other cues that occur as often but are more easily identified. Cue reliability "can be expressed numerically as the ratio of the number of cases in which a cue leads to the correct conclusion over the number of cases in which it is available" (Bates and MacWhinney, 1989, p. 41). For instance, preverbal position of a noun is highly reliable as an indicator of agency or instrumentality in English, but much less so in Italian. Conflict validity "is the number of competition situations in which [a] cue "wins," divided by the number of competition situations in which that cue participates" (Bates and MacWhinney, 1989, pp. 41,42). For instance, preverbal position is highly associated with agency/instrumentality in French in general, as is true of English. However, there is a very highly restricted set of structures in which it is very strongly associated with theme or goal in French (sentences containing "clitic pronouns," such as *Jean la mange*, John is eating it). Thus, because of these structures, preverbal position has a high overall cue availability and reliability but a low conflict validity in French (i.e., where preverbal position conflicts with case marking, case marking determines thematic role). Kail (1989) found that French-speaking subjects relied much less on word order in assigning agency/instrumentality to stimuli such as (38)–(40) than did English speaking subjects, and she attributed this difference to the difference in conflict validity scores of this word order cue in the two languages. Bates and MacWhinney (1989) review a variety of studies in several languages that indicate that these different types of cues interact to determine the assignment of aspects of sentential semantic meanings such as thematic roles in ways that are broadly consistent with these principles.

Mathematical models of the PDP type have been developed that incorporate this approach to sentence comprehension (McDonald and MacWhinney, 1989; MacWhinney, 1989; McClelland and Kawamoto, 1986; McClelland, St. John, and Taraban, 1989). The proponents of these models maintain that there is no such thing as the elaborate syntactic structures or their associated parsers that we have been discussing. Rather, a PDP-type mechanism integrates these relatively superficial cues and assigns a set of thematic roles (or other sentential semantic features). The prosyntax and antisyntax positions are frequently related to very large issues in human cognition and neurobiology, such as whether humans have a highly developed specialized set of cognitive and neural mechanisms that are specialized for the acquisition and use of natural language, or employ a much less specialized set of mechanisms that learn languages in a trial-and-error sort of way.

It is premature to take a strong position on these large and weighty matters. At present, these types of psycholinguistic models and their PDP formalizations have been applied to a very small number of sentence structures. More standard models that recognize the existence of syntactic structures and a parser are the only models that deal with many of the psycholinguistic phenomena described in the previous section. In addition, one can raise questions about results obtained in experiments that mix together both grammatical and ungrammatical sentence, as is the case in many studies reported in Bates and MacWhinney (1989). On the other hand, these models do offer formal, verifiable theories of aspects of sentence processing within a finite range of sentence structures, and have achieved some accurate simulations of processing data within this domain. They may, at the least, be seen as an important elaborated account of how nonsyntactic comprehension mechanisms may work.

Aside from these PDP-type models that challenge the appropriateness of parser-type models of sentence comprehension, some researchers have argued that the parser operates differently than we have described above. We began our discussion of how the parser might operate by citing several preference and garden path phenomena in understanding locally syntactically ambiguous sentences. We argued that these effects in sentences such as sentence (17) and sentence (20) (repeated here for the reader's convenience) were due to the parser following a principle we called miminal attachment.

(17)   The horse raced past the barn fell.

(20)   John hit the girl with a book.

Several researchers have argued, however, that these garden path and preference effects are not due to how the parser operates at all, but rather to the effects of discourse structure upon sentence processing.

Crain and Steedman (1985), Altmann and Steedman (1988), and others have argued that interpretation preferences and garden path effects are due to the role of discourse structure in interpreting sentences. According to these researchers, the effects we have described are artifacts of presenting sentences out of context. Their analysis is that biases such as those seen in (17) and (20) are not due to attachment preferences but rather to listeners' attempts to achieve "referential success." Referential success refers to the ability to assign all items mentioned in a sentence to specific individuals in a discourse (for more discussion of discourse and its processing, see chapter 9). In sentence (20), for instance, attaching *the book* to *the girl* implies that the context has identified more than one girl and that the sentence is referring to the girl with the book (of the girls mentioned in the context). Since presenting the sentence in isolation does not establish a context with more than one girl, the sentence is preferentially interpreted as attaching *the book* to *hit*. Evidence supporting this analysis would come from showing that context reverses preferences such as those seen in sentences like (17) and (20) in isolation. There is evidence that context changes many of these effects, and does so while sentences are being processed (Altmann and Steedman, 1988; see chapter 9).

In a similar vein, there are results in the literature that indicate that there are effects of verb structure and meaning on attachment (e.g., Ford, Bresnan, and Kaplan, 1982; Taraban and McClelland, in press; see Tyler, 1989; Frazier, 1989; Tanenhaus and Carlson, 1989; and Stowe, 1989; for discussion). For instance, Holmes (1987) showed that there is a more marked garden path effect in (41) than in (42):

(41)   The reporter saw her friend was not succeeding.

(42)   The candidate doubted his sincerity would be appreciated.

The relevant difference between the sentences is that, although a garden path could be created in both these sentences, *saw* is a verb that usually takes a direct NP object, whereas *doubt* is a verb that usually takes a sentential complement. If minimal attachment operated independently of the nature of a verb, there should be an identical garden path effect in both (41) and (42). Holmes argued that the reduced garden path effect in (42) indicates that the nature of the verb affects the parser's first-pass attachments.

This evidence that both context and lexical structure affects how constituents are attached to developing syntactic structures argues against the claim that a parser is a mechanism that operates independently of other sentence-processing mechanisms (i.e., it affects the claim that the parser is "encapsulated" in a certain way, as Fodor [1983] might claim; see chapter 1 for a brief discussion of the notion of encapsulation as it applies to language processors). However, these findings do not imply that there is no such thing as a parser. Even researchers who doubt the appropriateness of invoking principles such as minimal attachment to explain garden path and preference phenomena in sentences like (17) and (20) generally agree that what is at issue is not whether there is a syntactic processor that is involved in sentence comprehension, but how much its initial operations are entirely determined by purely syntactic information as opposed to being affected by other types of linguistic information (see the final discussion in Altmann and Steedman,1988, for instance). In addition, the interpretation of the data indicating that there are context and lexical effects on parsing remains controversial. Ferreira and Clifton (1986), Clifton and Ferreira (1987), Frazier (1987b), and others have argued that at least some garden path effects remain in effect despite strongly disambiguating context. Frazier (1987) argued that the existence of a garden path effect at all in (42) is evidence in favor of the operation of minimal attachment. Altogether, research in psycholinguistics provides reasonable evidence for the existence of a parser—a set of operations that constructs a syntactic structure—although what it takes as its input may be broader than the narrowest models of its operations originally claimed.

Altogether, there is evidence for both syntactically based sentence comprehension processes and other mechanisms that use means other than the construction of a full syntactic representation of a sentence to understand propositions. All these mechanisms can be affected in aphasia.

DISORDERS OF SENTENCE COMPREHENSION

There could be many reasons why a patient might fail to understand the propositional content of a sentence. We would expect that patients who fail to understand crucial single words, especially verbs, would have trouble understanding propositional meaning. We would also expect that some patients might have disturbances affecting their ability to assign thematic roles or other aspects of propositional meaning despite good single word processing. Moreover, we might expect there to be patients with disturbances of the various mechanisms that yield propositional meaning—the lexico-pragmatic, syntactic, and heuristic routes and processes we have been discussing.

There is good evidence that many patients do in fact fail to understand aspects of sentences. For instance, the Token Test (DeRenzi and Vignolo, 1962) has been used in many studies of aphasic populations. The Token Test examines a patient's ability to carry out commands such as "Touch the small red circle and the large blue square," varying the number of items to be manipulated, the number of adjectives modifying each item, and, in the last section of the test, the syntactic structure of the command. When a patient has good single word comprehension, abnormal performance on tests such as the Token Test indicates that he or she has a problem in comprehending sentences. Studies have shown that aphasic patients with good single word comprehension (at least for the words on this test) perform worse on the Token Test than normal controls and nonaphasic patients with either right or left hemipshere lesions (DeRenzi and Fagliolini, 1978).

Though results such as these indicate that many patients do have trouble with sentence comprehension, it is impossible to say on the basis of the Token Test just what parts of the sentence comprehension process are affected in a patient. In many sections of the Token Test, the patient's problem may be due to the fact that many propositional meanings are derived lexico-pragmatically for each sentence, making the selection of the one meaning compatible with the structure of the sentence difficult. This difficulty may be related to a short-term memory problem, as discussed below. Poorer performance on the final section of the Token Test has often been taken to indicate a disturbance affecting the use of syntactic structures in sentence comprehension, but this conclusion may be incorrect. Errors on this section may result from misinterpreting the meanings of subordinate conjunctions or being unable to carry out actions in the order required by a command when that order is opposite from the spoken order of clauses in the test item. These difficulties in determining the reason(s) for a disturbance of sentence comprehension measured on the Token Test indicate the kinds of considerations that must be taken into account in fractionating the various sources of a sentence comprehension deficit in an individual patient. I will now discuss these disorders, focusing first on disorders of syntactic comprehension mechanisms and then turning to other types of sentence comprehension impairments.

Disorders of Syntactic Comprehension

The greatest amount of work in the area of disturbances of sentence comprehension has gone into the investigation of patients who can understand at least some aspects of propositional meaning through lexico-pragmatic or heuristic means but whose use of syntactic structure to assign meaning is not normal (Caplan 1991a). Caramazza and Zurif (1976) first investigated the question of syntactic comprehension in aphasic patients. They tested patients with Broca's, Conduction, and Wernicke's aphasia on a sentence-picture matching test, using the four types of sentences illustrated in (43)–(46):

(43)   The apple the boy is eating is red.

(44)   The boy the dog is patting is tall.

(45)   The girl the boy is chasing is tall.

(46)   The boy is eating a red apple.

The patients were scored on the number of errors they made in selecting the correct picture among a set of four. Broca's and Conduction aphasic patients made almost no errors when pictures with incorrect adjectives or verbs were used as foils. Their errors were confined to pictures representing reversals of the thematic roles of the nouns in the sentences (so-called *syntactic foils*). Moreover, these patients only made errors on sentences such as (44) and (45), in which the syntax of the sentences either indicated an improbable event in the real world or in which the thematic roles are reversible. In the semantically irreversible sentences (43) and (46), these patients made no more errors than normal subjects. Caramazza and Zurif interpreted the results as indicating that some patients (those with Broca's and Conduction aphasia) cannot construct syntactic structures. They claimed that these patients relied upon lexico-pragmatic and heuristic routes to determine the meaning of a sentence.

However, to base such conclusions on these results is premature. One problem in interpretation involves the possibility of these results being based on how patients cope with the picture matching task used in this research. Sentence-picture matching requires the use of nonsensical picture foils to depict "reversed" thematic roles in semantically irreversible sentences. Patients may have performed better on the irreversible sentences than the reversible ones by simply rejecting such foils (Grodzinsky and Marek, 1988). To answer this objection requires more careful experimental controls. For instance, an answer to Grodzinsky and Marek's concerns would be the demonstration that the dissociation between interpretation of reversible and irreversible sentences is maintained in tasks such as object manipulation, that do not require processing of implausible foils (see also Caramazza, 1989). Research has moved in these directions, but the results are still incomplete. For instance, though many patients have been shown to have difficulty with reversible sentences using tasks such as object manipulation (see, e.g., Caplan, Baker, and Dehaut, 1985), none have also been tested for their ability to do this task with irreversible sentences. Caplan et al. (1985) found no effects of semantic plausibility in object-manipulation performances by aphasic patients, but the plausibility effects reported in that study were quite different from those discussed by Grodzinsky and Marek (1988). Thus, though many patients have been shown to have syntactic comprehension deficits, there is no proof that any of these patients have these deficits in the face of normal ability to comprehend constrained sentences. It is extremely likely, however, that disturbances of syntactic comprehension do, in fact, exist in patients who can understand sentences using nonsyntactic comprehension mechanisms.

Whether or not syntactic comprehension disturbances are isolated occurrences or part of a larger picture of comprehension impairments that also affect other routes to sentence meaning, recent studies have begun to shed light on the details of disturbances of the syntactic comprehension mechanism. I shall briefly review some of the contemporary literature, beginning (somewhat immodestly) with work carried out by myself and my colleagues. This work provides a general framework within which syntactic comprehension disturbances can be approached.

Caplan and his colleagues (Caplan et al., 1985; Caplan and Hildebrandt, 1988a,b) explored the nature of disturbances in the process of syntactic comprehension along linguistic lines, and have developed a general theory of the basic abnormalities that underlie such disturbances. Caplan et al. (1985) studied a large number of aphasic patients using an object-manipulation task requiring subjects to enact thematic roles in the nine sentence types (47)–(55).

(47)   Active (A): The elephant hit the monkey.

(48)   Passive (P): The elephant was hit by the monkey.

(49)   Cleft-subject (CS): It was the elephant that hit the monkey.

(50)   Cleft-object (CO): It was the elephant that the monkey hit.

(51)   Dative (D): The elephant gave the monkey to the rabbit.

Table 7.1
Mean Correct Scores for Different Sentence Types Achieved by Three
Aphasic Populations in an Enactment Task*

Pilot Study		Experiment 2		Experiment 3	
CS	3.9	A	4.4	A	4.1
A	3.9	CS	4.2	CS	4.0
P	2.8	D	3.2	P	3.2
D	2.8	P	2.9	D	2.9
CO	2.4	C	2.7	C	2.8
OS	1.9	CO	2.6	CO	2.7
DP	1.8	OS	2.3	OS	2.1
C	1.5	DP	2.0	DP	1.9
SO	1.2	SO	1.3	SO	1.4

Reproduced with permission from Caplan et al. (1985, p. 314).
* The maximal possible score for each sentence type is 5. Sentence types
that are bracketed are not significantly different from each other; sentence
types that are not bracketed are significantly different from each other.

(52) Dative passive (DP): The elephant was given to the monkey by
the rabbit.

(53) Conjoined (C): The elephant hit the monkey and hugged the
rabbit.

(54) Subject-object relative (SO): The elephant that the monkey hit
hugged the rabbit.

(55) Object-subject relative (OS): The elephant hit the monkey
that hugged the rabbit.

The authors report three studies of 56, 37, and 49 patients in which
they carried out several analyses of the patients' performances.

First, in each study they determined the relative difficulty of each
sentence type. For the most part, the same sentence types produced
the highest mean correct scores in each study, as shown in table 7.1.

Caplan et al. drew several conclusions from this pattern of
performance. First, they argued that these results indicate that syntactic structure influences sentence interpretation in aphasia. Sentences with "canonical" thematic role orders—the usual asignment
of agent and theme to the pre- and postverbal nouns in English and
French sentences with NP-VP or N-V-N word order—were consis-

tently easier than those with deviations from canonical thematic role order [cf. A (47) vs. P (48); CS (49) vs. CO (50); D (51) vs. DP (52); and C (53) and OS (55) vs. SO (54)]. The number of thematic roles assigned by a verb also affected performance: D sentences (49) were more difficult than A sentences (42) and DP (52) harder than P sentences (48). Sentences with two verbs were harder than those with one verb, when canonical word order was controlled [C (53) and OS (55) vs. A (47) and CS (49); SO (54) vs. CO (50)]. These results have since been replicated in several other languages, including Italian (Baruzzi and Caplan, 1985) and Japanese (Hagiwara and Caplan, 1990).

Caplan et al. argued that these results reflected the relative complexity of these different sentence types. They argued that the determinants of complexity were largely the syntactic features of the sentence. They suggested that the presence of a noncanonical thematic role order, a third thematic role, or a second verb, were elementary structural features of a sentence that contribute to the complexity of a sentence.[7] To a considerable extent, the relative complexity of a sentence type could be predicted from the number of these features that occur in a sentence.

Nonsyntactic factors also affected performance. Chief among these factors was the length of a sentence; e.g., D sentences were harder than A sentences [(51) vs. (47)]. However, sentence length could not have been the sole determinant of sentence complexity because sentences of equivalent length differed with respect to the number of correct interpretations, e.g., CS (49) vs. CO (50); C (53) and OS (55) vs. SO (54). In fact, in a related study, Butler-Hinz, Caplan, and Waters (1990) showed that, independent of length, sentences in which a verb assigned three different thematic roles were more difficult for group of 20 patients with closed head injuries than sentences in which the verb assigned only two different thematic roles. These authors compared these patients' enactment of dative sentences containing three thematic roles (e.g., *The monkey pushed the elephant to the tiger*) with that of transitive sentences containing two thematic roles but the same number of NPs (e.g., *The monkey pushed the elephant and the tiger*). Though performance on the active versions of these sentences did not differ, the passive versions of the first of these sentence types were significantly harder than the passive versions of the second of these sentence types. This finding suggests that the assignment of three different thematic roles to three NPs is more demanding of processing requirements than the assignment of two thematic roles to three NPs, independent of sentence length.

The finding that the complexity of the syntactic form of a sentence affects aphasic patients' comprehension abilities needs to be explained. One explanation of this finding is to say that one aspect of patients' problems in the domain of syntactic comprehension is a reduction in the resources that are available for this process. Further analysis of the data in the study of Caplan et al., and in other studies, provides considerable evidence that this is the case.

Caplan et al. reported the results of a clustering analysis of their patients, based on the similarity of patients' performances on individual sentences. Examination of the mean correct scores of each of the resulting clusters of patients on each of the nine sentence types showed that, as the mean correct score of patients declined on the test as a whole, performance declined on all the sentence types, and lower scores tended to occur on the sentence types with overall lower scores for the group as a whole. This relationship between performance on the test as a whole and performance of each subgroup of patients can be attributed to two factors: (1) increased processing demands of certain sentence types and (2) progressive diminution in the resources available for syntactic comprehension in each of the patient groups identified by the clustering analysis. The observed relationship between performance on the test as a whole and performance of each subgroup of patients would not be expected if patients' performances were determined solely by impairments of specific parsing or interpretive operations. Additional evidence for the importance of processing resource reductions in determining performance on this task was found in a principal components analysis, which showed a first factor that was equally positively weighted for all sentence types and that accounted for approximately 60% of the total variance of patient clustering. Given these analyses, the differences in mean correct scores of different sentence types seem to primarily reflect the processing resources associated with the comprehension of each of these sentence types.

Studies of the syntactic comprehension abilities of individual patients also shows that reductions in processing resources are important determinants of a patient's performance on syntactic comprehension tasks. The evidence for this comes from the finding that a patient may understand a sentence containing either of two syntactic features, but not one containing both. For instance, Hildebrandt, Caplan, and Evans (1987) reported a patient, K.G., who could understand sentences that contained the empty NP **PRO**, and sentences that contained a pronoun, but not a sentence that contained both (see below). This type of pattern strongly suggests that the patient could accomplish all the operations related to co-indexing both **PRO** and pronouns, but did not have the mental processing resources needed to carry out the combination of co-indexation operations required by the presence of both these referentially dependent NPs in a single sentence. When the combined complexity of concurrent parsing operations exceeds the processing capacity of these patients, the ability to perform individual parsing operations breaks down.

In addition to this reduction in the processing resources available for syntactic comprehension, patients may also have disturbances affecting specific parsing operations. In fact, a series of double dissociations has been demonstrated with respect to patients' abilities to interpret different aspects of syntactic structure (Hildebrandt, 1987; Hildebrandt et al., 1987; Caplan and Hildebrandt, 1988a, 1988b, 1989). These studies focus on patients' abilities to assign referential dependencies, both overt referentially dependent items (pronouns and reflexives) and empty referentially dependent NPs (the various types of empty NPs specified in Chomsky's theory, discussed above).

Using an object-manipulation test, the investigators observed isolated disturbances of patients' abilities to assign referents to different referentially dependent items (for details of methodology and interpretation, and for discussion of other cases, see Caplan and Hildebrandt, 1988a). Table 7.2 summarizes the results of six patients' performances.

Two of these patients had difficulties with all empty referentially dependent NPs, but showed a double dissociation between co-indexation of reflexives and pronouns. A.B. showed an impairment in co-indexing pronouns but did well on reflexives; C.V. showed the opposite pattern of performance. Four patients had selective difficulties with co-indexing particular empty NPs. J.V. had difficulty with sentences containing **NP-trace**, but did well on sentences containing **PRO** and **wh-trace**. G.S. did well on sentences with **NP-trace** but poorly on sentences containing **PRO** and **wh-trace**. G.G. experienced difficulty with sentences containing both **PRO** and **NP-**

Table 7.2
Correct Scores (%) Achieved by Six Aphasic Subjects on Different Sentence Types in an Enactment Task

Sentence Type	Patient					
	A.B.	C.V.	J.V.	G.S.	G.G.	K.G.
Subject control (John promised Bill to jump)	33%	25%	100%	50%	18%	53%
NP-raising (John seemed to Bill to be jumping)	42%	42%	33%	100%	0%	33%
Object relativization (The man who the woman kissed hugged the child)	17%	0%	93%	25%	100%	25%
Pronouns (The girl said that the woman washed her)	83%	23%	92%	92%	100%	100%
Reflexives (The girl said that the woman washed herself)	42%	100%	100%	92%	100%	100%

Data in part from Caplan and Hildebrandt (1988a).

trace—subject control and raising structures. K.G.'s deficits affected all empty NPs, but not all sentences containing empty NPs were equally affected. He was worse on sentences containing **trace** than those containing **PRO**. Object relativization was worse than subject relativization. The most general characterization of K.G.'s deficit is that he had trouble when a noun could not unambiguously be assigned a thematic role until after a subsequent noun received a thematic role.

These patterns of performance constitute double dissociations— different patients do better on certain sentence types than others. Because the sentence types on which patients perform well and poorly can be grouped together with respect to the types of referentially dependent NPs they contain, these results indicate that patients can have selective difficulties with aspects of syntactic processing. These deficits can be quite restricted. Because of the selectivity of the deficits, especially in cases that show disturbances of particular empty NPs, nonsyntactic causes for these performances seem unlikely: other than the particular co-indexation operation(s) associated with these different referentially dependent NPs, task demands are identical across sentence types. These performances thus strongly suggest that quite specific parsing operations exist and can be disrupted. We have suggested that the dissociations we observed are best accomodated within Chomsky's theory of syntactic structures and an associated parser (Caplan and Hildebrandt, 1988a, 1988b). However, studies of specific parsing impairments are in their infancy, and the range of specific parsing impairments and the ultimate implications of these deficits for the nature of linguistic representations and parsing operations are unknown.

Another observational technique used to explore the nature of disturbances affecting the syntactically based route to sentence meaning has been to compare patients' abilities to interpret semantically reversible sentences with their abilites to judge the well-formedness of sentences. Linebarger et al. (1983a) were the first to show that some patients (four agrammatic Broca's aphasic patients in their study) retained the ability to indicate whether sentences were correct or syntactically ill formed, despite performing at chance on tests of comprehension of reversible active, passive and locative sentences. These judgments can, at times, be made correctly for sentences that are not properly interpreted. For instance, Linebarger (1990) reported that some patients can correctly indicate that (56) is illformed, but not match sentences like (57) and (58) to pictures with thematic role reversal foils.

*(56)   The woman was watched the man.

(57)   The woman was watched by the man.

(58)   The woman was watched.

Linebarger and her colleagues interpreted these results as indicating that these patients can assign syntactic structures, but not map them onto propositional semantic features. This interpretation suggests that the process of assigning the syntactic structure of a sentence is at least partially independent of the process of using that syntactic structure to interpret a sentence.

Linebarger and her colleagues noted that her patients were not able to make grammaticality judgments in all sentence types, however. They found that their patients had trouble judging sentences with tag questions like (59) and (60) as ungrammatical, despite being able to make correct judgments regarding many other syntactic anomalies.

*(59)   The boy went to the drugstore, didn't they?

*(60)   The boy went to the drugstore, don't he?

Linebarger and her colleagues suggested that the difficulty these patients had in making grammaticality judgments in sentences like (59) and (60) reflected the memory requirements of processing these sentences. In (59) and (60), the listener has no indication that there will be an element that occurs late in the sentence that will have to agree in number with a previous noun or verb. The listener must search through a representation of the sentence in memory to see if the agreement features are correct, without ever having a marker encouraging him or her to keep the original noun or verb in mind. This contrasts with structures such as relative clauses and interrogatives, where there are indications that a noun occurring at a given point in the sentence will be relevant to syntactic processing of a later portion of the sentence (see discussion of gap hunting, above). The patients of Linebarger et al. did well on sentences of the latter type. For instance, they were able to reject sentences such as (61) as ungrammatical (Linebarger, 1990).

*(61)   How many did you see birds in the park?

The contrast between the sentence types on which the patients did well and poorly in this grammaticality judgment task led Linebarger and her colleagues to suggest that the problem these patients had was likely to be due to a reduction in working memory capacities in their cases.

Linebarger (1990) also argued that the pattern of grammaticality judgment abilities in these patients reflects what she called the "first-pass operations" of the parser. Her claim was that the parser operates to construct hierarchically organized syntactic structures, which are later interpreted semantically. When the incoming sentence yields a violation of the structures that parser can build, a patient can detect the violation and judge the sentence to be ungrammatical. Linebarger argued that patients' performance on this task could thus provide evidence as to what the output of first-pass parsing is. For instance, Linebarger argued that her patients' correct rejection of sentences such as (61) implies that they are sensitive to constraints on the movement of constituents and, therefore, that the first-pass parser is bound by these constraints.

However, as Linebarger herself indicates (Linebarger, 1990), these analyses of the causes of the discrepancies found across sentence types are debatable. It is very difficult to know what a patient bases a grammaticality judgment on. For instance, if patients take the phrase *how many* to be an NP and attempt to assign a thematic role to every NP in a sentence, they may rule out sentence (61) on the grounds that there are more NPs than argument structure slots in the subcategorization frame of the verb in the sentence (*see* is a transitive verb that only assigns two thematic roles). If this is how the patients rejected (61), their rejection of this ill-formed sentence does not imply that they base their judgments on the output of a first-pass parsing process that rules out sentences on the basis of the constraints on movement of constituents.

The results published by Linebarger have been subject to great scrutiny and numerous interpretations by other researchers. Two major forms of explanation—a linguistic account of the patterns of judgment capacities, and a psychological account of these patterns—have been pursued in this work. In both cases, researchers have concentrated on patients who omit function words and bound morphemes in their speech—so-called agrammatic aphasics (see chapters 6 and 8)—in an effort to ascertain whether these patients have particular types of syntactic comprehension problems.

The linguistic account has attempted to interpret the pattern of judgments made by these patients in terms in terms of the nature of the syntactic categories that can be used to make grammaticality judgments. One analysis has maintained that these patients are capable of judging grammatical well-formedness on the basis of the content words (nouns, verbs, and adjectives) but not function words (determiners, prepositions, etc.) in a sentence (Zurif and Grodzinsky, 1983). Linebarger (Linebarger et al., 1983b; Linebarger, 1990) has argued strongly against this interpretation of her results, on the grounds that her patients were able to judge the ill-formedness of sentences such as (62), which is determined only by erroneous function words.

*(62)   Have you do the homework problem?

Several researchers have proposed modified versions of a "function word" account of syntactic comprehension problems in

agrammatic patients (see Rizzi, 1985; Friederici, 1881, 1982; Grodzinsky 1990, for examples). I cannot review all these suggestions in
detail here. At present, all of these analyses run into difficulties
accounting for aspects of the performances of agrammatic patients
on syntactic comprehension or grammaticality judgment tasks, or
both (see Linebarger, 1990, Schwartz et al., 1985, 1987; Martin et al.,
1989; Caplan and Hildebrandt, 1986, 1988b; Caplan, 1987a, in press,
for discussion of various problems with these accounts).[8]
    The second approach to characterizing the syntactic comprehen-
sion disturbance found in some agrammatic patients is in terms of
psycholinguistic processes. As noted, Linebarger and her colleagues
(see Schwartz et al., 1985, 1987) have suggested that these patients
are impaired at using the results of a syntactic analysis to determine
aspects of sentence meaning. In support of this analysis, Schwartz,
Linebarger, and their colleagues cite the fact that their patients were
able to judge the ill-formedness of sentences such as (63), below, but
not the anomalous nature of sentences such as (64).

* (63)   Who did the teacher smile?

* (64)   It was the little boy that the puppy dropped.

In (63), the ill-formedness is created by a syntactic violation—*smile*
is an intransitive verb and cannot assign two thematic roles. In (64),
the anomaly is created by a violation of real-world probability—
puppies are unlikely to drop boys. The fact that patients could detect the ill-formedness of (63) suggests that they built the relevant
syntactic structures. The fact that they did not detect the anomaly
in (64) suggests that they could not use more complex syntactic
structures to assign thematic roles. (It is unlikely that these patients
were unaware of the fact that puppies do not usually drop boys.)
    Studies combining judgments of grammatical well-formedness
and semantic anomaly with sentence-picture matching tasks have
thus greatly added to our knowledge regarding patients' sensitivity
to syntactic structure, at the same time as they have considerably
increased the complexity of the picture of what goes wrong in a
patient with a syntactic comprehension disorder. Despite many
remaining uncertainties regarding the interpretation of patients'
performances on these tasks, several conclusions appear reasonably
firm at present. It does appear that disorders affecting the construction and use of syntactic structures disorders can be very selective,

both in the sense that they can affect comprehension of certain types of sentences containing particular syntactic elements and requiring particular parsing operations in a given task, and in the sense that they affect performance differently on different tasks. In addition, it seems very likely that some patients retain a sensitivity to some features of syntactic form and can base their judgments of the well-formedness of a sentence on this knowledge base, but cannot use these aspects of sentence form to understand a sentence (or, at least, to respond correctly on a given task that requires comprehension, such as sentence-picture matching). Many hypotheses have been formulated regarding what linguistic representations and aspects of sentence parsing and interpretation are impaired in patients with syntactic comprehension disorders. No single generalization appears to hold true of all patients or even of all patients with a given clinical syndrome (such as agrammatism). Rather, the analyses that have been developed for both single cases and various groups of patients illustrate a range of possible disturbances of syntactic comprehension that must be explored in each individual patient.

Before turning to other types of sentence comprehension disturbances, we should note that the question has been raised of whether the disturbances we have been describing reflect impairments of unconscious, obligatory, sentence processing or of the conscious, more controlled use of the products of unconscious sentence processing. Tyler (1985, in press) has looked at disorders of sentence comprehension along these lines. Using a word-monitoring task to investigate on-line processing of syntactic and propositional semantic codes, she identified patients who showed the normal effects of syntactic and semantic anomalies upon word monitoring in sentences, but who could not report either syntactic or semantic anomalies verbally at the end of the presentation of a sentence. One patient, for instance (D.E., also discussed in chapter 6), showed an increase in reaction times when a word that he had to monitor for created a violation of verb subcatgerorization structure [as in monitoring for the word *guitar* in (65)].

*(65)   The woman slept the guitar.

However, the same patient was unable to indicate that this sentence was ill formed or anomalous. Tyler suggested that this pattern of performance indicated that syntactic and propositional semantic codes were being automatically activated normally on-line but could not be used by off-line controlled processes.

Given these findings, it is possible that all the results reported above that involve off-line measures (enactment tasks, sentence-picture matching tasks, grammaticality and anomaly judgments) could be documenting deficits that are restricted to controlled processes that arise after sentences have been understood. However, while this is possible, it seems very unlikely that all the patients described in all the studies we have reviewed were able to assign and interpret syntactic structures normally in an unconscious fashion, but were limited in their ability to use these structures and interpretations in later controlled stages of processing. Because of their high degree of specificity, it is reasonable to think that many, if not all, of the patterns of abnormal performance described above reflect failures of the unconscious processes associated with parsing. Tyler's results, however, indicate that more work is needed to prove that this is the case and to document the range of deficits found in the unconscious on-line processes related to sentence comprehension.

The Role of the Function Word Vocabulary in Parsing

Studies of aphasic patients have been related to another question regarding syntax-processing mechanisms: Is there a special role for certain vocabulary classes in parsing procedures? Several parsing theories (mostly of a slightly older vintage, such as Kimball, 1973) have proposed that the construction of phrase markers is driven by minor lexical categories. According to these models, the pattern-action rules that create syntactic representations are mostly, or entirely, triggered by function words and morphological affixes. Data from aphasia have been thought to be relevant to this claim.

Some aphasiologists have investigated the co-occurrence of syntactic comprehension disturbances and omission of function words in the speech of a class of patients known as "agrammatic" aphasic patients. Agrammatism is a disturbance of speech production in which, clinically, patients omit a disproportionate number of affixes and freestanding "function words" (see chapters 6 and 8). Agrammatic patients have a variety of other disturbances in processing function words (Rosenberg et al., 1985; Friederici, 1982). In particular, Bradley, Garrett, and Zurif (1980) presented evidence that the recognition of function words is abnormal in agrammatic aphasics. Caramazza and Zurif (1976), Schwartz et al. (1980b), Grodzinsky (1986), and others have shown that these patients often have syntactic comprehension disturbances. Some researchers have concluded that the syntactic comprehension disturbances seen in these patients are due to specific impairments in activating function words. However, the relationship of these disturbances affecting function words to the syntactic comprehension impairments of agrammatic patients is not clear. Bradley's data have been subject to both reanalysis and nonreplication (Gordon and Caramazza, 1982), so that the implications of the original data are not as clear as had been thought at first. No patients have been described in whom a disturbance affecting function words has been related to a comprehension impairment for structures containing the affected items. Some agrammatic patients do not have syntactic comprehension disorders (Nespoulous et al., 1988) and some patients without agrammatism have syntactic comprehension disorders that are indistinguishable from those seen in agrammatic patients (Zurif and Caramazza, 1976; Caplan et al., 1985; Schwartz et al, 1987; Martin, 1987). Overall, there is no credible evidence from studies of language pathology that function words provide a critical input to the parser.

The Independence of Recognizing and Producing Syntactic Structures

Finally, studies of aphasic patients are relevant to the question of whether there is a single mechanism that computes syntactic structure in both input and output tasks. Again, the discussion focuses on the fact that patients with expressive agrammatism often have syntactic comprehension disturbances (Heilman and Scholes, 1976; Schwartz et al., 1980; Grodzinsky, 1986; Caplan and Futter, 1986; among others). Several authors have argued that the co-occurrence of deficits in sentence production and comprehension seen in these patients indicates that there are "central" or "overarching" syntactic operations, used in both comprehension and production tasks (Berndt and Caramazza, 1980; Zurif, 1984; Grodzinsky, 1986).

However, though deficits in syntactic comprehension frequently co-occur with expressive agrammatism, it does not appear that the two are due to a single functional impairment. Patients with agrammatism show a wide variety of performance in syntactic comprehension tasks. As noted above, several patients with expressive agrammatism have shown no disturbances of syntactic comprehension whatsoever (Miceli et al., 1983; Nespoulous et al., 1984; Kolk and van Grunsven,1985) and some patients with syntactic comprehension disorders that are indistinguishable from those seen in agrammatic patients do not have expressive agrammatism (Zurif and Caramazza, 1976, Caplan et al., 1985, Schwartz et al., 1987, Martin, 1987). To the extent that disturbances of syntactic comprehension and expressive agrammatism can be assessed in terms of degree of severity, there seems to be no correlation between the severity of a syntactic comprehension deficit and the severity of expressive agrammatism in an individual patient. These data constitute an argument against the view that there is only one impairment producing expressive agrammatism that necessarily entails a disturbance of syntactic comprehension. They are consistent with a model that has separate mechanisms dealing with the construction of syntactic form in input- and output-side processing, and with the view that these mechanisms can be separately disturbed.

The Use of Simplified Syntactic Structures (Heuristics) in Sentence Comprehension

Patients who do not assign propositional meanings on the basis of syntactic structures are limited to the lexico-pragmatic and heuristic routes to these aspects of meaning. Heuristics have been studied by analyzing the systematic errors that patients make in syntactic comprehension tests (i.e., tests that use reversible sentences). Our studies have reported error types for many sentence types in object manipulation tasks, where subjects are free to assign any interpretation they wish to the sentence (Caplan and Futter, 1986; Caplan et al., 1986b; Caplan and Hildebrandt, 1988a). Errors made by patients usually respect basic aspects of sentence structure and meaning, such as the number of thematic roles assigned by a verb, the number of propositions expressed in a sentence, and the distinction between referentially dependent NPs and referential expressions. We have found that what we have called "strictly linear interpretations," in which thematic roles are assigned to sequential NPs in canonical order (agent-theme-goal in English), are the most common error type regardless of the syntactic structure of a sentence. In addition, patients appear to be sensitive to the relevance of some minor lexical items for thematic role assignment, such as a *by* phrase.

We have provided a linguistic analysis of the structures which underlie these errors (Caplan and Hildebrandt, 1988a). The error patterns we have documented can all be accounted for by the application of simple interpretive rules to linear sequences of major lexical categories. The most common erroneous responses in English-speaking aphasic patients can result from the application of the following rules to the sequence of nouns and verbs in a sentence:

(1) In sequences of the form N-V-N or N-N-V, assign either the immediately preverbal noun or the first noun in the sentence the role of agent and assign the remaining noun the role of theme.

(2) In sentences with a verb requiring three arguments, assign the first noun the role of agent, the second noun the role of theme, and the third noun the role of goal.

(3) In a sentence with two verbs each of which has two argument places, use rule 1 iteratively around each verb.

(4) Assign the noun in the sequence *by*-N the thematic role of agent.

These rules only mention the linear sequences of major lexical categories—nouns and verbs—and one lexically specified preposition (*by*) as the syntactic structures to which interpretive algorithms apply. We have not found it necessary to postulate hierarchically organized phrase markers as the structures to which interpretive rules apply to yield erroneous interpretations. Moreover, the interpretive rules themselves are very simple; they assign thematic roles on the basis of the absolute position of a noun in a sentence, simple precedence relations among items specified in a linear sequence of categories, and a few lexical items (such as *by*). These structures would result from the operation of lexical identification processes, coupled with a memory system which maintains lexical items and their associated grammatical categories in linear sequences. In other languages, patients appear to make use of other readily available cues (declensional morphology, subject-verb agreement) in generating erroneous responses (Smith and Mimica, 1984; see Bates and Wulfeck 1989, for review).

The most significant feature of these heuristics is that they are closely related to normal syntactic operations. Linear sequences of major lexical categories and associated morphological markings are precisely those representations which we indicated were the input to the parser in English (see above). One possibility is that the mechanism which generates these structures is related to look-ahead mechanisms in a parser (Marcus, 1980; Berwick and Weinberg, 1984). Adaptive heuristics thus may be derived from aspects of the normal parser. Alternatively, or in addition, heuristics may make use of what Chomsky calls the primitive conceptual basis for syntax (Chomsky, 1981). In either case, patients' adaptations to parsing impairments make use of a subset of the primitive items and operations found in normal parsing operations; they do not consist of behaviors based on other cognitive systems, such as spatial arrays, pragmatic factors, etc. We conclude that patients retain elementary operations within the domain of parsing, and that their first attempts to deal with tasks that normally involve the parser make use of these retained abilities. These heuristics are exceptionally resistant to disturbance after brain damage. In the study of Caplan et al. (1985), only the most severely impaired subjects were unable to make use of at least some of them.

The Use of Nonsyntactic Mechanisms in Aphasic Sentence Comprehension

We have been discussing disorders affecting the ability to use syntactic structures to assign aspects of sentence meaning. Are there patients who cannot use any syntactic mechanisms at all—either a full parse or simplified syntactic structures—to assign these aspects of meaning? Such patients would be restricted to the use of lexical semantic, pragmatic, and possibly discourse cues to the assignment of features of meaning such as thematic roles, etc.

There is evidence that semantic features of single words play a disproportionately important role in determining the sentence comprehension abilities of some aphasic patients. For instance, Schwartz et al. (1980b) presented the results of sentence comprehension tests in five agrammatic patients that showed that these patients were largely unable to use either syntactic structures or heuristics based on word order to assign thematic roles. As a group, these patients tended to assign the thematic roles of agent and theme randomly in both reversible active and passive sentences. In several tests of sentence *production*, these patients were unusually influenced by the animacy of nouns in sentences in the assignment of thematic roles, taking animate nouns to be agents and inanimate nouns to be themes, regardless of the thematic roles depicted in pictures that the patients had to describe (Saffran, Schwartz and Marin, 1980; see discussion in chapter 8). The results for both comprehension and production of simple active sentences are displayed in figure 7.11.

Schwartz et al. claimed that these results indicated that these patients assigned thematic roles entirely on the basis of animacy. However, the data regarding the effects of animacy were obtained in production, not comprehension, tasks. Moreover, as Caplan (1983) pointed out, even the analysis of these patients' sentence production is suspect. If these researchers were correct in their analysis, assignment of thematic roles to nouns would have been random in I/I sentences (since neither noun is animate), and assignment of thematic roles to nouns in I/A sentences would have been consistently incorrect (since the animate noun incorrectly would have been taken as the agent). This was not what was found. The group as a whole assigned agency to the first noun in I/I sentences about 86% of the time, and to the first noun in I/A sentences about 50% of the time. This pattern is more in keeping with the idea that both linear order and animacy affected the patients' assignments of thematic roles to nouns.

Similar interactions between lexical semantic features of words and syntactic markers for thematic roles have been described in other studies of aphasic patients, some of them involving sentence comprehension (Smith and Mimica, 1984; Smith and Bates, 1987; Bates, Friederici, and Wulfeck, 1987; see Bates and Wulfeck, 1989, for review). These studies thus show that nonsyntactic factors do appear to influence the assignment of sentential semantic meanings in aphasic patients to a greater degree than they do in normal subjects. They do not show that patients make no use of any syntactic information, however. On the contrary, what has been found are complicated interactions between lexical semantic factors, such as the animacy of nouns, and simple aspects of sentence form, such as word order, subject-verb agreement, and case markings, that determine the assignment of thematic roles.

However, some patients whose sentence comprehension is very impaired may not use any aspects of syntactic structure to determine aspects of sentence meaning. For instance, the patients in the

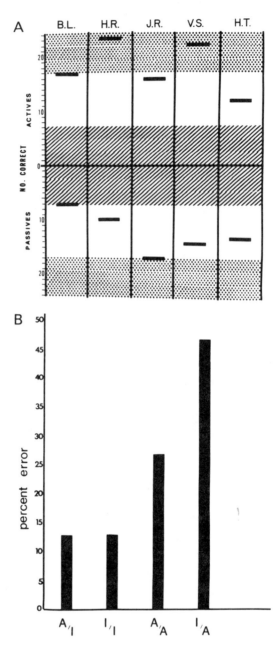

Figure 7.11
Performance of agrammatic patients on a sentence comprehension test (A) and a sentence production test (B), illustrating failure to use word order in comprehension and reliance on animacy in sentence production. (Reproduced with permission from Schwartz et al., 1980b, p. 260 (A) and from Saffran et al., 1980, p. 276 (B).)

most impaired groups identified by clustering analyses in the study of Caplan et al. (1985) (see above) showed random assignment of thematic roles to nouns in simple active, cleft-subject, passive, and cleft-object sentence types, and virtually no correct responses to the other, more complex, sentences used in that study. These patients did not seem to be using even linear word order to determine thematic roles. Thus, it appears that all syntactically based comprehension strategies may be affected in some patients. However, we do not know if patients who make no use of even syntactic heuristics can use lexical semantic features, such as animacy of nouns, to assign sentential semantic features such as thematic roles. To answer this question, we would have to test patients such as those in the worst groups in the study of Caplan et al. for their ability to assign thematic roles in sentences in which the animacy of lexical nouns was varied. To my knowledge, this has not been done, and we do not know if such patients could make use of any nonsyntactic information to assign thematic roles.

Conversely, whether all aphasic patients show a disproportionate effect of lexical semantic meanings on sentence comprehension, or whether only moderately impaired patients do so, is not clear at present. That is, whether the lexico-pragmatic route ever operates in isolation or whether it has a pathologic influence on sentence comprehension in patients who have only very mild syntactic comprehension deficits is unknown.

The answers to these questions have theoretical as well as clinical implications. If the lexico-pragmatic route can survive in isolation and can also not become disproportionately important in determining meaning for some sentence types in the face of impairments of the syntactic comprehension mechanism, a model of sentence comprehension that postulates that the lexico-pragmatic and syntactic mechanisms are inseparable (such as the model proposed by Bates and MacWhinney, discussed above) would be hard to maintain. If, however, disturbances of sentence comprehension always involve some interaction between the operation of the lexico-pragmatic and syntactic routes to sentence meaning, the interactive model receives support. Clinically, what influences a patient's comprehension of aspects of sentence meaning is clearly important information for clinicians and other persons who interact with a patient to have.

Do Patients Lose the Ability to Assign Sentential Semantic Meanings?

To this point, we have been discussing patients who seem to assign thematic roles to nouns in at least some sentences. Is it possible for a patient to retain the meanings of words but lose the notion of thematic roles and other sentential semantic features, or to be totally unable to assign these features to the words in sentences? Such a patient would be very severely communicatively impaired.

Evidence that this is the case would require several findings. First, the patient must not show any systematic assignment of a sentential semantic feature, such as agency, to any noun in a sentence. This requirement is met if a patient shows completely random performance in assigning agency to the simplest sentences in enactment or sentence-picture matching tasks, regardless of the presence of cues such as word order, declension, agreement, animacy, and soon. To date, to my knowledge, no such patient has been described. Even if such performance were to be found, however, it would not be enough to show that a patient had lost the notion of thematic roles or could not assign them at all. It is possible that a patient who chooses randomly between pictures in a sentence-picture matching task is assigning thematic roles randomly, rather than not assigning them at all. A second finding that would support the view that such a patient did not assign thematic roles at all would be that the patient did not distinguish between sentences and unstructured lists of words in comprehension tasks. For instance, such a patient might continue to put objects into random contact with each other in enactment tasks or to point to pictures randomly in picture matching tasks when given lists of words as well as all types of sentences. This would constitute an absence of what might be called a "sentence superiority effect" in these tasks, and would suggest that thematic roles were not being assigned in sentences. Such results have not been reported.

Despite absence of this type of data, one paper in the literature has entertained the possibility that some patients tested may have lost the concept of thematic roles altogether. This is the study by Schwartz et al. (1980b), discussed above. The researchers' conjecture is based on the view that their patients interpreted sentences randomly. As we have seen, this was not shown to be the case for irreversible sentences. To date, there is no patient described whose performance clearly indicates that he can understand single words but not extract thematic roles from sentences. Like so many other deficits that researchers and clinicians might expect to exist (see chapter 2, for instance, for a discussion of the as yet unsuccessful search for a "true" Wernicke's aphasic patient who can accomplish acoustic-phonetic processing but not recognize spoken words), this devastating disturbance has proved hard to find.

The Role of Short-Term Memory in Sentence (and Discourse) Comprehension

Research on memory has provided considerable evidence for a verbal short-term memory system (STM) which is involved in memory tasks, such as free recall and serial probe recognition, in which subjects must retain small amounts of information over brief delays. Evidence both from studies of normal subjects (Waugh and Norman, 1965; Postman and Phillips, 1965; Glanzer and Cunitz, 1966) and of brain-injured patients (Milner, 1966; Shallice and Warrington, 1970; Warrington and Shallice, 1969) suggests that this memory system is separate from other longer-term memory systems such as episodic (Tulving, 1972) and semantic (Rumelhart, Lindsay, and Norman, 1972) memory. Although there is considerable debate about the exact nature and structure of the verbal STM system, one important characteristic of this memory system is that representations are maintained in STM in a phonological form. Auditorily presented items are entered into a phonological store directly (Greene and Crowder, 1984; Salame and Baddeley, 1982; Baddely and Vallar, 1984a; Baddeley, Lewis, and Vallar, 1984), while printed items are entered through a process of subvocal rehearsal (Baddeley, 1966 a,b; Baddeley, Thompson, and Buchanan, 1975). There is a progressive diminishing of the strength of the phonological representations in the phonological store over a period of a few seconds. A second important feature of STM is that the strength of these representations can be increased through the use of articulatory rehearsal processes.

Some researchers have argued that phonological STM is involved in the initial assignment of structure and meaning to a sentence. A characteristic statement of this view is that of Clark and Clark (1977). Their claim, closely related to earlier work by Fodor, Bever, and Garrett (1974), was that parsing is carried out on a clause-by-clause basis and that material is held in STM until it is structured and interpreted semantically. The preliminary phrasal packager of Frazier and Fodor's "sausage machine" parsing model (Frazier and Fodor, 1978) also suggests a role for STM in parsing. However, the speed of the parsing process suggests that it does not make much use of look-ahead, and researchers have largely abandoned the view that a great deal of lexical material is held in STM as part of the look-ahead required by a parser.

Despite this, the view that STM is important in sentence comprehension has not been totally abandoned. A slightly different model that assigns a role to the STM system in sentence comprehension maintains that some lexical items are held in a phonological STM in phrase markers when parsing is difficult (Caramazza and Berndt, 1985; Vallar and Baddeley, 1984b; Baddeley, Vallar, and Wilson, 1987).

A quite different point of view has been articulated by several other researchers (Warrington and Shallice, 1969; Saffran and Marin 1975; McCarthy and Warrington, 1987a,b, 1990; Caplan and Waters, 1990). They postulate no role for STM in parsing but argue that phonological memory systems are involved in processes that arise after sentence meaning is assigned. These processes include mapping propositional content onto motor actions, mapping propositional content onto long-term memory to verify the truth or plausibility of a proposition, checking the meaning derived from the syntactic processing of a sentence against meanings derived lexico-pragmatically, and other reasoning and learning processes (updating semantic and long-term memory) based on propositional content.

Data from brain-damaged patients are relevant to these models. Researchers who maintain the view that STM is used in comprehending more complex sentences have pointed to a variety of sentence comprehension disturbances found in patients with STM limitations (Caplan et al. 1986b; Vallar and Baddeley, 1987). Sentence length has been shown to affect certain comprehension tasks in some patients who do not show disturbances of syntactic comprehension (Schwartz et al., 1987, document this pattern and call it the P2 pattern of sentence comprehension imapirment). However, in an extensive and detailed analysis of the comprehension abilities of all the STM patients in the recent neuropsychological literature, Caplan and Waters (1990) argued that the comprehension deficits found in these patients do not prove that STM limitations lead to syntactic comprehension deficits. In fact, case studies show that patients with STM impairments can have excellent syntactic comprehension abilities (McCarthy and Warrington, 1984; Butterworth Campbell, and Howard, 1986). One such patient of ours, B.O., had a short-term memory span of two to three items. However, B.O. showed excellent comprehension of syntactically complex, semantically reversible sentences, even including those containing long-distance dependencies that spanned considerably more than three words in which STM limitations would be expected to have clear effects if STM were required for long-distance co-indexation (Waters, Caplan, and Hildebrandt, 1991). Thus data from B.O. and other STM patients provide strong evidence against any role of STM in parsing itself.

On the other hand, the data from STM patients are compatible with the view that phonological memory systems are involved in processes that arise after sentence meaning is determined on the basis of sentence structure. Many STM patients show comprehension disturbances that seem STM-related. B.O. had particular problems understanding sentences that contained three or more noun phrases, especially if these were proper nouns. McCarthy and Warrington (1987a, 1990) reported two STM patients who were unable to map commands onto actions when the task involved a pragmatically unpreferred arrangement of objects. Vallar and Baddeley (1987) reported an STM patient who could not detect discourse anomalies involving referential dependencies (see chapter 9 for a discussion of this case). These data suggest that STM patients show deficits in a variety of situations in which the ability to review the initial analysis of a sentence could be useful (see Caplan and Waters, 1990, for discussion). Whether these deficits are an invariable consequence of STM limitations, and whether disturbances in comprehension arise in different ways for written and spoken sentence and discourse comprehension, remain to be established.[9]

SUMMARY

Sentences convey aspects of meaning beyond those implicit in single words. These aspects of meaning arise from the combination of individual word meanings in the syntactic structure of a sentence. Some of these aspects of meaning can also be inferred from a combination of word meaning and real-world knowledge, and some sentences can be understood by applying heuristics to assign their structure. Many patients fail to extract these aspects of meaning when the full syntactic structure of a sentence must be assigned, and these disturbances of "syntactic comprehension" have been investigated in considerable detail. These patients rely on lexico-pragmatic and heuristic means of understanding sentence meaning. In some cases, even heuristic mechanisms may fail. Short-term memory disorders do not seem to lead to disturbances of syntactic comprehension but to affect patients' abilities to review a sentence, leading to increased difficulties when a patient has not understood a sentence or needs to refer to its form to accomplish some other task. Disturbances of sentence comprehension are common, potentially important clinically, and reasonably easy to diagnose. Since some have been shown to be remediable (see chapter 10), they should be sought as part of the diagnostic evaluation of every aphasic patient.

NOTES

1. As we shall see below, Chomsky's theory maintains that noun phrases leave **traces** when they move. Since these **traces** remain in S-structure, thematic roles can be assigned at S-structure as long as they are assigned to **traces** of moved NPs, not the lexically specified noun itself. In fact, thematic roles are assigned in the same fashion at all levels of syntactic structure and logical form in this theory, but at times are assigned to syntactic elements that are not pronounced (see discussion of empty categories, below).

2. Many, if not all, phrase structure rules are done away in some modern versions of this theory (see Lasnick and Uriagereka, 1988, for discussion), while other theories of syntactic structure eliminate transformations and have nothing but "generalized" phrase structure rules (Gazdar et al., 1985). We are presenting only one (simplified) version of Chomsky's model here.

3. In English, words like *him* or *himself* do restrict the range of possible entities in the real world to which they refer to those that are single males, and, in other languages, similar words restrict the possible entities in the real world to which they refer to those for which the words have a particular grammatical gender or number, or both. However, the meaning of a word like *him* or *himself* is far less specific than that of word like *boy*.

4. Note that the fact that PDP models do not pose such a threat to these models does not imply that the particular model we have outlined in the greatest detail—that developed by Chomsky—is correct. This model is particularly abstract in certain respects, and it is possible that a less abstract model will prove to be adequate and better in some ways.

5. Most of the evidence for how the parser operates that I shall review is based upon experiments and observations made with written sentences. Sometimes these sentences are presented for short periods of time, or are

presented in a word-by-word fashion, or a subject has a limited time to respond to a presented stimulus. These conditions more closely approximate the conditions of comprehending spoken sentences inasmuch as the input cannot be inspected at leisure before a response is made, but they are still not the same as presenting a sentence auditorily. In particular, spoken sentences have intonational contours that affect parsing, which are only partially related to written punctuation marks. Thus, some caution must be exercised in accepting these results as evidence upon which to build theories of spoken sentence comprehension. However, many of the results to be presented here are also found for spoken sentences in informal observations. For the time being, until there are more studies of spoken sentence comprehension, we will rely on these studies for data pertinent to how the parser operates.

6. Parsers that operate via pattern-action rules are among the simplest types of parsers that are now implemented in computer programs. A review of several other types of parsers can be found in Shieber (1985).

7. Hagiwara and Caplan (1990) found that violations of thematic role order canonicity (the usual order of thematic roles in a given sentence structure in a language) were more costly than violations of thematic role markedness (the most common thematic role order for that structure in the languages of the world in general), suggesting that language-specific factors are more important than language-universal factors in determining the processing resource requirements of a sentence's structure.

8. For instance, Grodzinsky (1990) has suggested that agrammatic patients who show disturbances of syntactic comprehension are unable to utilize function words that are not attached to S nodes, but are able to use those that are so attached to assign syntactic structures and use them to interpret sentences. Grodzinsky (1990) considered passive constructions to be a test of this hypothesis. He argued that the preposition *by* in a passive sentence is attached to the topmost S node, and therefore that agrammatics with syntactic comprehension disorders will be sensitive to its presence. This will lead to their being able to make grammaticality judgments correctly in passive sentences. It will also lead to their assigning the thematic role of agent to the object of the preposition *by*. He also argues that agrammmatic patients cannot co-index **traces** and therefore tend to assign agency to the subject of passive sentences. Therefore, assigning the thematic role of agent to the object of the preposition *by* will lead these patients to a random assignment of the role of agent to either the subject of the sentence or the object of *by* in passive sentences. He claims that these predictions have been verified in two studies (Grodzinsky, 1988; Grodzinsky and Pierce, 1987). However, there are problems with these results and this account of agrammatic syntactic comprehension disorders. In Grodzinsky and Pierce's study of grammaticality judgments, the only sentences in which the preposition *by* appeared were well-formed passive sentences, all the ill-formed passive sentences were created by substituting the preposition *with* for the preposition *by*, and almost no other sentences contained the preposition

with. Under these circumstances, subjects can simply indicate that any sentence containing the preposition *with* is ill formed and any sentence containing the preposition *by* is well formed, without assigning any structure to the sentence whatsoever. Similarly, though agrammatic patients with syntactic comprehension disorders do tend to assign agency randomly to either the subject of the sentence or the object of by in passive sentences, they also make random assignments of agency and theme to the subject of passive sentences in which the by phrase has been eliminated (e.g., *The woman was watched;* see Martin et al., 1989). This makes it unclear whether their random performance on full passive sentences is related to their use of the *by* phrase.

9. Research with normals has centered on the role of STM in sentence processing (e.g., anomaly detection, Baddeley, 1979; Baddeley, Eldridge, and Lewis, 1981; semantic acceptability judgment, Kleiman, 1975; change detection, Levy, 1975; 1977; Slowiaczek and Clifton, 1980). In contrast to the work with patients, most research with normals has assessed written as opposed to auditory sentence comprehension. In general, these data suggest that STM is involved in tasks which require the subject to refer back to the verbatim form of the item after a sentence has already been assigned a meaning (Waters, Caplan, and Hildebrandt, 1987).

8 Sentence Production

We indicated in chapter 7 that sentences convey information that is not expressible through single words. This information includes thematic roles, attribution of modification, and other semantic values. Information of this sort may be called "sentential semantic information." In addition to sentential semantic information, sentences convey information regarding aspects of discourse, such as what information is new and what is old in a sentence, what the topic of the sentence is, and so forth. Both sentential semantic and discourse-level information affect the form of sentences. The two aspects of sentence form that they affect that will be considered here are the syntactic structure of a sentence and its intonational contour.

Given the many processes that occur in the production of even the simplest sentences, it is not surprising that language disorders almost always show up in sentence production in spontaneous speech and conversational settings. We have dealt with disturbances that involve the production of simple and complex words in earlier chapters. Disturbances of accessing words from concepts (chapters 3 and 4), developing the sound pattern of words and preparing lexical phonological representations for articulation in sentences (chapter 4), and constructing morphological forms (chapter 6) can disrupt aphasic patients' attempts to produce sentences. In this chapter, we are concerned with aspects of sentence production that are more narrowly related to sentence-level structures: accessing lexical items in relationship to the construction of syntactic form and inserting lexical items into sentences, the generation of syntactic structure, and the production of intonational contours.[1]

MODELS OF SENTENCE PRODUCTION

The Generation of Syntactic Form

The process of formulating the structure of a sentence presumably begins with an intention to communicate a message (see chapter 9). Among the many aspects of messages that are to be conveyed to a listener are the sentential semantic functions mentioned above and discussed in somewhat greater detail in chapter 7. I am concerned here with the processes that occur while the speaker encodes this sentential semantic information into appropriate sentence forms. I shall concentrate on the encoding of thematic roles, and touch briefly on other aspects of sentence meaning.

In essence, thematic roles convey information about the participants in activities in the world. I have repeatedly characterized this information as expressing "who did what to whom" and, though the nature of the information conveyed by thematic roles is in fact considerably more subtle than this, this is a reasonable way to begin to think of thematic roles. In chapter 7, I indicated that this information is conveyed by the interaction of the meanings of individual words and the syntactic structures in which words are located. I gave a sentence like (1) as an example of the importance of syntactic structure in determining thematic roles. In (1) the underlined noun phrase (NP), not the italicized NP, plays the role of agent of the main verb, because of the structure of the sentence.

(1)   The dog that chased *the cat* drank the milk.

Let us consider in slightly more detail the way in which syntactic structures and lexical items interact to convey thematic roles. We shall focus on the role of verbs in determining thematic roles. Verbs have what we may call an intrinsic meaning: the meaning of the verb *hit* includes the notion of a forceful collision between two objects, while the meaning of the verb *scratch* includes the notion of contact between two objects that results in one of them becoming slightly marked. However, in addition to their intrinsic meanings, verbs also specify the initiators, recipients, and other participants in the actions or states designated by their intrinsic meanings. For instance, both *hit* and *scratch* contain the information that someone (or something) initiates the action of verb and someone (or something) receives that action. This information is the same for both *hit* and *scratch.* We shall call it information about the thematic roles related to a verb.

Information regarding the thematic roles specified by a verb does not affect the choice of the lexical item corresponding to the intrinsic meaning of the verb itself (if one wants to talk about scratching, one will have to use the verb *scratch*). However, it does affect the choice of other words in a sentence. To use the verb *scratch* requires that the speaker indicate who is scratching and who is being scratched. In other words, the choice of a verb commits the speaker to specify the persons or objects involved in the thematic roles associated with the verb. Moreover, there are very specific constraints regarding the order in which the words expressing thematic roles can be produced. Some of these come from the syntax of the language (see chapter 7), but others are due to the verb itself. For instance, both the verbs *send* and *return* have three thematic roles (agent, theme, and goal), which can be expressed as in the (a) versions of sentences (2) and (3). However, only *send* allows for the b) versions of these sentences. (The asterisk * indicates that a form is ungrammatical.)

(2a)   The mayor sent a gift to the general.

  b)   The mayor sent the general a gift.

(3a)   The mayor returned a gift to the general.

 *b)   The mayor returned the general a gift.

We will say that the verb *send* allows two "argument structures" to express its thematic roles; that is, it can be followed by an NP and a prepositional phrase or by two NPs. The verb *return* allows only one argument structure—a noun phrase followed by a prepositional phrase.

Information regarding the argument structures associated with a verb is part of what Levelt (1989) calls the "lemma" of the verb—the syntactic and semantic features of a verb (see chapter 4). We indicated in chapter 4 that a word's lemma is activated at an early stage of the processes involved in accessing a "word" from a concept. It has been suggested that the process of constructing the syntactic form of a sentence is based upon information registered in the lemmas of words (Levelt, 1989). According to this model, concepts activate lemmas which in turn require that certain syntactic structures be constructed.

Let us work through a simple example. Suppose the speaker wishes to convey the information that a particular cat scratched a dog. The concepts CAT, DOG, and SCRATCH become active, along with the information about thematic roles that the cat is agent and the dog is theme. We shall call this information "message-level" information. The concepts CAT, DOG, and SCRATCH activate the lemmas [cat], [dog], and [scratch]. In the lemma for [scratch] is the information that two thematic roles are required by this verb and that the argument structure of the verb [scratch] includes one internal argument and one external argument (for discussion of internal and external arguments, see chapters 6 and 7). The message-level information associates the role of agent with [cat] and the role of Theme with [dog]. At this point, the conceptual message has been converted into lemmas, and the thematic roles required by the lemma for the verb filled with other lemmas. The first stage in converting a thought to a sentence has been accomplished.[2]

The second stage of the process consists of creating a syntactic structure to express this set of lemmas and arguments. We saw in chapter 6 that the thematic roles assigned by a verb are related to the argument structure of a verb. The internal argument of the lemma [scratch] will be filled by the lemma [dog], because the internal argument is the theme of the verb. Similarly, the external argument will be filled by the lemma [cat], because the external argument is the agent of the verb. All that remains to be done is for the external and internal arguments to be mapped onto syntactic structures. If there is no reason not to do so, the external argument will be mapped onto the grammatical role of subject and the internal argument onto the grammatical role of object. As indicated in chapter 7, subject and object are specifications of the particular place in a syntactic structure where an NP is found. The syntactic structure of the sentence is thus completed, insofar as the specification of thematic roles is concerned.

Discourse-level factors and other influences enter into the sentence planning process. In the example given, for instance, if discourse factors make the speaker wish to focus attention on *a dog*, one way to do so would be to use the passive form (*A dog was scratched by the cat*). In this case, the relationship between the internal and external arguments of the verb is more elaborate. In chapter 7, we indicated that Chomsky's theory of syntax maintains that *a dog* is still assigned to the internal argument of *scratch* in an underlying "D-structure," but is moved to its final position in "S-structure." (Other theories of syntactic structure do not postulate movement of this sort in passive sentences.) In all theories, the external argument of *scratch* is realized in a *by* phrase, in which the preposition *by* assigns the thematic role of agent to its object. If no special considerations of this sort apply and the most common syntactic form for expressing thematic roles is chosen by default, or if *the cat* is chosen to begin the sentence for some positive reason, the active form is developed.

The final syntactic form of a sentence is also determined by the syntactic forms available in a given language. In English, for instance, the subject of a sentence is expressed by the position of a NP in relationship to a verb; that is, English is a language in which grammatical roles are largely mapped onto word order. English is a so-called subject-verb-object language, in which the NP that precedes the verb is its subject and the NP that follows the verb is its object. Other "word order" languages have different basic word orders (e.g., Japanese has a basic subject-object-verb order). Yet other languages, such as German or Serbo-Croatian, express grammatical roles largely through the use of case markers. In German, NPs are marked as "nominative," "accusative," etc., and are much freer to occur in different positions without thereby playing different grammatical roles. These language-specific "choices" of syntactic forms determine the final form of a sentence.

It remains unclear exactly how all these sources of information interact during the process of planning syntactic form. Kempen (1988; Kempen and Hoenkamp, 1987) and Levelt (1989) present a computational model of this process, according to which conceptual information activates lemmas that in turn activate syntax-building procedures. The theory maintains that lemmas are converted into phonological representations as soon as they are accessed. This feature of the theory has been confirmed in experimental work by Lindsley (1975, 1976). It allows for an interesting interaction between lexical access and the generation of syntactic structure. Suppose, for instance, that in expressing the thought that THE CAT SCRATCHED A DOG, the lemma [dog] is activated before the lemma [cat] for some reason (perhaps dictated by the discourse). The early activation of the lemma [dog] leads the speaker to begin the sentence with the words *a dog*. If the speaker begins with the NP *a dog*, he will have to use a particular syntactic form to express the thematic roles specified at the message level, such as the passive.

The possibility that differential ease of lexical access for different words may affect syntactic structure has been explored in a number of experiments. Prentice (1967), Turner and Rommetveit (1968), Flores d'Arcais (1975), Perfetti and Goldman (1975), Bock and Irwin (1980), Bock and Warren (1985), Sridhar (1988), and other researchers have used a variety of experimental techniques to show that a number of features of a noun can make it more or less accessible. Extralinguistic factors (such as whether a word was just presented before a subject has to start a sentence), discourse factors (such as whether a speaker has just been asked a question about an item that plays a role in the sentence he or she is about to utter), conceptual factors (such as whether an item is animate or human, or is definite or indefinite), perceptual factors (such as whether an item is large or brightly colored), and others, have all been shown to lead to speakers' putting words in either subject position or early in a clause or phrase. Levelt (1989) argues that ease of phonological access or production also affects the positioning of a word in a sentence, citing the results of experiments by Bock (1986a). This latter finding indicates that there is some feedback from the process of lexical phonological activation to that involved in inserting words into syntactic structures.

The discussion above suggests that the generation of the syntactic form of a sentence takes place in two stages. The first stage assigns lemmas to thematic roles around verbs. The second stage converts these representations into surface syntactic structures. There is interesting evidence that these two stages of sentence planning exist. The evidence also speaks to the relationship between these two stages and the insertion of the lexical phonological forms of words into syntactic structures. The evidence comes from analyzing spontaneously occurring speech errors.

Garrett (1975, 1976, 1978, 1980, 1982) studied a corpus of several thousand naturally occurring speech errors and suggested a model of the sentence production process based on the most frequent types of errors in speech production. Four types of errors that he considered to be especially revealing as to the nature of sentence production are the following:

(1)   Semantic substitutions, such as "boy" for "girl," "black" for "white," etc. These errors only occur with the content word vocabulary and certain prepositions.

(2)   Word exchanges, such as "he is planting the garden in the flowers" for "he is planting the flowers in the garden." These exchanges affect words of similar categories (nouns exchange with nouns, adjectives with adjectives, verbs with verbs), and also only affect the content word vocabulary. In addition, as would be expected by these constraints, word exchanges do not affect words within a single phrase. For instance, exchanges of the form "this is a room lovely" for "this is a lovely room" do not occur.

(3)   Sound exchanges, such as "shinking sips" for "sinking ships." Sound exchanges also affect the content word vocabulary. Sound exchanges usually affect adjacent words. They therefore are primarily phrase-internal and frequently affect words in different categories within the content word vocabulary, as in the example illustrated.

(4)   "Stranding" errors, as in "he is schooling to go," for "he is going to school," in which the suffix "ing" has been "stranded" in its original position and the verb stem to which it was originally attached has been moved elsewhere in the sentence. The elements which are "stranded"–i.e., that are left in their syntactic positions–are affixes; it is the content words that are moved.

The stages of sentence planning identified in Garrett's model are illustrated in figure 8.1. The first level is termed the "message" level. This is not a linguistic level, strictly speaking, but rather consists of the elaboration of the basic concepts which a speaker wishes to talk about. The first truly linguistic level is the "functional level." At the functional level, lexical items are found for concepts. At this stage, the speaker has accessed the lexical semantic representation of a word (part of its lemma) but not its phonological representation. In addition, the functional level contains information about aspects of meaning that are related to sentences, such as thematic roles. As with lexical semantic information, this sentential semantic information is not related to the form of the sentence at this stage of processing. These "functional argument structures" do not, for instance, require that a sentence take a particular syntactic form, such as the active or the passive. They correspond to the first stage of sentence production described above.

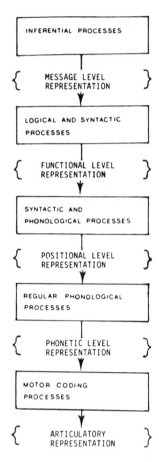

Figure 8.1
Garrett's model of the stages involved in speech production. (Reproduced with permission from Garrett, 1984, p. 174.)

It is at the "positional level" that information about the form of words and sentences is specified. At the positional level, the syntactic form of a sentence is produced, and the phonological forms of words are inserted into their appropriate positions in the syntactic structure of the sentence. An important feature of Garrett's model is that syntactic structures contain function words and bound morphemes at the point when they are accessed, that is, at the point when the positional level of representation is created. Because the phonological forms of function words are not inserted into the positional-level representations, as is true of the phonological forms of content words, function words are only subject to certain types of errors. The positional level corresponds to the second stage of sentence generation described above. Following the creation of the positional level, the phonological form of words is specified in greater detail to yield a phonetic level of representation, which is ultimately transformed into a series of commands to the vocal apparatus.

The types of errors that Garrett has documented in normal speech can be attributed to disturbances arising at these different levels as follows. Word exchanges and word substitutions arise at the functional level. Since the representations at the functional level only specify content words, these errors only apply to content words. Sound exchange errors arise during the insertion of content words into syntactic structures at the positional level. The fact that sound exchanges occur primarily between adjacent words suggests that the process of inserting the phonological form of content words into syntactic structures takes place on a phrase-by-phrase basis. Function words are not subject to sound exchanges because they are already present in the structures at the positional level. The stranding errors, in which function words and bound morphemes are stranded while the content words and stems are moved, also arise during the creation of the positional level, when content words are misordered. The fact that bound morphemes remain in place while stems move is one piece of evidence suggesting that the syntactic structures accessed during the creation of the positional level of representation already contain bound morphemes and function words in their final position. (For a more detailed discussion of speech errors in relationship to a model of syntactic generation, see Levelt, 1989, chapter 7).

In summary, the evidence from speech errors strongly supports a two-stage model of the generation of syntactic form. It also suggests that the insertion of nouns, verbs, and adjectives into syntactic structures takes place in a different fashion from that of function words and morphological affixes. Garrett's model of sentence production maintains that the second stage of generation of sentences—the creation of syntactic form—is closely tied in some way to accessing function words and morphological affixes. We shall see that these models are directly relevant to understanding aspects of aphasic disturbances in sentence production.

The Generation of Intonational Contours

Sentences are spoken with a variety of intonational contours. There are several determinants of intonational contour. The first input into intonation is the sound patterns of individual words. As discussed in chapter 2, words consist of sequences of phonemes that vary in sonority, constriction, manner of articulation, nasality, etc. These aspects of phonemes make for alternations in the pitch and intensity of the sounds produced by the vocal apparatus. In addition, words have internal variation in the relative prominence of different sonorant peaks. In English, these differences reflect lexical stress patterns; in other languages, they reflect lexical tonal patterns. These variations in the prominence of sonorant aspects of word-sound patterns are also mapped onto articulatory gestures. Both the segmental (phonemic) and word-level patterns of stress or tone are part of the input into the mechanisms that generate intonational contours. In English, intonational contours build upon these patterns, by adding prominence to those syllables that are already stressed lexically. An important feature of this process is that morphemes that do not receive lexical stress—function words and level II affixes (see chapter 6)—do not receive sentence-level intonational stress.

We noted in chapter 4 that postlexical phonological rules change word-level phonological features by processes such as cliticization, resyllabification, etc. These processes create "phonological words," such as /wanna/ from want to, etc. Intonational contours are added to these phonological words created by postlexical phonological processes.

The second input into intonational contours is the syntactic structure of the sentence. Syntactic structures provide the basis for grouping the words of a sentence together into phonological phrases. Selkirk (1984) and others have emphasized the fact that phonological phrases are not the same as syntactic phrases. For instance, in the sentence in (4a), the syntactic phrases are those indicated in b) while the phonological phrases are those indicated in c).

(4a)   The man who watched the dog that ate the bone walked away slowly.

b)   [[The man who watched [the dog that ate the bone]] walked away slowly].

c)   /The man / who watched the dog / that ate the bone/ walked away slowly.

The relationship between syntactic phrases and phonological phrases can become complex, but a simple rule that relates the two in many instances is as follows: A phonological phrase consists of all the phonological words up to and including the one that is the head of a syntactic phrase. In c), for instance, *the man* is the head of the syntactic phrase *the man who watched the dog that ate the bone. The man* is therefore a phonological phrase. On the other hand, *the dog that ate the bone* cannot function as a phonological phrase, even though it is a syntactic unit (see chapter 7 for discussion of the syntactic structure of relative clauses).

A variety of rules apply to phonological words and phonological phrases to create aspects of intonation. For instance, there is a rule in English that shifts lexical stress to avoid the occurrence of two stressed syllables in a row in adjacent words. For example, lexical stress falls on the second syllable of *sixteen'* and the first syllable of *dia'monds*. The rule changes the stress pattern on *sixteen'* to *six'-teen* in the phrase *six'teen dia'monds*. Rules such as this are subject to a number of complex constraints. For instance, the change to *six'-teen dia'monds* does not occur if the two words are in separate phrases, as in (5):

(5)   When Susan turned sixteen', diamonds were what she wanted for a gift.

Another rule affecting intonation is the "nuclear stress rule" (Selkirk, 1984). Roughly, this rule adds an extra stress to the last word in a phrase. This rule applies after the stress retraction process described above has already applied. Thus, the sequence of words in

(6a) undergoes the changes indicated in b)—d), where "x" indicates an increment of stress:

```
          X   X           X
```
(6a)   Sixteen diamonds disappeared.

```
        X       X           X
```
  b)   Sixteen diamonds disappeared. (Stress retraction has applied.)

```
              X           X
        X     X           X
```
  c)   Sixteen diamonds disappeared. (nuclear stress has applied to the NP and verb phrase [VP].)

```
                          X
              X           X
        X     X           X
```
  d)   Sixteen diamonds disappeared. (Nuclear stress has applied to the sentence.)

Stress retraction is one mechanism that serves to induce a regular alternation between stressed and unstressed syllables in English utterances—a phenomenon known as "isochrony." There is considerable debate over whether isochrony is reliably found in spoken English; it appears to occur in at least some speech situations (Pike, 1945; Kelly and Bock, 1988; Jassem, Hill, and Witten, 1984).

Aside from the intonation contours determined by the creation of phonological words and phonological phrases, and the adjustments of lexical stress as a result of processes such as avoidance of two adjacent lexically stressed syllables and the nuclear stress rule, two other major factors determine intonational contour.

The first is the illocutionary force of a sentence. There is a characteristic intonation associated with declarative sentences, questions, etc. For instance, sentence (7) can be a statement if spoken with a falling intonation, or a question if intonation rises at the end of the sentence.

(7)   My daughter ate the spinach.

Many different moods can be conveyed through changes in the melody of a sentence (see Levelt, 1989, chapter 10, for discussion).

The second major factor that affects intonational contour is emphasis. A speaker can choose to focus upon any word in a sentence by adding emphatic stress to that word. In fact, emphatic stress can even be added to a syllable that does not contain lexical stress in an effort to make lexical identity clear (as in "I said ABduct, not ADduct"). Emphatic stress is superimposed upon the intonational contours determined by the factors described above.

As noted in chapter 4, intonational factors affect the realization of lexical phonological form. In chapter 4, we discussed cliticization, flap formation, segment deletion, and other adjustments to segmental lexical phonetic values that occur as a consequence of the creation of phonological words and phrases. The "higher-order" aspects of intonation we have been discussing (stress retraction, nuclear stress, intonation reflecting illocutionary force, emphatic stress) also affect the realization of lexical phonology. As noted in chapter 4, all these aspects of phonology eventually coalesce into movements of the vocal tract.[3]

Despite the intimate connection between intonational contour and lexical phonology, data from speech errors suggest that the two processes are separate at some planning stage(s). The evidence is that intonational stress is usually left behind when words exchange. For instance, there are errors such as (8) and (9):

(8)   The child gave the mother the CAT → The child gave the cat the MOTHER (Levelt, 1989).

(9)   Seymour sliced the salami with a KNIFE → Seymour sliced the knife with a SALAMI (Fromkin, 1973).

Nuclear stress remains in place in most word exchange errors, indicating that this aspect of intonational contours is planned separately from lexical access or lexical insertion into syntactic structures. Conversely, emphatic stress tends to move with the word to which it is attached in word exchanges, suggesting that it is linked directly to specific lexical items (Fromkin, 1973; Stemberger, 1985). This is an intuitively understandable finding, since nuclear stress arises in relationship to the creation of phonological phrases, while emphatic stress is associated with highlighting specific words.

In summary, a wide variety of factors determine sentence intonation contours, which in turn affect the realization of lexical phonological forms. Many aspects of planning intonational contours appear to be separate from the processes involved in accessing words or inserting lexical phonological representations into phrase markers.

The Time Course of Planning Syntactic Form and Intonational Contours

Sentence structure and intonational contours are expressed through their effects on sequences of words. This raises the question of how far the speaker must "look ahead" to plan syntactic form and intonational contours.

Several researchers have argued that such look-ahead is limited. Experimental results by Lindsley (1975, 1976) and Kempen (Kempen and Huijbers, 1983; Kempen and Hoenkamp, 1987) indicate that accessing the phonological form of the first noun in a sentence occurs before the form of the verb in the sentence is accessed. We presented several arguments in chapter 4 to the effect that look-ahead was also limited in the planning of phonological words. Together, these results indicate look-ahead is limited in planning phonological forms of words and inserting them in sentence structures.

However, several of the phenomena we have discussed above suggest that some look-ahead occurs in planning intonation. Stress retraction requires that the stress pattern be known for the word following the word being uttered. Stress retraction is cumulative, so considerable look-ahead may be needed in some situations. For instance, in (10), taken from Levelt (1989), stress has been retracted on *abstract* and then on *sixteen*, because of the stress pattern on *paintings*.

(10)   six'teen ab'stract paint'ings.

In general, isochrony would benefit from look-ahead at the phonological level.

Planning the overall intonational contour of a sentence is another process that must require some look-ahead, since some patterns involve both a rise and then a fall in pitch, and the final level of pitch influences the degree of the rise. In addition, the existence of anticipatory duplications of phonemes and other segmental elements in speech errors requires some look-ahead. We should note that such errors are quite rare and are always phonological phrase–internal. Overall, as Levelt (1989) has argued, phonological look-ahead can be limited to a few words in most cases.

Syntactic look-ahead is a more complex matter. How much of the structure of a sentence is planned before lexical items are accessed and/or inserted into phrase markers remains unclear. Similarly, it is not known how much of a sentential semantic representation is formulated before syntactic planning begins. Garrett's model, reviewed above, suggests that a fair amount of the semantic representation relevant to sentence form is constructed before syntactic structures are activated, but that lexical insertion into phrase markers takes place on a phrase-by-phrase basis. Levelt (1989) has suggested that look-ahead at the syntactic level can be limited if sentence structure is planned on the basis of information in the lemmas of words as they are activated. The reader is referred to Levelt (1989) for discussion of these issues.

DISORDERS OF SENTENCE PRODUCTION

As I indicated at the beginning of this chapter, problems in producing sentences are ubiquitous in aphasic patients. This is partly because, when patients have disturbances with the production of single words, these problems almost always surface in sentence production as well. Phonemic paraphasias, apraxia of speech, anomia, semantic paraphasias, circumlocutions, abnormal generation of morphological form, and other abnormalities of speech output affecting the production of words in naming, repetition, and reading tasks often are also found in the conversational speech of patients. Though there are many unanswered questions regarding the relationship between the disturbances seen in single word processing and those found in sentence production, we may assume that many disorders affecting the production of many vocabulary elements in sentences are related to disturbances of the processing of the same items in isolation.

However, in addition to disturbances that carry over from the production of single words to the production of sentences, many patients have problems in the sentence planning process itself. These patients have impairments of their ability to produce particular types of vocabulary elements in sentences despite an ability to perform a wide variety of tasks with these same vocabulary items in isolation, to use certain types of syntactic structures to convey particular propositional semantic features, or to produce intonational aspects of sentences. I shall discuss disturbances of sentence production under four headings: (1) problems affecting the production of grammatical elements, (2) problems affecting the generation of syntactic form, (3) problems affecting the production of thematic roles, and (4) problems affecting the production of appropriate intonational contours. Before turning to these issues, I shall mention one or two methodological points.

Aphasiologists have attempted to understand disturbances of sentence production by examining both patients' spontaneous speech and their performances on more constrained sentence production tasks. These tasks include story narration, story completion, picture description, sentence completion, anagram solution, reading, and repetition. Each of these tasks requires speech production (or, in the case of anagram solution, some processes related to the structuring of sentences), but the input to the speech planning and production system varies. It may consist of a set of guidelines regarding the semantic structure of a story or sentence (in story narration and picture description), a frame that restricts the syntactic structures that can be used (in sentence and story completion), or phonological information (in repetition).

In general, most studies of sentence production have relied heavily upon analysis of conversational speech and storytelling, and have made much less use of more highly constrained tasks in which the particular form of a sentence that would be produced on a particular trial is highly restricted in a normal population. It appears that the degree of structure in a discourse context affects patients' abilities to produce particular syntactic structures (Ostrin, Schwartz, and Saffran, 1983; Ulatowska et al., 1981, 1983a). In general, unconstrained discourse situations are more difficult for patients, who are less likely to produce complex syntactic forms in these circumstances. It therefore may be said of the existing literature that it does not establish the existence of selective impairments in the production of syntactic form when the maximal abilities of patients are examined, which would only arise if the sentence production tasks set for the patients were highly constrained. In addition, the existing literature does not look for the relationship between the patient's ability to produce a particular syntactic structure in a constrained setting and his or her ability to produce that structure in successively less constrained situations. Current research is beginning to address these issues.

Most of the research into disturbances of sentence production has centered on clinical aphasic syndromes such as agrammatism, paragrammatism, jargonaphasia, and others. In keeping with my effort to relate aphasic disturbances to stages of language processing, I will attempt to analyze the sentence production disturbances of aphasic patients in relationship to models of the sentence production process. This effort will lead us to consider the deficits seen in these syndromes, but the focus is on the nature of sentence production abnormalities found in aphasic patients, not on a characterization of the disturbances associated with a particular syndrome.

Disturbances of Production of "Grammatical" Vocabulary Elements

I indicated in my discussion of sentence generation that there is good evidence that different mechanisms underlie the production of different vocabulary elements in English (and many other languages). The different production mechanisms apply to two major categories of vocabulary elements, which we have called "major" and "minor" syntactic categories. These vocabulary classes are also called "content" and "function" words. Content words consist of nouns, adjectives, verbs, many adverbs, and perhaps some prepositions; function words are exemplified by articles, pronouns, auxilliary verbs, other prepositions, possessive adjectives, and a few other items. Function words and the morphological affixes (or "bound morphemes") appear to be accessed at a stage of processing that is somehow closely related to the creation of sentence structure. There are two aphasic disturbances that affect the production of function words—agrammatism and paragrammatism. Because of the link between production of these vocabulary elements and the generation of sentence structure, it is appropriate to investigate the nature of these disturbances and to see whether they engender disturbances of sentence form.

We begin with agrammatism, a disorder of speech production that has attracted a good deal of attention in the past decade (Goodglass, 1976, 1990; Kean, 1977, 1982, 1985; Menn and Obler, 1990; Badecker and Caramazza, 1985, 1986; Caplan, 1986, 1991b; Miceli et al., 1989). In the clinical classification of aphasia, agrammatism is considered a component of the syndrome of Broca's aphasia. The most noticeable deficit in agrammatism is the widespread omission of function words and affixes and the greater retention of content

Table 8.1
Different Patterns of Omission of Function Words and Bound Morphemes in Two Agrammatic Patients

	I Correctly Supplied	%	II Incorrect Morpheme (Substitutions)	%	III Omission	%	Total I + II + III
Definite articles	61	94	—	—	4	6	66
Indefinite articles	6	86	1	14	—	—	7
Possessive adjectives	5	100	—	—	—	—	5
Other determiners	2		—	—	—	—	2
Lexical adjectives	16	100	—	—	—	—	16
Other adjectives	—	—	—	—	—	—	—
Personal pronouns	15	100	—	—	—	—	15
Impersonal pronouns	6	100	—	—	—	—	6
Other pronouns	5	100	—	—	—	—	5
Nouns	90	98	1	1	1	1	92
Progressive auxiliaries	22	73	—	—	8	27	30
Other auxiliaries	3	60	1	20	1	20	5
Copulas	16	94	1	6	—	—	17
Other empty verbs	1		—	—	—	—	1
Lexical verbs	66	96	—	—	3	4	69
Subordinating conj.	2		—	—	—	—	2
Clause internal coord.conj.	6	86	—	—	1	14	7
Clause-initial coord.conj.	32	100	—	—	—	—	32
Infinitive markers	6	86	—	—	1	14	7
Case & locative prep.	10	91	1	9	—	—	11
Other prepositions	1		1	—	—	—	2
Derived adverbs	2		—	—	—	—	2
Other adverbs & particles	13	100	—	—	—	—	13
(Other words)	(3)		—				(3)
Total "content" words	173	97	1	1	4	2	178
Total "function" words	216	92	4	2	15	6	235
Bound Morphemes							
Noun plural markers	3		—	—	—	—	3
Possessive markers	—	—	—	—	4	100	4
Verb past tense markers	7	78	—	—	2	22	9
-ing progressive markers	24	92	—	—	2	8	26
3rd person singular markers	7	58	1	8	4	33	12
Total bound morphemes	41	76	1	2	12	22	51

Reproduced with permission from Menn (1990, p. 122, 125).

Table 8.1
Continued

	I Correctly Supplied	%	II Incorrect Morpheme (Substitutions)	%	III Omission	%	Total I + II + III
Definite articles	22	47	3	6	22	47	47
Indefinite articles	7	44	—	—	9	56	16
Possessive adjectives	1	8	2	15	10	77	13
Other determiners	—	—	—	—	1		1
Lexical adjectives	13	93	1	7	—	—	14
Other adjectives	1		—	—	—	—	1
Personal pronouns	8	33	—	—	16	67	24
Impersonal pronouns	2	40	—	—	3	60	5
Other pronouns	1		—	—	—	—	1
Nouns	133	96	3	1	3	2	139
Progressive auxiliaries	—	—	—	—	2		2
Other auxiliaries	—	—	—	—	3		3
Copulas	2	13	—	—	14	87	16
Other empty verbs	1		—	—	—	—	1
Lexical verbs	39	76	6	12	6	12	51
Subordinating conj.	—	—	—	—	2		2
Clause internal coord.conj.	10	71	—	—	4	29	14
Clause-initial coord.conj.	4	67	—	—	2	33	6
Infinitive markers	—	—	—	—	—	—	—
Case & locative prep.	5	19	1	4	21	78	27
Other prepositions	—	—	1	17	5	83	6
Derived adverbs	2		—	—	—	—	2
Other adverbs & particles	5	83	—	—	1	17	6
(Other words)	(5)				(2)		(7)
Total "content" words	188	91	9	4	9	4	206
Total "function" words	70	36	7	4	115	60	192
Bound Morphemes							
Noun plural markers	13	87	—	—	2	13	15
Possessive markers	2		—	—	2		4
Verb past tense markers	5	56	—	—	4	44	9
-*ing* progressive markers	1		—	—	2		3
3rd person singular markers	24	92	—	—	2	8	26
Total bound morphemes	45	78			12	21	57

words. This disparity is always seen in the spontaneous speech of patients termed *agrammatic*, and often occurs in their repetition and writing as well. Analyses of agrammatic speech are shown in table 8.1. Contemporary work deals with the exact delineation of the class of items that are affected in this condition, the abnormalities of processing that give rise to these disturbances, and the ancilliary symptoms that are associated with these abnormalities.

The class of words that are affected in agrammatism has been described in two quite different frameworks. The first is a psychological framework, and the second is linguistic. According to the psychological account, the words that are affected in agrammatism are those that belong to the closed class of vocabulary elements. This set consists of all the vocabulary elements of English other than nouns, verbs, adjectives, and derived adverbs. An adult speaker does not learn new elements of this set, in contrast to the ability to learn new nouns, verbs, and adjectives. The linguistic approach to the characterization of agrammatism has been explored by several researchers. Kean (1977) first enunciated a theory of the vocabulary elements affected in agrammatism in relationship to linguistic theory. Kean proposed that the class of elements affected in this syndrome be defined in terms of aspects of their sound pattern. The rules for assignment of stress to words, phrases, and sentences in English assign stress to phonological words—stems and roots of nouns, adjectives, and verbs—and ignore function words and certain affixes (level II affixes; see chapter 6). Kean suggested that agrammatics tend to omit items that are not phonological words. One of the principal pieces of evidence which Kean took as support for her analysis is that agrammatism affects both freestanding function words and inflectional affixes. She emphasized the point that these different elements accomplish quite different functions syntactically and semantically, but have in common the feature that they are all "phonological clitics," elements that do not affect stress placement in English. Other linguistic descriptions, mainly proposed in reaction to Kean's theory, have also been suggested (Rizzi, 1985; Lapointe, 1983; Grodzinsky, 1984). I shall not pursue these different linguistic descriptions here, but simply point out that they exist. The reader is referred to Grodzinsky (1990) for a review of the evidence supporting these different accounts. I shall call the vocabulary items affected the "function word and bound morpheme vocabulary."[4]

Many studies of agrammatic patients (Goodglass, 1973; Luria, 1973; Tissot, Mounin, and Lhermitte, 1973; Miceli et al., 1983, 1989; Menn and Obler, 1990; Berndt, 1987; Parisi, 1987) have shown that patients with agrammatism can have different patterns of retention of the function word and bound morpheme vocabulary. For instance, one Italian patient showed preservation of freestanding function words but produced incorrect verbal inflections (Miceli et al., 1983). In contrast, one agrammatic English patient correctly inflected verbs (Goodglass, 1976). M.M., a French patient studied by Nespoulous and his colleagues (Nespoulous et al., 1988) had trouble producing auxiliary verbs and certain pronouns in French (the "weak" forms of pronouns—*le, la, lui*,—but not the "strong" forms—*il, elle, moi, toi*), but considerably less trouble producing other function words. These limited impairments indicate that there are many patterns of speech, all of which have traditionally been included in the category known as agrammatism.

Because of the variation in the speech production of patients who have been called agrammatic, it is unclear whether agrammatism should be considered a "syndrome" (see Badecker and Caramazza, 1985, 1986; Miceli et al., 1989; Caplan, 1986, 1991b, for discussion). Patients with agrammatism do have in common the fact that they make more omissions of function words and bound morphemes than content words and, on this basis, it may be reasonable to group them together into a single broadly defined category. This is especially true if it can be shown that this disturbance arises at a particular stage of sentence planning. The most obvious stage of sentence planning at which these disturbances might arise is the "positional" stage of processing in Garrett's model (or its equivalent in other models), since this is the stage of processing at which the function word–bound morpheme vocabulary is accessed. Clearly, however, if all patients with agrammatism have impairments at this level of processing, their impairments differ noticeably from each other with respect to the function words and bound morphemes that are affected.

In the discussion of whether agrammatism deserves to be considered a syndrome, a number of interesting efforts have been made to see whether at least some of the interindividual variation in agrammatism can be explained. The results of these efforts have led to the identification of several factors that account for variation in agrammatism by affecting patients' abilities to produce particular vocabulary items in particular tasks. However, these general factors do not account for the entirety of the observed variation; accordingly, the question of whether all agrammatic patients should be considered to have different forms of the same deficit is unresolved at present.

One factor that makes for variation in the manifestations of agrammatic speech is the patient's overall severity. We have referred to the overall severity of a deficit as a factor that is important in determining the level of abnormal performance in many disturbances, ranging from alexia (chapter 5) to syntactic comprehension (chapter 7). Most agrammatic patients have been studied on different protocols, and many have been primarily studied with respect to spontaneous speech, which is very hard to quantify. Therefore, data on which to base quantitative judgments regarding level of severity are scarce. Nonetheless, referring to the original reports on agrammatic patients, it is clear that the patients described vary from quite mild to much more severely impaired, and that the number of closed class items produced varies as a function of a patient's overall severity (Menn et al., 1990).

The ability to produce particular affixes and function words also seems to depend upon the nature of particular items. De Villiers (1974) reported that seven agrammatic patients she studied tended to produce the same function words in spontaneous speech. She also reported that the function words that these patients tended to produce were not those that children produced at the earliest stages of spoken language development (table 8.2). Apparently, there is something that makes the production of particular closed class items difficult after certain types of brain damage in adults, but it is not exactly the same as whatever determines the ontogenetic sequence of production of these elements.

There have been several linguistic and psycholinguistic investigations of agrammatic patients that give more specific clues regarding the origin of some of the variation observed in the production of inflectional morphology by agrammatic patients. A well-known example of this variation is the report by Goodglass and Berko (1960) of the ability of 21 agrammatic aphasic patients to produce the suffix $-s$. In English, the suffix $-s$ can mark the plural, the third person singular present tense inflection of verbs, and the possessive. These are so-called "morphological" facts about this ending. In addition, the phonological form of the suffix $-s$ varies systematically regard-

Table 8.2
Difficulty Ordering of Morpheme Production for Nonfluent Aphasics
Compared to the Acquistion Order for These Morphemes

Morphemes	Order of Difficulty in Aphasia	Order of Acquisition in Children (de Villiers, Method 2)
Progressing -*ing*	1	2
Plural -*s*	2	1
Contractible copula	3	6
Uncontractible copula	4	7
Articles *a* and *the*	5	5
Past regular -*d*	6	4
Past irregular	7	3
Third person regular -*s*	8	8

Reproduced with permission from de Villiers (1974, p. 128).

less of the morphological use to which it is put. When −*s* follows an unvoiced stop-consonant, it is unvoiced (*he hits; two cups; Jack's tie*); when it follows a voiced consonant or a vowel, it is voiced (*he runs; two ties; John's cup*); and when it follows voiced affricates, such as "ch," it is produced in a syllabic form, with the sound of a reduced vowel as part of the suffix, (*he watches; two churches; Mitch's glasses*).

Goodglass and Berko found that the possessive and third person singular forms of −*s* were more frequently omitted than the plural, that the third person singular inflectional ending was omitted about as frequently as the possessive, and that the patients had more trouble producing the nonsyllabic forms (e.g., bats, cubs) than in producing the syllabic form of the suffix (e.g., churches) regardless of the morphological role the suffix played. There are several approaches to explaining these observations. Kean (1977) pointed out that, in normal subjects, "stranding errors" affect inflectional affixes more often than derivational affixes. She argued that this suggested that inflected affixes are more likely to be separated from their stems and roots, and she suggested that the greater problems with the possessive and third person singular forms than with the plural form may be due to the former being treated by agrammatic patients as inflectional and the latter as derivational affixes, with the inflectional affixes that are more easily separated from their stems by normal speakers being more likely to be omitted by agrammatic speakers.[5] Kean (1977) also pointed out that the differential susceptibility of syllabic and nonsyllabic affixes to omission can be explained linguistically in terms of the sonorance hierarchy (see chapter 4). The syllabic form of −s, /əs/, is more sonorant than either of its nonsyllabic forms, /s/ and /z/. Kean suggested that this feature affects agrammatic patients' tendency to omit a word-boundary affix: more sonorant elements are less likely to be omitted.

Goodglass (1973) took a different approach to explaining the variation in producing affixes that he and Berko documented. He suggested that it is possible to integrate data from a number of experiments to define a class of words that are less "salient" and therefore more difficult for an agrammatic patient. Salience is the "psychological resultant of stress, of the informational significance, of the phonological prominence, and of the affective value of a word" (Goodglass, 1973, p.204). Function words have low information and affective value, and are consequently more vulnerable to omission than other vocabulary elements. Phonologically prominent suffixes are better produced. In other work, Goodglass (1976) showed that function words following phonologically stressed words were better produced by agrammatic patients. Stress itself, even when it applies to a syntactically complex item like a negative auxiliary, makes it significantly easier for an agrammatic patient to produce a word. Goodglass argued that these elements combine into a single factor—salience—that determines performance. I noted above that a wide variety of factors can affect the accessibility of particular words in sentence production. "Salience" may be a term that refers to the amalgamation of these factors. However, we should note that the factors included in Goodglass's concept of salience are only some of those that have been investigated as determinants of word accessibility in agrammatic sentence production.[6]

Other aspects of the variation found among different agrammatic patients can be accounted for in other ways. Kean (1977) has proposed that agrammatic patients are constrained to produce real words. The presence of inflection on Italian main verbs (Miceli et al., 1983) may thus be explained by the fact that Italian verb roots are not lexical items and require inflections to be real words. A paper that made this point dramatically was Grodzinsky's (1984) report of several Hebrew-speaking agrammatic patients. The vowels in Hebrew words are determined by inflectional and derivational morphological considerations. For example, the word for a single male child is /YELED/, for a single female child /YALDA/, and in the plural the corresponding forms are /YILADIM/ and /YILADOT/. The three consonants /Y-L-D/ form a root, into which the markers for gender and number are interpolated. These markers consist of vowels (and a terminal consonant), and the particular vowel patterns are used in many words in the language: the various forms of the word for "dog," whose triconsonantal root is /K-L-V/, are /KELEV/, /KALVA/, /KILAVIM/ and /KILAVOT/. As Grodinsky (1984) pointed out, a patient who omitted the inflectional and derivational morphemes carried in this "vowel tier" would not be able to say anything, because the triconsonantal roots are unpronounceable. In fact, what Grodzinsky found his patients did was to omit freestanding function words, but substitute vowels from within the appropriate set of morphological items.

Yet other aspects of variation in the production of function words and bound morphemes may reflect little-understood attentional and control mechanisms, as is shown by a further study of the patient mentioned above, M.M. Realizing that M.M. had trouble mainly with certain words (auxiliary verbs and weak pronouns), Nespoulous et al. (1988) presented a written sentence to M.M. and highlighted these difficult words with a rose-colored magic marker. M.M. then read these highlighted words and the content words in the sentences correctly, but began to omit other function words. When both the original and the second set of affected function words were highlighted in subsequent trials, M.M. began to omit yet other function words. M.M. never omitted content words (nouns, verbs, or adjectives) in any of these experiments. Therefore, his impairment seemed to be limited to function words, but the extent of the impairment was not limited to the particular subset of function words he omitted in spontaneous speech. More detailed testing showed that other function words were affected, under particular task conditions. Nespoulous et al. suggested that the overt pattern of M.M.'s performance reflected a number of deficits—one related to function words as a whole, and one making for particular difficulty with a subset of function words—that are affected by attentional and control processes.

We thus see that several factors— the sonorance hierarchy, the status of an affix with respect to derivational or inflectional mor-

Table 8.3
Co-occurrence of Omissions and Substitutions of Function Words and
Bound Morphemes in Individual Patients

Error Types	Patients					Patients (Total)	Controls
	N.S.	J.F.	K.C.	D.I.	K.P.		
Open class							
Category	3	4	7	2	1	17	3
Subcategory	6	2	9	5	—	22	2
Omission	—	1	12	4	—	18	1
Addition	—	—	—	—	—	—	1
Closed class							
Category	—	—	—	—	—	—	1
Subcategory	5	4	6	5	1	21	5
Omission	4	6	8	6	5	29	9
Addition	—	—	1	2	—	3	1
Inflexional	7	9	18	18	4	56	9
Constructional	3	4	12	6	8	33	5
Residue	5	2	12	6	2	27	2
Totals	33	33	85	53	21	226	39

Reproduced with permission from Butterworth and Howard (1987, p. 13).

phology, the lexical status of a root or stem, the salience of a lexical item, attentional and control processes— go at least some way toward accounting for parts of the variation found in agrammatism. Some of these factors are better understood than others; notions like salience, attention, and control are harder to define with respect to sentence production tasks than the first three factors listed above. More research into these and other possible factors that make for variation in agrammatic output is needed.

To this point, we have discussed agrammatism as an example of a disturbance in which function words and bound morphemes are omitted. It has been known for some time that omissions of these elements rarely (if ever) occur in isolation, but are often accompanied by substitutions of morphological elements and freestanding function word vocabulary items (see table 8.3). Patients in whom substitutions predominate, and whose speech is fluent, are often said by clinicians to have a different syndrome known as "paragrammatism." The notion that paragrammatism is fundamentally different from agrammatism is under renewed attack, as recent observations have rediscovered and reemphasized the fact that the two patterns are not easily distinguished. Menn and Obler (1990) noted that all of the patients studied in their extensive cross-linguistic project on agrammatism showed both omissions and substitutions of function word and bound morpheme vocabulary elements. Heeschen (1985) also documented the co-occurrence of omission and substitution of freestanding function words and morphological elements in so-called agrammatism, and de Bleser (1986) pointed out that this co-occurrence had also been noted by many classic aphasiologists.

Agrammatism and paragrammatism may in fact reflect fundamentally similar disturbances of production of the function word and bound morpheme vocabularies. Grodzinsky (1984) argued that the fundamental problem in both agrammatism and paragrammatism is the mis-selection of the appropriate element from a set of morphological items. Grodzinsky suggested that omission of elements in agrammatism simply reflects a preference for phonologically empty elements of these morphological sets, whenever such elements exist, constrained by the requirement that lexical items be produced.

There are relatively few detailed studies of the patterns of substitution of function words and morphemes in paragrammatism. The studies that do exist show a considerable variety of patterns of substitutions (similar to the variety of patterns of omission seen in different agrammatic patients). We have already noted that some patients with both omissions and substitutions in their speech make substitutions primarily in a subset of the bound morphemes in their language, such as the patient reported by Miceli et al. (1983) who made many substitutions in verb suffixes. The clinician can anticipate seeing a wide variety of different profiles of substitution of function words and bound morphemes in different patients.

In some patients, there seems to be some systematicity to the pattern of substitutions. Lapointe (1983) analyzed the production of infinitives and gerunds in English agrammatic patients in relationship to the morphological stucture of the English verbal system. Infinitives and gerunds are the basic forms in the entire verbal system and, Lapointe argues, they are produced because they are the first to be accessed by patients with limited resources available for accessing verb forms. In other cases, substitutions are closely related to the inferred target. Miceli, Giustolisi, and Caramazza (1990) reported that one of their patients, who made both omission and substitution errors on bound morphemes, produced verbal affixes closely related to the intended affix when he made errors. In almost all cases, errors are "paradigm internal," that is, they do not violate the word formation and even the syntactic processes of the language. Thus, in a language like Italian that has several verb declensions marked by different thematic vowels, substitutions of verb affixes almost always respect the declension of the verb root. In Hebrew, substitutions of the vowels in words are always appropriate to the type of word being produced; shifts from one morphological paradigm to another and purely phonological errors do not occur with any frequency. It thus appears that many constraints on word formation processes are respected in both paragrammatism and agrammatism.

What is the origin of these disturbances in producing function words and bound morphemes? There seem to be two broad sources of these impairments, at least for agrammatism. Some patients who omit function words and bound morphemes have disturbances affecting the production or processing of these items in isolation (see chapter 6). This suggests a primary disturbance of lexical access on the production (output) side for these elements. The second major category of agrammatic patients is those who have trouble with function words and bound morphemes in sentence production but not in isolation. We shall consider these impairments in turn.

Several well-known studies by Bradley and her colleagues (see Bradley et al., 1980) suggested that agrammatic patients might have disturbances affecting their ability to access visually presented function words. Some researchers have also argued that the co-occurrence of syntactic comprehension disorders with expressive agrammatism reflected a "central" disturbance in the processing of function words and bound morphemes (Zurif, 1984).[7] These arguments are now discredited by studies that failed to replicate the original results of Bradley et al. and by reports of cases with expressive agrammatism but not comprehension deficits (see chapter 7). However, though these analyses are no longer convincing, it is still likely that some patients with agrammatism have disturbances affecting the processing of function words and bound morphemes at the single word level. Many patients with agrammatism have deep dyslexia (see chapter 5), and cannot read function words and bound morphemes aloud. Others, such as patient F.S. (chapter 6) have problems repeating some morphological forms. In cases such as this, several authors have suggested that the omission of function words and bound morphemes seen in sentence production is related to these processing disturbances at the single word level.

In other patients, however, agrammatism occurs only in relationship to sentence planning and production, without any disturbance of processing function words or bound morphemes in isolation. Caramazza and Hillis (1988) present a patient of this sort, and M.M., the patient mentioned above, also appears to have had trouble with auxiliary verbs and weak pronouns only when he had to produce sentences. M.M. had no trouble reading or repeating these words in isolation or in recognizing them as words in a lexical decision task, but he tended to omit them often in speech, repetition, and reading, when dealing with sentences. In fact, in certain situations, M.M. sometimes realized that a sequence of words was a sentence, and only then began to have trouble with these function words. For instance, Nespoulous et al. (1988) tried an experiment in which they asked M.M. to read words written vertically, one to a page. M.M. did so perfectly, turning the pages over and reading each word, until he quite suddenly realized that the sequence of words formed a sentence. From that point on, he had difficulty with the items in these affected groups of words.

Overall, these studies indicate that patients can have disturbances affecting closed class vocabulary elements in sentence production tasks. It is rare for these disturbances to occur in isolation, but a few patients with fairly restricted disturbances of this sort have been described.

Disturbances of Generating Syntactic Form

We have been discussing disturbances patients have in producing function words and bound morphemes. These disturbances would be expected to affect the construction of syntactic structure, if the mechanism involved in generating syntactic structure requires that lexical access for function words and bound morphemes be normal. This might be true whether the disturbance in producing function words and bound morphemes arose both in single word and sentence production tasks or only in sentence production tasks. It might also be true regardless of whether the disturbance appears as primarily one of omission of function words and bound morphemes, one of substitution of these vocabulary elements, or one of both omission and substitution.

Though all these possibilities exist in theory, observations of aphasic patients suggests that there are different disturbances of sentence form generation in cases with primarily omission and primarily substitution of these elements, that is, in agrammatism and paragrammatism. Paragrammatism differs markedly from agrammatism in that paragrammatic speech is typically fluent and syntactically varied, while agrammatic speech is typically hesitant and syntactically impoverished. For this reason, I shall discuss these two conditions separately, keeping in mind the fact that virtually all patients who have one of these disturbances of production of function words and bound morphemes have both, and that the different patterns of syntactic production found in different cases are most clearly seen in patients whose production is more clearly characterizable as agrammatic or paragrammatic.

It has been suggested by several researchers (Kean, 1982, Caplan, 1985, Schwartz, 1987) that some forms of agrammatism may be associated with or even be due to disturbances affecting the construction of the positional level of sentence representation (in Garrett's model of sentence production). In support of this view is the fact that disturbances in producing syntactic structures are extremely common in agrammatic patients. Goodglass et al. (1972) documented the syntactic constructions produced by one agrammatic patient and found virtually no syntactically well-formed utterance. All the agrammatic patients studied in a large contemporary cross-language study showed some impoverishment of syntactic structure in spontaneous speech (Menn et al., 1990). The failure to produced complex NPs and embedded verbs with normal frequency were the most striking features of the syntactic simplification shown by these patients.

Studies of sentence repetition by agrammatic patients also document their syntactic planning limitations. Ostrin (1982) reported the performance of four agrammatic patients in repeating sentences with a variable number of NPs, prepositional phrases (PP), and adjectives modifying nouns. She found that the patients had a strong tendency to repeat either a determiner and a noun (the man) or an adjective and a noun (old man), but not both (the old man). She characterized this finding as showing that the presence of a determiner as a prenominal modifier was not independent of the presence of an adjective in the same position in these patients. Similarly, in sentences with both an NP and a PP in the VP (*The woman is showing the dress to the man*), the patients showed a similar tendency to produce either the NP or the PP but not both. However, the patients' multiple attempts to repeat the target sentences often produced all the elements of the sentence, one on each attempt. Ostrin suggested that these results indicated that the patients retained the entire semantic content of the presented sentence but could not produce all the elements they retained. She suggested that these patients have a reduced number of "planning frames" that they can use. In general, this analysis is in the same spirit as those that have suggested that the problem in agrammatism involves a failure to construct syntactic structures, though some of the details of all these proposals differ slightly.

A second study of the repetition abilities of six agrammatic subjects introduces other considerations into the analysis of what is wrong with these patients. Ostrin and Schwartz (1986) had their patients repeat semantically reversible, semantically plausible, and semantically implausible sentences in the active and passive voice. They found that errors differed for plausible, reversible and implausible sentences. Errors to plausible sentences were primarily lexical substitutions. Many errors to implausible sentences reversed the thematic roles in the sentence to render the resulting utterance plausible. The patients tended to retain the order of nouns and verbs in the presented sentence, and made many errors that the authors analyze as efforts to produce passive forms ("mixed morphology errors" such as *The bicycle is riding by the boy* for *The bicycle is riding the boy*). The authors argue that the performances of their patients reflected a tendency on their part to produce plausible sentences from an incomplete memory trace that contained the grammatical roles (subject, object) of the noun phrases in the presented sentence.

The production of one particular type of function word, prepositions, is of particular interest and bears on the relationship of omissions to syntactic planning. The facts that there are a limited and fixed number of prepositions and that they do not enter into word formation processes productively (see chapter 6) mark prepositions as members of the function word vocabulary. However, some prepositions have semantic content that is intuitively similar to that of open class words; for instance, locative prepositions express relationships that are somewhat similar to the relationships expressed by some verbs. Similarly, other prepositions are the heads of their syntactic phrases, as is true of nouns and verbs. Thus prepositions share some features of the open class vocabulary. In fact, Garrett (1982) has found that the spontaneous speech errors affecting prepositions made by normal subjects have features of the errors made on both open and closed class vocabulary elements.

Studies of the production of prepositions by agrammatic patients indicate that different types of prepositions show greater or lesser susceptibility to omission. Friederici (1982) reported that 12 agrammatic aphasic patients were better at supplying prepositions with lexical content (such as *under* in *The dog is under the table*) than prepositions that are entirely determined by the verb of a sentence and play little semantic role (such as *for* in *He hopes for a nice present*) in a sentence completion task. Ostrin (1982) reported that there were more omissions of the latter type of preposition and more substitutions for the former type in a sentence repetition task. These results are broadly consistent with the view that some agrammatic patients have difficulty with the production of syntactic structures, and that the omission of function words is related to that problem: prepositions with greater semantic similarity to open class words are better produced than those that play a more syntactic role.

Despite these impairments in sentence production in agrammatic patients, it is not clear that these disturbances affecting syntactic forms are related to these patients' omission of function words and bound morphemes. First, there is no clear connection between the disturbances in production of function words and bound morphemes seen in individual patients and their syntactic abnormalities. Second, though many agrammatic patients show severe reductions in the production of syntactic structures, not all patients do so. Miceli et al. (1983), Berndt (1987) and others, have documented patients who omit disproportionally high numbers of function words and bound morphemes but who produce an apparently normal range of syntactic structures.

It may be that the distinction between agrammatic patients whose agrammatism reflects a failure of accessing function words and bound morphemes in single word tasks and agrammatic patients whose problems only arise in sentence production is important in understanding the relationship of omission of grammatical elements to syntactic simplification. It is possible that the agrammatic patients that do not show syntactic simplification are agrammatic patients whose disturbances affect the production of function words and bound morphemes in isolation. It is perhaps not to be expected that syntactic aspects of sentences would be affected in these cases. A more specific and restricted claim based on Garrett's model is that those agrammatic patients whose omission of function words and bound morphemes only occurs in sentence production and not in single word processing tasks will have disturbances affecting the construction of syntactic structures (Caplan, 1986, note 2).

There are few data on this point, but the two agrammatic cases I am aware of whose single word processing has been examined in detail and shown to be normal both have significant reductions in the syntactic structures they produce. M.M. (Nespoulous et al., 1988) has almost no embedded structures and very few elaborated NPs in his speech, and M.L. (Caramazza and Hillis, 1989) was even more impaired in the production of syntactic structures, with a mean length of utterance of less than 1.5 words and almost no well-formed sentences at all. It may be that certain forms of agrammatism *are* accompanied by significant disturbances in the production of syntactic phrases because the disturbance affecting the function word/bound morpheme vocabulary elements arises at a stage in sentence planning intimately connected to the elaboration of syntactic structures.

Turning to paragrammatic patients, several studies suggest that the syntactic production of these patients differs from that found in agrammatic patients. For instance, Butterworth and Howard (1987) described five paragrammatic patients who each produced many "long and complex sentences, with multiple interdependencies of constituents (p. 23)," such as those shown in table 8.4. In addition, their patients also correctly inflected neologisms (see table 8.4), indicating that they were sometimes able to access and use the correct inflection even when a lexical item was not retrieved (see also Caplan et al., 1972, for discussion of this phenomenon). However, paragrammatic errors do include substitution errors, affecting closed class items, as noted above. Errors in paragrammatism include (but are not restricted to) errors in tag questions, illegal noun phrases in relative clauses, and illegal use of pronouns to head relative clauses

Table 8.4
Examples of Paragrammatic Errors

Blends

Patients

N.S. Isn't look very dear, is it?
ISN'T   VERY DEAR, IS IT?
Doesn't LOOK VERY DEAR, does it?

J.F. I mean they don't get very wet through
THEY DON'T GET VERY WET
THEY DON'T GET   WET THROUGH

K.C. I'm very want it
I'M VERY keen on IT
I   WANT IT

D.J. I've got a publican
I'VE GOT A pub
I am a   PUBLICAN

Controls

I.R. They were all had pleasant sandy beaches
THEY WERE ALL   PLEASANT SANDY BEACHES
THEY   ALL HAD PLEASANT SANDY BEACHES

D.G. The father's imagination is tends to frequent the bar
THE FATHER's IMAGINATIONS IS   fre-
quenting THE BAR
THE FATHER's IMAGINATION   TENDS TO FRE-
QUENT   THE BAR

(Butterworth and Howard, 1987). A particular type of error that has often been commented on in paragrammatism is a "blend", in which the output seems to reflect two different ways of saying the same thing (see table 8.4). These features of the speech of paragrammatic patients are not found in agrammatic patients—at least not with the same frequency as in paragrammatism—and they suggest that there are differences in the ability of these different patients to construct syntactic structures.

Very few studies of paragrammatic patients' performances on more constrained sentence production tasks have been undertaken. However, one well-known result based on a more constrained test —anagram solution—also indicates differences in the ability of fluent paragrammatic and nonfluent agrammatic patients to construct syntactic structures. Von Stockerdt (1972; von Stockerdt and

Table 8.4
Continued

Inflected Neologisms
Patients

J.F.　with a pair of /ɪDɪsɪz/ or whatchemecallem
(correct: pluralization of noun)
J.F.　this person is /raʊndʒɪŋ/
(progressive aspect of verb)
J.F.　you get /dæbd/ up
(Past participle)
N.S.　put over two /baɪlz/ the were /sneɪkt/ in
(Pluralization of noun; past participle)
N.S.　Mr. Lavender, he did drive all the /aɪənvɔlz/
(pluralization of noun)
K.C.　when she /wɪksəz/ a /zen/ from me
(third singular present tense; singular noun)
K.C.　I was /pleɪzd/ to see the other /dŋkjumen/
(past participle; singular noun)
D.J.　There's a bloke trying to sell /peɪtɔz/
(pluralization of noun)
D.J.　She then /dɪfraɪdɪd/ that . . .
(past tense)
K.P.　You see nice /peɪpəneəz/
(pluralization of noun)

Reproduced with permission from Butterworth and Howard (1987, pp 19–20, 24).

Bader, 1976) found that paragrammatic patients solved anagram tasks according to syntactic constraints whereas agrammatic patients solved them using semantic constraints. Paragrammatic patients have not been tested as much as agrammatic patients on repetition, picture description, and story completion tasks, to ascertain whether they use both basic and more complex syntactic structures to convey specific propositional and discourse-level semantic features. The common belief is that they are much more capable of using a wide range of syntactic structures for these purposes than agrammatic patients, but make errors in their use.

Butterworth (1982, 1985, Butterworth and Howard, 1987) has argued that the syntactic and morphological errors in paragrammatism result from the failure of these patients to monitor and control their own output. If this is correct, the basic locus of the syntactic errors in paragrammatism may differ from those in agrammatism. Agrammatism would reflect a disturbance of one basic aspect of the sentence-building process—the construction of syntactic form—while paragrammatism would result from a disturbance of control mechanisms that monitor the speech-planning process. This analysis assumes that normals often generate erroneous utterances unconsciously, and that these errors are filtered out by control processes. Butterworth has argued that this is indeed the case.

Several studies indicate that aphasic patients' abilities to utilize syntactic devices to convey aspects of sentence meaning depend upon the devices commonly used in their language. Bates and her colleagues have studied the abilities of patients to produce simple sentences in a language that makes extensive use of word order and little use of declensional or inflectional morphology (English), a language that makes extensive use of declensional morphology (German), a language that makes heavy use of inflectional agreement (Italian), and a language that uses both inflectional and declensional forms (Serbo-Croatian) (see Bates and Wulfeck, 1989, for a review of these studies). In each case, the patients tended to produce structures that incorporated the most commonly used syntactic markers in the language, and had difficulties producing sentences that required the use of less commonly used devices. This finding indicates that the "canonicity" of a structure or a grammatical device—the degree to which it is used in a particular language—influences the ability of a patient to employ that device to express aspects of sentential meaning. These disturbances have been most clearly described in agrammatic patients, and it remains to be seen whether they affect patients with primarily paragrammatic output, as well as patients with other types of aphasic disturbances (such as various forms of anomia, phonological disturbances, etc.).

Disturbances Affecting the Realization of Thematic Roles

Several researchers have suggested that there is a more "profound" disturbance of sentence production in certain patients. This disturbance has been said to affect the patients' ability to use the basic word order of English to convey propositional features such as thematic roles. Saffran et al. (1980b) presented data regarding the order of nouns around verbs in sentences produced by five agrammatic patients describing simple pictures of actions. The authors noted a strong effect of animacy upon the position of the nouns around the verbs (see chapter 7, figure 7.11). The authors suggested that thematic roles were not mapped onto the canonical noun-verb-noun word order of English, and that animacy determined the position of nouns around verbs in these patients. They concluded that agrammatic patients have either lost the basic linguistic notions of thematic roles (agency, theme) or else cannot use even the basic word order of the language to express this sentential semantic feature. They argued that this more profound deficit cannot be related to problems with the function word–inflection vocabulary, and, therefore, that agrammatic patients have more than one impairment affecting sentence planning and production. Though Caplan (1983) argued that the data in the study of Saffran et al. did not support the authors' contention that animacy alone determined word order in the patients' responses, this report raises the question of whether the basic linguistic notions of thematic roles are always preserved in aphasia and whether patients always try to use some sort of structure to convey them. It is possible that some very severely affected patients lose these concepts or do not attempt to convey them. At the least, it appears that some agrammatic patients tend to assign agency to animate items, even where the task calls for the assignment of another thematic role to an animate noun (see chapter 7 for further discussion).

The ability to produce utterances that convey thematic roles is closely linked to the ability to produce verbs. Many agrammatic patients have particular difficulties with the production of verbs. These difficulties do not entirely consist of trouble in producing the correct inflectional and derivational forms of a verb in a given context. They also affect the ability to produce verbs themselves, resulting in omissions, paraphrases, and nominalizations of verbs such as those shown in table 8.5.

Two recent studies have investigated this disturbance of verb production in agrammatic patients, with similar results. Miceli et al. (1984) compared five agrammatic, five anomic, and ten normal subjects on tests requiring naming objects (the Boston Naming Test: Kaplan, Goodglass, and Weintraub, 1976) or actions (the Action Naming Test: Obler and Albert, 1979). They found that the agrammatic patients were better at naming objects than actions, while the anomic patients and normal controls showed the opposite pattern. The agrammatic patients' difficulties in naming actions did

Table 8.5
Examples of Errors Affecting the Production of Verbs

(A) *Short excerpts from discourse showing function word and inflectional omissions:*

   (1) ah . . . Monday . . . ah. Dad and P.H. [the patient's name] and Dad . . . hospital. Two . . . ah. doctors . . . and ah . . . thirty minutes . . . and yes . . . ah . . . hospital. And, er Wednesday . . . nine o'clock. And er Thursday, ten o'clock . . . doctors. Two doctors . . . and ah . . . teeth. Yeah . . . fine

   (2) My mother died . . . uh . . . me . . . uh fi'teen. Uh. oh. I guess six month . . . my mother pass away. An' uh . . . an'en . . . uh . . . ah . . . seventeen . . . go uh High School. An'uh Christmas . . . well. uh. I uh . . . Pitt'burgh

(B) *Omission of main verbs:*

(Patient attempts to describe the picture of a girl presenting flowers to a teacher)

   (1) The young . . . the girl . . . the little girls is . . . the flower

   (2) The girls is . . . going to flowers

(C) *Nominalizations used instead of verbs:*

(Same situation as in B)

   (1) The girl is flower the woman

   (2) The girl is . . . is roses. The girl is rosin

(Picture of a man taking a photograph of a girl)

   (3) The man kodaks . . . and the girl . . . kodaks the girl

(D) *Semantic ill-formedness:*

(Picture of a man painting a house)

   (1) The painter washed the paint . . .

(Picture of a cat peeping out from behind an armchair)

   (2) The cat leans the sofa up . . .

(Picture of a boy giving a valentine to a girl)

   (3) The boy put the valentine into this girl

Reproduced with permission from Badecker and Caramazza (1985, pp. 107–109).

not appear to arise at the level of achieving the concept of the action, since many erroneous responses were nouns, phrases, and nominalizations that were related to the intended verbs. Miceli and his colleagues concluded that their agrammatic patients had a sort of anomia for verbs—a disturbance separate from the other aspects of their output.

What relationship does a disturbance affecting verbs have to the rest of a patient's language abilities? Given the crucial role that verbs play in sentences, one would expect that a disturbance affecting the ability to use information regarding verbs would severely affect many other aspects of sentence production and comprehension. In at least one instance, McCarthy and Warrington (1985) have argued that this is the case. Their patient, R.O.X., had a severe disturbance in naming actions and matching verbs to pictures. The authors argued that this disturbance was the result of a category-specific degradation of the meaning of verbs that also resulted in almost no production of verbs in speech and in difficulties in syntactic comprehension. However, the relationship between an inability to produce verbs and other abnormalities in the speech of agrammatic patients is not always so clear. In the study of Miceli et al., patients' inabilities to produce verbs were only partially responsible for the shortened phrase length found in their speech, since the overall correlation between the noun-verb ratio and phrase length in the five agrammatic patients was not high. It thus appears that some agrammatic patients have a disturbance affecting their ability to produce verbs, and that this disturbance can affect their ability to accomplish some sentence processing tasks such as spontaneously producing a normal range of syntactic structures, but that some patients can build at least some phrasal structures despite poor verb production while others cannot produce normal phrase structure despite relatively good verb production.

Disturbances Affecting Intonational Contours

Many patients have difficulty producing prosodic aspects of speech. In many cases, these disturbances are secondary to motor output disorders (Monrad Kohn, 1947; Kent and Rosenbek, 1983). Recent work has begun to investigate disturbances affecting duration of segments and pauses, pitch, and other aspects of the speech signal related to prosody, many of which show up in the production of single

words (Kent and Rosenbek, 1983; Gandour and Dararananda, 1984).
In this section, we consider aspects of these disturbances that appear
to be related to the production of intonational contours relevant to
the structure of phrases and sentences.

Two reports in the recent literature describe acoustic correlates of
these disturbances in a reading-aloud task. Danly and Shapiro (1982)
examined prosodic capacities of patients with Broca's aphasia, and
Danly, Cooper, and Shapiro (1983) those of Wernicke's aphasic patients. Both these studies measured speakers' fundamental frequency (F_0), one of the principal determinants of intonational contour.
Several aspects of F_0 were measured that are normally present in
speech: the decline in F_0 from the beginning of an utterance to its
end; the sentence-final fall in F_0; the frequency and determinants of
resetting of F_0; the relationship between sentence-initial F_0 (known
as P_1) and sentence length; and the presence of so-called continuation rises in F_0, which indicate that the utterance is not complete.
In addition to these measurements of F_0, sentence-final segment
lengthening was also measured.

Five patients with Broca's aphasia were found to have a sentence-
final drop in F_0 that was larger than that found in normal controls.
These patients also showed some declination in F_0 as the utterance
progressed, but only for short utterances and only in some trials.
There was frequent resetting of F_0, and the degree of resetting was
greater than that found in normal controls. Resetting of F_0 occurred
as frequently at minor syntactic boundaries (prepositional phrases)
as at major boundaries (relative clauses), unlike the finding in normals that the strength of a syntactic boundary correlates well with
the presence of F_0 resetting. Continuation rises also occurred at
minor boundaries more often than was true of normals. There was
no higher P_1 for longer sentences than for shorter sentences, and
sentence-final segment lengthening was not present. Emmorey
(1987) reported similar results in agrammatic patients with respect
to the production of pitch and segment duration as a function of
producing compound nouns (*black'board*) and noun phrases *black
board'*). None of six testable Broca's aphasic patients were able to
use pitch (F_0) contours as indicators of the difference between these
forms, and only two of these patients could use duration of the
words or of the interword silent period for this purpose. All these
authors concluded that these patients retained some aspects of
intonational contour but not others. Danly and Shapiro argued

that the overall existence of a sentence was coded into intonational contours, but not specific aspects of syntactic structure.

Many results were similar in five patients with Wernicke's aphasia studied in a second report (Danly et al., 1983). Sentence-final F_0 fall was exaggerated. Four of the five patients showed normal declination in F_0. Interestingly, this normal F_0 declination occurred regardless of whether or not the patient made many paraphasias or produced neologisms. There was more frequent resetting of F_0 in the patients than in normal subjects, especially in sentences of intermediate length. As with the patients with Broca's aphasia, resetting of F_0 occurred as frequently at minor syntactic boundaries (prepositional phrases) as at major boundaries (relative clauses), unlike the finding in normals. Continuation rises were more common than in normals, and also occurred at minor boundaries more often than was true of normals. Unlike the Broca's aphasic patients, there was a higher P_1 for longer sentences than for shorter sentences. In addition, these patients showed greater variability in F_0 than controls. The authors concluded that these patients also retained most aspects of intonational contour but did not use intonation to encode specific aspects of syntactic structure. In addition, the finding that F_0 declination did not correlate with the presence of paraphasias and neologisms suggested that the planning of intonational contour and segmental phonological values is under separate control.

Shapiro and Danly (1985) extended some of these observational techniques to the study of patients with right hemisphere lesions. They reported that patients with anterior and central right hemisphere lesions showed abnormally low F_0's and an abnormally small range of F_0, leading to less variability in F_0 than in normals. Patients with posterior right hemisphere lesions had the opposite pattern. These patterns occurred regardless of the emotion associated with a sentence. The authors argued that these patterns represented a primary disturbance of intonation in right hemisphere–damaged patients that differed as a function of lesion location in the hemisphere. However, this conclusion has been questioned by both Ryalls (1986) and Colsher, Cooper, and Graff-Radford (1987). These authors argue that the variability in F_0 that Shapiro and Danly found could have resulted simply from the overall level of setting of F_0 : a higher level of F_0 allows for more variation in F_0 and a lower level allows for less. Emmorey (1987) also failed to find any differences between normals and right hemisphere–damaged patients on her tests. Overall, the evidence that patients with right hemisphere lesions have impairments in generating linguistically relevant prosody is weak.

Right hemisphere–damaged patients do have trouble, however, in using prosody to confer emotional state. Ross and Mesulam (1979) have described right hemisphere–damaged patients whose abilities to express happiness, sadness, and other emotions through intonational contours is virtually nonexistent. These authors have used the term "aprosodia" to refer to this condition. This is a potentially confusing usage, since it is important to distinguish between the ability to use intonation and prosody in the fashion required by the language code to convey aspects of the structure and meaning of words and sentences, and the ability to use these features of speech to convey emotional states.

Overall, these results indicate that the generation of linguistically determined prosody can be impaired. A variety of acoustic correlates of intonation exist, and the ability to produce these individual correlates dissociates, as least as far as production of F_0 and segmental lengthening is concerned. It appears that the ability to produce intonational contours is impaired more frequently and more severely in patients with disturbances affecting the production of segmental phonological values, but the two abilities do appear to be separate to some degree. The ability to produce intonational contours does seem to correlate strongly with the ability to produce syntactically well-formed structures: no patients have been described who produce completely syntactically correct sequences of words with inappropriate intonational contours. However, some mild Wernicke's aphasic patients (and possibly some right hemisphere–damaged patients) do seem to have minimal but definite impairments in intonation that might not reflect disturbances in producing syntactic structures. The range of specific impairments in the production of intonational contours largely remains to be explored.

SUMMARY

I have described some of the more common disturbances of production of sentence form seen in aphasia. As everywhere in this text, I have tried to relate these patterns to the functional architecture of the language processing system. Briefly, we have found that patients with agrammatic speech show different patterns of omission of function words and inflectional morphemes, some of which are explicable on the basis of linguistic and psycholinguistic principles. Many agrammatic patients have problems constructing normal syntactic structures, and the range of syntactic structures that are constructed varies greatly. Whether these restrictions are in any way related to the patterns of omission of function words and bound morphemes found in individual cases is not clear. In addition, some agrammatic patients omit verbs or make other errors on verbs that may entail disturbances in realizing thematic roles. Studies on paragrammatism indicate that patients of this sort typically also have disorders of syntactic structure, but do produce many well-formed complex syntactic structures. It has been suggested that their errors arise at a quite different stage of speech planning than the syntactic simplifications seen in agrammatism, one involving the control of the process of constructing syntactic form. Finally, many patients have disturbances affecting their ability to produce intonational contours on the basis of syntactic structures and sentence meaning. When these disturbances affecting the construction of sentence form are added to those that arise in single word production, patients' speech may become abnormal in quite complex ways.

NOTES

1. I do not discuss written sentence production because not enough is known about it and its disorders.

2. The information that the cat in question is a particular one whereas the dog is just any dog is also available to the speaker, but I shall not concentrate on this aspect of meaning at this point. It is discussed in chapter 9.

3. In addition to these factors, the determinants of vocal tract movement also include emotional state (anger, sadness, etc.), attitude (irony), and others. It is quite amazing how many different aspects of information are expressed through a single production system.

4. Some authors (e.g., Badecker and Caramazza, 1985) have argued that the failure of linguistically oriented aphasiologists to choose among these various definitions of the vocabulary elements affected in agrammatism is an argument against the coherence of the category "agrammatism" itself. This seems an odd conclusion (Caplan, 1986). It would be analogous to saying that, because there are controversies about the nature of semantic representations, we cannot speak of disturbances of lexical semantic processing; because there are controversies about how written word forms are represented, we cannot speak of disturbances of activation of written word forms, etc. It is, of course, quite reasonable to hope that future research will provide evidence that one or another of the various characterizations of

affected elements will be shown to characterize the deficit found in specific patients or groups of patients, but the fact that present theories are only an approximation to the data and are all subjects of scientific controversy is not a reason to reject them altogether.

5. Kean's division of these affixes into these categories requires that "semantic" affixes, such as plural markers, be classed as derivational. This is a controversial analysis. It is justified on the ground that plural markers are not related to "syntactic" facts such as agreement, but it is not justifed on the ground that derivational morphology tends to create new categories of words from existing simple words. (See chapter 6 for discussion of these questions.)

6. The factor of salience does not apply to all agrammatic patients, according to Goodglass. He claims that some agrammatic patients have a problem at a more conceptual level of language involving relationships between words, statements, and concepts. However, Goodglass postulates that salience is the factor that influences the performance of those agrammatic patients who do not have this "conceptual" form of the syndrome.

7. Zurif (1984), who has made this argument, claimed that the "central" disturbance affecting these vocabulary elements is due to disruption of an access procedure that is operative when these items are activated on the basis of their syntactic functions (as opposed to their semantic meanings). He thus specified two access mechanisms for these elements, only one of which is affected in agrammatism. The evidence for this claim is based upon results obtained by Bradley et al. (1980), and this theory is thus substantially weakened by the failure to replicate the findings of Bradley et al.

9 Comprehension and Production of Discourse

To this point in this book, we have dealt with single words, morphologically complex words, and sentences. In this chapter, I venture beyond the single sentence, into the realm of discourse. This is a vast area, and I shall only touch upon some of the many topics and issues that fall in this domain. The discourse level is the level of language that relates each item and proposition to what has gone before. It captures the organization of sentences into higher-order structures that express the topics in a discourse, and the flow of information from topic to topic. The structure of a discourse is therefore closely linked to the intentions and attentional state of the participants in a discourse. I review theories of discourse structure and experimental research that deals with aspects of how discourse structures are processed, and then turn to disorders of discourse comprehension and production seen in brain-damaged patients.

THE STRUCTURE OF DISCOURSE

As noted above, discourse is a level of language structure. Like all the levels of linguistic structure discussed in this book, the level of discourse structure introduces new semantic features into language. Among these features are what the topic of a sentence or a portion of the discourse is, which ideas are leading ideas and which are subordinate, what information has previously been presented in the discourse and what has not, what information a speaker can assume the listener should know and what information has to be explicitly presented in a new sentence, and others.

Modern approaches see discourse structure as being related to the purpose of a discourse itself, that is, as an outgrowth of the intentions of the speakers and listeners. These intentions usually involve the desire to convey or receive information, to have certain actions performed, to ask questions, etc.[1] When people use language to realize these intentions, they must structure their linguistic productions in particular ways. A person who wishes to inform someone about the political events leading up to the American Civil War must produce propositions that describe those events. He or she must also produce those propositions in an organized fashion—it would be a good idea to produce them in chronological order, or in relationship to the roles of particular individuals, and not as a random list of statements. The listener who wishes to receive and understand this discourse has work to do too. He or she must understand each proposition and relate it to some part of the larger topic.

Discourse structures are somewhat different from the language structures have been discussed to this point in this book. The language-processing components that we have discussed up to now relate a set of linguistic forms (words and sentences) to various aspects of meaning—concepts and items in the world; modifiers of those concepts and items; and the actions, states, and events that relate those concepts and items to each other. These concepts are directly related to the forms of simple words and are encoded in the forms of derived words and sentences, in the sense that the literal meaning of a word or sentence is accessible from these linguistic elements without any other semantic process intervening. We know (or don't know) something about the word *dog*: that dogs are domestic mammals with certain physical and functional characteristics. Likewise, once we assign the syntactic structure of a sentence, we know how that structure affects sentential semantic values (e.g., we know that *the cat* is the agent of *ate* in *The cat that chased the mouse ate the cheese* once we know that it is the subject of *ate*). Discourse structures are not entirely of this sort. In discourse, a listener must make a wide variety of inferences on the basis of the propositions that are directly presented, in order to structure and understand the discourse.

It is rarely, if ever, the case that a speaker conveys every bit of information that is logically needed to relate the propositions in a discourse to each other. Rather, the speaker relies on the assumption that the listener already knows a great deal about the world and even, at times, about the topic under discussion, that he can refer back to material that has just been presented, that he can shift the focus of his attention from one topic to another and then return to the first topic, etc. Making these assumptions allows the speaker to omit certain statements (those he or she believes the listener already has access to), and requires the speaker to use a variety of cues to indicate where the focus of attention is in the discourse. The listener, in turn, assumes that the speaker is assuming that he or she (the listener) can access long-term memory, keep track of what has been said, shift attention, etc., and the listener further assumes that the speaker is structuring the discourse and making use of linguistic devices that reflect his or her (the listener's) ability to keep up with the discourse. Speakers and listeners thus follow a complex set of rules regarding how a discourse can be structured.

Let us look at a very simple example of how these factors affect what is produced in a discourse. Suppose a speaker produces passage (1).

(1)   John and Mary went to Lily's last night. They were happy they did. They found the food delicious and were still raving about the dessert a day later.

The listener will naturally infer several things: that Lily's is a place where John and Mary ate; that they liked the food they had there, etc. None of these propositions is actually stated in (1). A listener infers them, or something like them, because he or she seeks to impose semantic coherence on the entire discourse in (1). Passage (1) is coherent, not because all these propositions are spelled out, but because the speaker is making the safe assumption that they can be inferred by the listener on the basis of what he or she knows about the world.

Researchers have investigated some of the basic principles that underlie the structure of discourse. Research by Grice (1975), Searle (1969), and others (e.g., Sperber and Wilson, 1986) has identified principles that guide utterances, such as: "Be informative," "Do not present information the listener can be expected to already have," etc. In passage (1), these principles have applied to allow for the omission of the propositions we filled in above.

These principles apply to more than just what can be left out of a discourse and what must be part of one. Many features of discourse are influenced by principles such as these. For instance, one widely studied discourse feature is the use of so-called indirect directives—utterances such as (2) that have the form of questions but are in fact requests for action.

(2)   Man at table: Can you pass the salt?

Utterance (2), rather than an utterance in the form of a command, is used as a request for action in social situations calling for a certain level of politeness. Utterance (3) is not an appropriate response to (2), but response (4), which involves no utterance at all, is:

(3)   Second man at table: Yes.

(4)   Second man at table: [passes the salt].

Examples such as (2) indicate that the principles enunciated by Grice, Searle, and others mediate the relationship between *intentions* and the utterances in a discourse. This relationship is part of the larger subject of pragmatics. Pragmatics, broadly conceived, is the study of the relationship between behavior and intentions. It extends to the study of social interactions, and includes the analysis of many nonverbal phenomena. Within the area of language use, pragmatics involves analysis of a wide variety of phenomena, such as the effect of the social status of the participants in a discourse on linguistic forms; the relationship between the setting of a discourse and the linguistic features of the discourse; the use of metaphor; the association between gesture and utterances, etc. (for reviews of aspects of pragmatics related to language, see Bates, 1976; Horn, 1988; Sperber and Wilson, 1986; Murphy, 1990). In this book, I will not be dealing with much of the larger field of pragmatics. It is important however, to touch on those aspects of pragmatics that relate the intentional and attentional states of the speaker and the listener to the meanings of words and sentences and the relationship of propositions in a discourse.

Let us pursue this approach to discourse by considering the following dialogue (adapted from Grosz and Sidner, 1986):

(5)   Man at railroad ticket counter: What track is the next train to Detroit?
Ticket agent: Track 12, but it's a local. The 1:45 will get you there sooner.

A response to the question posed by the first speaker could simply involve indicating the location of the next train to Detroit. However, the respondent provides more information—the fact that the next train is a local and that a later train will arrive in Detroit earlier. This information is not perceived as being out of place; on the contrary, it is perceived as being directly relevant to the first speaker's question.

What part of the first speaker's question is the additional informa-tion provided by the ticket agent relevant to? Certainly not the prop-ositional content of that question: the first speaker's question does not request information about the nature of the next train to Detroit or about whether later trains arrive in Detroit sooner. Rather, the additional information advanced by the second speaker is relevant to the inferred intentions of the first speaker. These inferred inten-tions include, roughly, the propositions (1) that the first speaker asked about the location of the next train to Detroit because he wished to go to Detroit and (2) that he probably wished to arrive in Detroit as soon as possible. Reasoning based on real-world knowl-edge does enter into establishing these inferred intentions: the tic-ket agent presumably believes that a man who enquires about the next train to Detroit probably wants to get there as soon as possible. But these assumptions based on real-world knowledge pertain to the intentions behind the first man's utterance, not its propositional content. Given these inferred intentions, the ticket agent's response is completely appropriate. If these inferences are wrong —if, for in-stance, the first speaker was inquiring about the location of the next train to Detroit because he wanted to meet someone who he thought was on that train—the additional information in the ticket agent's response is irrelevant.

Let us pursue this line a little further by imagining several con-tinuations of this interchange. Suppose the ticket agent was correct in his inferences. Then the dialogue might continue somewhat as in (6).

(6)   Man: Thank you. One ticket on the faster train, then, please [man hands over credit card].

Suppose, however, that the ticket agent has made the wrong infer-ence. Suppose the man wanted to meet someone on the next train to Detroit. hen the dialogue might continue as in (7).

(7)   Man: Thank you very much [man leaves and proceeds to track 12].

These scenarios illustrate two fundamental points about dis-courses. First, discourses are actions that are related to the inten-tions of the speakers. In (5) and (6), the first man's intention is to get to Detroit as soon as possible. In (5)–(7), it is to meet someone on the next Detroit train. In (5) and (6), the first man's intention is such that his next statement and his actions no longer deal with the topic of the first sentence (the next train to Detroit). In (5)–(7), the first man's intention is such that his next statement and his action does deal with the topic of the first sentence (the next train to Detroit).

Second, these scenarios indicate that coherent discourse is related to the intentions of the participants and to which of these intentions are being attended to at any point in time. The discourse has both an "intentional" and an "attentional" structure. Both these structures are created by the participants in the discourse and evolve as the discourse evolves. The intentional and attentional structure of a discourse can never be known in advance, even by the initiator of a discourse. In scenarios (5) and (6) and (5)–(7), for instance, the intentional and attentional structure of the discourse changes dramatically when the ticket agent offers information about another, potentially more attractive, train. The attention of the participants in the discourse is now drawn to this faster train. This shift in attention has consequences for the linguistic content of the subsequent discourse. It allows the speaker in (6) to use the term "the faster train" to refer to the 1:45 train. The ticket agent knows exactly which faster train he should provide a ticket for—the one that occupies the focus of attention in the present part of the discourse.

Grosz and her colleagues (Grosz and Sidner, 1986; Grosz, Pollack, and Sidner, 1989) have developed a computer-based model of discourse that includes these three different levels of structure: the linguistic form of the utterances in a discourse, the speaker's and listener's intentions, and the speaker and listener's attentional state. In this model, discourses are divided into "discourse segments" that correspond to different intentions of the participants in the discourse. For instance, in dialogue (5), each utterance constitutes a discourse segment with its own intentions. The intentions associated with different discourse segments are related. For instance, the intention associated with the ticket agent's utterance in (5)—roughly, that the first speaker should come to know that there is a train that will arrive in Detroit before the one that leaves next on track 12—is related to the inferred intentions of the first speaker that have been set up by his initial utterance—roughly, that he wishes to get to Detroit as soon as possible. Boundaries between discourse segments are indicated in a variety of ways. In most cases, there are linguistic signs of these boundaries, including overt cue words (such as *by the way*, *incidentally*, etc.); changes in verb mood, tense, and aspect markers; intonational contours; etc. In many cases, however, the structure of the discourse is based upon the inferred intentions of the participants in the discourse. Grosz and her colleagues set up different "focus spaces" in a computer program corresponding to these different discourse segments. These focus spaces are placed in a vertical "stack," in which the topmost space is the one currently being attended to by the participants in the discourse. An illustration of the way Grosz and her colleagues approach the division of a discourse into discourse segments and establish the relationships between different segments is given in table 9.1 and figure 9.1.

The discourses we have just considered—passages (5) and (6) and (5)–(7) and the one illustrated in figure 9.1—have a fairly complex set of intentional and attentional states. This is the case for most, but not all, discourses. One type of discourse that does not have as complex an intentional structure is a narrative or a text, such as that presented in (1) above. In this type of discourse, there is little, if any, turn-taking, and the intentional states of the speaker and listener— to convey and receive information—remain essentially unchanged throughout the entire discourse. For this reason, it is possible to analyze the structure created by the propositions in a narrative or a text, without continually changing the intentional structure of the discourse. Several researchers have proposed models of the structure of narratives and texts that rely entirely on relations between the propositions in these discourses. I shall briefly present the model of this aspect of this type of discourse developed by Kintsch and van Dijk (1978; van Dijk and Kintsch, 1983), which has been used a great deal to analyze discourse function in brain-damaged patients.

According to this model, there are at least three different levels of structure in a text or narrative. The highest level of a text is its "schematic" structure—roughly, the flow of topics in a discourse. The second level groups together sequences of utterances that share a common topic. This level is frequently called the "macrostructure" of a discourse. The most elemental level of a discourse is that at which sentences are related to each other locally. This level of structure is often called the "microstructure" of a discourse. Kintsch and van Dijk (1978; van Dijk and Kintsch, 1983) propose various rules that map the microstructure of a discourse onto its macrostructure. I begin with a description of this lowest level of discourse structure, and work up to the highest level.

Table 9.1
A Segment of a Task-Orient Dialogue

DS1	(1)	E:	First you have to remove the flywheel.
	(2)	A:	How do I remove the flywheel?
	(3)	E:	First, loosen the two allen head setscrews holding it to the shaft, then pull it off
	(4)	A:	OK.
DS2	(5)		I can only find one screw. Where's the other one?
	(6)	E:	On the hub of the flywheel.
	(7)	A:	That's the one I found. Where's the other one?
	(8)	E:	About ninety degrees around the hub from the first one.
	(9)	A:	I don't understand. I can only find one. Oh wait, yes I think I was on the wrong wheel.
	(10)	E:	Show me what you are doing.
	(11)	A:	I was on the wrong wheel and I can find them both now.
DS3	(12)		The tool I have is awkward. Is there another tool that I could use instead?
	(13)	E:	Show me the tool you are using.
	(14)	A:	OK.
	(15)	E:	Are you sure you are using the right size key?
	(16)	A:	I'll try some others.
	(17)		I found an angle I can get at it.
DS4	(18)		The two screws are loose, but I'm having trouble getting the wheel off
DS5	(19)	E:	Use the wheelpuller. Do you know how to use it?
	(20)	A:	No.
	(21)	A:	Do you know what it looks like?
	(22)	A:	Yes.
	(23)	E:	Show it to me please.
	(24)	A:	OK.
	(25)	E:	Good, Loosen the screw in the center and place the jaws around the hub of the wheel, then tighten the screw onto the center of the shaft. The wheel should slide off.

Reproduced with permission from Grosz and Sidner (1986, p. 186).

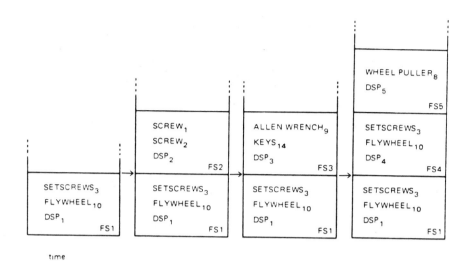

Figure 9.1
The evolution of the focus stack leading up to utterance 25 in table 9.1.
(Reproduced with permission from Grosz and Sidner, 1986, p. 191.)

Like many models of discourse structure, Kintsch and van Dijk assume that the input into the structure of a text are the propositions in the text. The ordered list of propositions that are extracted from sentences (and sentence fragments) constitutes the "text base" of the text. The microstructural level of organization of a text base has been most clearly related to continuity of reference, that is, to the continuing mention of items and actions from one proposition to another. This has been said to be "the most important single criterion for the coherence of text bases" (Kintsch and van Dijk, 1978, p. 366). The way continuity of reference is expressed linguistically reflects what several researchers have termed the "cohesion" of a discourse. Halliday and Hasan (1976) discuss several types of linguistic devices that can be used to express continuity of reference. These include the use of pronominals, substitution, ellipsis, conjunction, and lexical repetition. The following passages illustrate some of these devices making for cohesion.

(8) *Pronouns*: The colonel ordered the corporal to raise the flag, and he complied at once.

(9) *Ellipsis*: John asked Mary to help prepare the agenda for the meeting. She said she would be happy to.

(10) *Substitution*: We saw elephants, tigers, lions, and the new panda at the circus. The children were thrilled by the animals.

(11) *Lexical repetition*: To make hospital corners, lay a sheet out on the bed. Fold the ends of the sheet over the top of the bed. Tuck the ensuing flap under the mattress.

In (8), *he* refers to the corporal. In (9), what Mary would be happy to do is to help prepare the agenda for the meeting; the words *help prepare the agenda for the meeting* are omitted, but the continuity of reference is nonetheless clearly expressed. In (10), the term *the animals* is used to refer to the particular items mentioned earlier. In (11), the words *the sheet* are repeated. All of these devices establish continuity of reference and all are examples of cohesive devices.

The rules regulating the appropriate use of one or another cohesive device are complex, and I will not attempt to present them all in any detail. However, I will exemplify their use by briefly reviewing the way that pronouns establish co-reference.

As we saw in chapter 7, sentence-level grammar does not indicate what noun a pronoun refers to. This is determined by discourse factors. Consider the assignment of the antecedent of *they* in passage (1), repeated here for the reader's convenience.

(1) John and Mary went to Lily's last night. They were happy they did. They found the food delicious and were still raving about the dessert a day later.

If Lily is a person, "they" could refer, in principle, to any two of John, Mary, and Lily, or to all three, or to people not already mentioned in the discourse. However, the speaker can safely assume that the listener will take "they" to refer to John and Mary in both sentence 2 and sentence 3 of passage (1). How does this happen?

One theory maintains that pronominal reference is accomplished by logical inference. This view maintains that the pronoun *they* in the second sentence is related to *John and Mary* as part of the listener's effort to create a "mental model" of the discourse (Johnson-Laird, 1983). Nouns and pronouns specify entities in this mental model, and logical processes connect these entities, in much the same way as the inferences about Lily's being somewhere where John and Mary ate are made. There is good evidence that some pronouns are assigned antecedents by a logical, inferential approach, but other mechanisms also affect the interpretation of pronouns and other cohesive elements. A pronoun can be related to a noun phrase (NP) on the basis of an aspect of the structure of the sentences that contain the pronoun and the NP. For instance, a pronoun can be related to the immediately preceding NP or to a NP in the same grammatical position in a previous sentence. Another mechanism involves establishing the focus of a part of the discourse, and using that focus (or foci) to guide pronominal reference. The theory of discourse structure developed by Grosz and her colleagues relies exclusively on this method of relating pronouns to antecedents. These approaches are clearly relevant to determining the antecedent of *they* in the third sentence of (1), and probably play a role in determining the antecedent of *they* in the second sentence of (1) as well.

Devices that serve to make discourse cohesive help create a semantically coherent discourse. Aside from continuity of reference, one of the more important factors making for coherence is related to the notion of "topic." The topic of a sentence is described by van Dijk and Kintsch (1983) as an element from a representation in a text base that "is the starting point for the construction of the next propositional schema" (p.155). These authors go on to say that the existence of a sentence topic "accounts for the overlap defining semantic relatedness and, at the same time, the continuation with respect to the previous discourse" (p. 155). The topic of a sentence is usually signaled in some way. It may occupy a particular syntactic position, such as being the subject of a sentence in English, receive emphatic stress, etc.

Coherence and cohesion of sequences of sentences result in the second level of discourse, which van Dijk and Kintsch (1983) call the "macrostructure" of a discourse. The macrostructure of a discourse is an indication of what the discourse itself and its various parts are about. A second sense of "topic" (or "theme," "gist," etc.) is captured in the notion of the macrostructure of a discourse. The notion of macrostructure can be appreciated by considering the following passage (cited in van Dijk and Kintsch, 1983, p. 207):

(12)   We got up at four in the morning, that first day in the East. On the evening before, we had climbed off a freight train at the edge of town and with the true instinct of Kentucky boys had found our way across town and to the race track and to the stables at once. Then we knew we were allright.

A series of violent, bloody encounters between police and Black Panther Party members punctuated the early summer days of 1969. Soon after, a group of Black students I teach at California State College, Los Angeles, who were members of the Panther Party, began to complain of continuous harassment by law enforcement officers. Among their many grievances, they complained about receiving so many traffic citations that some were in danger of losing their driving privileges. During one lengthy discussion, we realized that all of them drove automobiles with Panther Party signs glued to their bumpers. This is a report of a study that I undertook to assess the seriousness of their charges and to determine whether we were hearing the voice of paranoia or reality. (Heussenstam, 1971, p. 32)

Proposition
No.   Proposition

1 (SERIES, ENCOUNTER)
2 (VIOLENT, ENCOUNTER)
3 (BLOODY, ENCOUNTER)
4 (BETWEEN, ENCOUNTER, POLICE, BLACK PANTHER)
5 (TIME: IN, ENCOUNTER, SUMMER)
6 (EARLY, SUMMER)
7 (TIME: IN, SUMMER, 1969)

8 (SOON, 9)
9 (AFTER, 4, 16)
10 (GROUP, STUDENT)
11 (BLACK, STUDENT)
12 (TEACH, SPEAKER, STUDENT)
13 (LOCATION: AT, 12, CAL STATE COLLEGE)
14 (LOCATION: AT, CAL STATE COLLEGE, LOS ANGELES)
15 (IS A, STUDENT, BLACK PANTHER)
16 (BEGIN, 17)
17 (COMPLAIN, STUDENT, 19)
18 (CONTINUOUS, 19)
19 (HARASS, POLICE, STUDENT)

20 (AMONG, COMPLAINT)
21 (MANY, COMPLAINT)
22 (COMPLAIN, STUDENT, 23)

23 (RECEIVE, STUDENT, TICKET)
24 (MANY, TICKET)
25 (CAUSE, 23, 27)
26 (SOME, STUDENT)
27 (IN DANGER OR, 26, 28)
28 (LOSE, 26, LICENSE)

29 (DURING, DISCUSSION, 32)
30 (LENGTHY, DISCUSSION)
31 (AND, STUDENT, SPEAKER)
32 (REALIZE, 31, 34)
33 (ALL, STUDENT)
34 (DRIVE, 33, AUTO)
35 (HAVE, AUTO, SIGN)
36 (BLACK PANTHER, SIGN)
37 (GLUED, SIGN, BUMPER)

38 (REPORT, SPEAKER, STUDY)
39 (DO, SPEAKER, STUDY)
40 (PURPOSE, STUDY, 41)
41 (ASSESS, STUDY, 42, 43)
42 (TRUE, 17)
43 (HEAR, 31, 44)
44 (OR, 45, 46)
45 (OF REALITY, VOICE)
46 (OF PARANOIA, VOICE)

Note. Lines indicate sentence boundaries. Propositions are numbered for ease of reference. Numbers as propositional arguments refer to the proposition with that number.

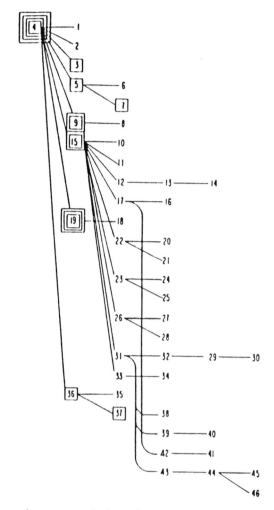

The complete coherence graph. (Numbers represent propositions. The number of boxes represents the number of extra cycles required for processing.)

Figure 9.2
Analysis of text. (Reprinted with permission from Kintsch and van Dijk, 1978, pp. 377–379. Copyright 1978 by the American Psychological Association.)

This passage makes use of pronominalization and other linguistic elements to achieve cohesion. It is coherent. But simply indicating the continuity of reference and sentence topics does not capture the entirety of the information conveyed by the passage. The passage is about something—the arrival of boys from Kentucky in an eastern city. This overall theme can be seen as a summary of this passage.

Macrostructural units are further organized into what Kintsch and van Dijk call "schemata" or "superstructures." For instance, a narrative, according to Kintsch and van Dijk (1978), typically consists of a setting, a complication, and a resolution. If a narrative becomes complex, there can be more than one complication, and new complications can be introduced before old ones are resolved. This approach to the structure of discourse has led to a model of discourse structure in which the individual propositions in the text base are viewed as the terminal elements in a tree, something like the syntactic trees described in chapter 7 (Mandler and Johnson, 1977). The highest node in the entire structure is a representation of the main event that the discourse depicts. These hierarchical structures can be quite complex, depending on the nature of the narrative. Figure 9.2 illustrates how Kintsch and van Dijk (1978) represent the text base, macrostructure, and superstructure of a short portion of a report of an experiment in social psychology.

In summary, discourse is a level of language structure, itself made up of several levels of structure. Discourses relate the items and propositional contents of utterances to each other in coherent ways, relying in part on the use of markers that create linguistic cohesion to do so. Discourse coherence also critically requires that the speaker and listener access shared real-world knowledge. Discourses are of different types; story-grammar models of narratives are the best-studied discourse structures in brain-damaged patients, but many other discourse types exist (conversations, instructions, etc.). The structure of a discourse is tied to the intentional and attentional states of the participants, and ultimately reflects the purposes of the discourse.

PROCESSING DISCOURSE STRUCTURES

The models of the structure of a discourse that we have been discussing—even those that include descriptions of the attentional states of the participants—are not in and of themselves models of how discourse is processed. Psychologists have begun to study this question, and have developed a variety of models of how discourse is comprehended and produced.

Several models involve sequential construction of different levels of discourse structure. Kintsch and van Dijk (1978; van Dijk and Kintsch, 1983) have suggested, for instance, that a listener processes a narrative or text to create the microstrucural, macrostructural, and superstructural levels in a sequence. They postulate that a certain number of propositions in a text base must be understood and retained in a memory store in order for higher-level discourse structures to be built. However, though there may be some role for a memory system in discourse comprehension (Glanzer, Dorfman, and Kaplan, 1981), any model of discourse processing that relies heavily on sequential construction of progressively higher levels of discourse structure is likely to be wrong. The evidence that such models are probably incorrect comes from data documenting the speed of discourse processing. I therefore will discuss experiments dealing with the speed of discourse processing in some detail.

Data regarding the effects of discourse structure on the interpretation of pronouns and other referentially dependent forms, and on the attachment of modifiers, provide some of the strongest evidence indicating that discourse processing occurs extremely quickly on the input side. I shall review a few of these studies to illustrate some of the results of this research.[2]

As we have seen many times, pronouns and many other referentially dependent items are linked to their antecedents on the basis of a variety of factors. One process involved in establishing the antecedent of a pronoun or one type of empty referentially dependent noun phrase (**PRO** in Chomsky's theory of syntax; see chapter 7) is based on logical inferences. Marslen-Wilson and Tyler (1987) reported a series of experiments designed to investigate how rapidly these inferential processes go on. In the simplest of these experiments, subjects heard a passage such as (13):

(13)   As Philip was walking back from the shop, he saw an old woman trip and fall flat on her face in the street. She seemed unable to get up.
   a) Philip ran toward . . .
   b) He ran toward . . .
   c) Running toward . . .

In (13), there are both discourse-based inferences and syntactic cues regarding the antecedent of the pronoun in the continuation fragment. In continuation a), the name *Philip* is repeated. In b), *he* agrees in gender with *Philip*. In continuation c), there are no syntactic cues as to the agent of *running*. The grammatical subject of *running* is a phonologically empty category of a sort we discussed in chapter 7 (**PRO**). Inferences alone establish *Philip* as the agent of the verbal gerund, *running*, in c).

Marslen-Wilson and Tyler investigated the effects that these different combinations of inferential and syntactic determinants of an antecedent have on subjects' on-line processing of these discourses. They presented passages like (13) with each of the continuations, a), b), and c), auditorily. After the word *toward*, subjects saw the pronoun *him* or *her* on a computer screen, and were required to read the word they saw aloud. *Him* is never a felicitous continuation, while *her*, which refers to the old woman both grammatically and logically, is an appropriate continuation for all the discourse fragments. The point of the experiment is that at the point that the target word appears on the screen, the establishment of who is doing the running is possible only on logical discourse grounds in fragment c), and on both logical and linguistic grounds in a) and b). Marslen-Wilson and Tyler argued that if logical inferences are slow to develop in discourse processing, there should be a significant difference between subjects' performances in passages a) and b), on the one hand, and c), on the other. In fact, no difference was found in errors or reaction times for reading the visually presented word (see table 9.2). Marslen-Wilson and Tyler concluded that subjects had already established *Philip* as agent of *running* by the end of the word *toward* in c) as well as in a) and b) and thus that logical inferences in discourse processing occur with the same speed as the linguistically based operations that are involved in establishing co-reference.

Another area in which discourse effects have been shown to occur very rapidly is the assignment of certain syntactic structures. Tyler and Marslen-Wilson (1977) used their sentence-fragment technique to study subjects' use of context to disambiguate syntactic ambiguities. They presented sentences such as (14) and (15) auditorily, followed by the word *is* or *are* in visual form.

(14)   If you walk too near the runway, landing planes . . .

(15)   If you've been trained as a pilot, landing planes . . .

Table 9.2
Reaction Times for Reading Different Stimuli in the Experiments by
Marslen-Wilson and Tyler (see text)

	Mean Naming Latencies (ms)		
	Appropriate Probe	Inappropriate Probe	Difference
Experiment on anaphora			
Type of anaphor			
Repeated name	379	429	50
Pronoun	385	434	49
Zero anaphor	384	420	36
Experiment on ambiguity			
Continuation			
is	440*	460*	
are	423*	438*	

* Approximate.
Reprinted with permission from Marslen-Wilson and Tyler (1986, pp. 50, 52).

In (14), landing planes is most likely to be a plural NP, while in (15) the same words are most naturally taken to be a nominal gerund. Thus, *are* is the most natural continuation for (14) and *is* the most natural continuation for (15). Subjects were required to read the visually presented word as quickly as possible. Reading latencies for the more natural continuations were significantly shorter than for the less natural continuations, indicating that discourse context affected subjects' analysis of the syntactically ambiguous sequence of words (see table 9.2).

A similar result was reported by Altmann and Steedman (1988). In chapter 7, we discussed parsing mechanisms (the process of assigning structure to a sentence), and noted that the parser must attach each incoming word to a phrase marker. We reviewed evidence that these attachments were constrained by principles, such as minimal attachment and late closure, that keep attachments local and minimize revisions of already-constructed phrase markers. We noted that minimal attachment is said to play a role in determining the preferred attachment of a phrase such as *with the gun* in sentences like (16).

(16)   The policeman shot the robber with the gun.

Attaching the phrase *with the gun* to the verb phrase (VP) (leading to the interpretation that the policeman used the gun) does not require any revision of the phrase marker that has been constructed, whereas attaching the phrase *with the gun* to the NP *the robber* (leading to the interpretation that the robber used the gun) does require a revision of the phrase marker that has been constructed. Frazier and others argue that this is why sentence (16) is more naturally taken to mean that the policeman used the gun. However, we noted that there is another interpretation of this effect, one based on discourse considerations.

Crain and Steedman (1985), Altmann and Steedman (1988), and others have pointed out that the interpretation of (16) in which the robber used the gun is infelicitous unless more than one robber has been specified in the previous discourse. If only one robber is under discussion, there is no need to indicate that the one who has been shot is the one with the gun. If there is no lead-in discourse for sentence (16), no individuals have been specified in the discourse prior to that sentence. To make the interpretation of (16) in which the robber had a gun a natural one, a listener would have to infer that there were several robbers, and that the policeman shot the one who had a gun. Intuitions indicate that this is not a simple inference to make. Crain, Altmann, and Steedman argue that this discourse factor underlies the preference for the first interpretation of (16).

To investigate this possibility, Altmann and Steedman (1988) created passages like (17) and (18):

(17)   A burglar broke into a bank carrying some dynamite. He planned to blow open a safe. Once inside, he saw there was a safe which had a new lock and a safe which had an old lock.

(18)   A burglar broke into a bank carrying some dynamite. He planned to blow open a safe. Once inside, he saw there was a safe which had a new lock and a strongbox which had an old lock.

These passages were followed by the sentences (19a) or (19b):

(19a) The burglar/ blew open/ the safe/ with the dynamite/ and made off/ with the loot.

   b)   The burglar/ blew open/ the safe/ with the new lock/ and made off/ with the loot.

Passage (17) is "NP-supporting": it mentions two safes and therefore establishes the discourse conditions necessary for a prepositional phrase PP to be attached to an NP. Continuation (19b) is an "NP-attached" continuation: *with the new lock* is naturally taken as a modifier of the NP *the safe*, not the verb *blew open*. Passage (18) is "VP-supporting": it mentions one safe and therefore establishes the discourse conditions under which PP is naturally attached to a VP. Continuation (19a) is a "VP-attached" continuation: *with the dynamite* is naturally taken as a modifier of the the the verb *blew open*, not *the safe*.

Subjects were shown passages (17) and (18) sentence by sentence and continuations (19a) and (19b) phrase by phrase (phrases are indicated by slashes), pressing a button as soon as they wished to see the next item (the so-called self-paced reading technique). The authors measured the time subjects took to read each successive phrase in (19a) and (19b). The results are shown in figure 9.3. There were two important findings. First, reading times were the same for all phrases up to the point at which the PP is displayed and then immediately differed. Second, the PP was read faster when it was congruent with context [the NP-attached PP (19b) was faster in the NP-supporting context (17) than in the VP-supporting context (18), and vice versa]. This pattern indicates that the effects of context affect the attachment of a PP while it is being processed.

In all these studies, information derived from context affects processing very quickly. Though not definitive, these results make any model that involves construction of higher levels of discourse only after a great deal of lower discourse structure is established unlikely.

These studies raise an issue that we have discussed in chapter 7: to what extent is processing of word and sentence form independent of higher-level processing? The results we have just presented have been taken as evidence that inferences based upon information available in the preceding discourse occur as rapidly as other more purely linguistic processes and affect psycholinguistic processing as soon as they become available. However, this conclusion has been questioned by some studies which indicate that there are some lexical and syntactic processes whose earliest stages are not affected by context.

One of the most frequently cited results in the psycholinguistic literature of this sort deals with the role of discourse context in disambiguating lexically ambiguous words (Swinney, 1979; Seidenberg

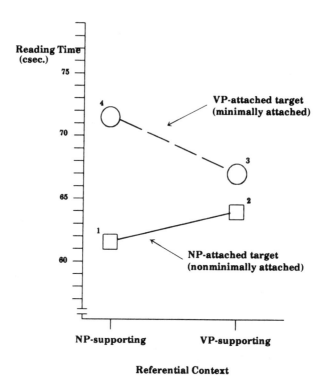

Figure 9.3
Reading times for the ambiguous prepositional phrase in NP-supporting and VP-supporting discourse context. (Reproduced with permission from Altmann and Steedman, 1988, p. 227.)

et al., 1982). In one experiment, Swinney used a "cross-modal lexical priming" technique to investigate this question. He presented passages such as (20) to subjects:

(20)   The guests were concerned about the appearance of the hotel lobby. There were spiders, ants, and other insects all over the floor. They were not surprised to find bugs in their room.

At the end of the word *bugs*, subjects performed a visual lexical decision task. They saw a letter string on a computer screen, and were required to say whether it was a word or not. On some occasions when a word was presented, it was related to one of the two senses of *bugs* (e.g., the presented word might be *insect* or *microphone*). The same task was repeated, with the visually presented word being shown at progressively longer intervals from the word *bugs*. Subjects' reaction times to identify the letter string as a word were significantly faster for words related to *both* senses of *bugs* (compared to unrelated words) when the visual stimulus appeared right after bugs. When the visual stimulus appeared more than 300 ms after the end of the word *bugs*, however, only a word related to the *contextually relevant* sense of *bugs* (i.e., *insect*, in this case) was responded to faster than control words. This pattern has been interpreted as indicating that the effects of context are not felt in the first stages of accessing lexical meaning, but serve to select one meaning over another within a few hundred milliseconds.

Fodor (1990) has also questioned the immediacy of the use of discourse information in assigning co-reference. He used the same types of materials as Marslen-Wilson and Tyler, but with the cross-modal lexical priming task just described. Subjects heard passages such as (13) with final sentences beginning as in the three fragments a)–c) and terminating with the pronouns *him* or *her*, and saw a letter string on a computer screen after each word in the continuation. Half the letter strings were words and half were not; the subject was asked to say which were which. Words related to *Philip* were identified faster at all points in fragments a) and b). However, words related to *Philip* were only identified faster after the final pronoun him in fragment c). Fodor interpreted these data as showing that the antecedent of a logically referential item [the subject of *running* in c)] is not activated by inferential processes at the the point where the gerund occurs.

It thus appears that as fast as inferencing based upon discourse information may be, processes such as the earliest stage of lexical semantic access and the determination of the antecedent of a pronoun based upon matches of syntactic markers may go on so quickly that they cannot be influenced by inferences based upon a discourse. However, these very fast processes are linked to recognition of words and extraction of the form and literal meaning of sentences as they are presented, not to the construction of the microstructure of a narrative. The argument from the speed of discourse processing to the conclusion that discourse representations are not constructed in a sequential fashion, as in the Kintsch and van Dijk (1978;–van Dijk and Kintsch, 1983) model, is not affected by the fact that some lexical and syntactic processes may go on faster than the construction of discourse representations.

The results we have just reviewed suggest that there is a temporal course over which discourse-based information becomes available in order to be able to interact with certain lexical and sentential processes. There are also results that suggest that there is a time course over which this information ceases to remain active or available for these purposes. A series of experiments by McKoon and Ratcliff (1980) and Dell, McKoon, and Ratcliff (1983) are relevant to this issue.

In a first experiment, McKoon and Ratcliff used a combined self-paced reading and priming technique to investigate aspects of co-indexation. They presented passages such as (21) visually, having the subject press a bar to make each successive sentence appear on a computer screen.

(21)   The burglar surveyed the garage set back from the street.
       Several milk bottles were piled at the curb.
       The banker and her husband were away on vacation.
   a) The_1 $burglar_2$ $slipped_3$ $away_4$ from the_5 street $lamp_6$
   b) The_1 $criminal_2$ $slipped_3$ $away_4$ from the_5 street $lamp_6$.
   c) The_1 cat_2 $slipped_3$ $away_4$ from the_5 street $lamp_6$.

The last sentence in these passages varied, containing either a repetition of a previously presented word (*burglar*), a superordinate term that referred to the same entity (*criminal*), or an unrelated word (*cat*). Following the last sentence, subjects were shown the previously presented word (*burglar*), a word from the same clause as that word (*garage*), or a word that had not appeared in the passage, and were asked to indicate as quickly as possible whether the word had or had not been in the passage. Reaction times for both *burglar* and *garage* were faster in completions a) and b) than in c). These results indicate two things: (1) that a superordinate term (modified by a definite article) activates a previously introduced NP to which it is related, and (2) other items in the sentence containing the "antecedent" of a definite NP are activated along with the antecedent.

Dell and his colleagues built on this result to chart the time course of activation of both the antecedent and a word in the same sentence as the antecedent. They used a combined priming and word-by-word forced-paced reading technique. This involved presenting the last words in these same passages to a new set of subjects word by word and having a test word appear—separated from

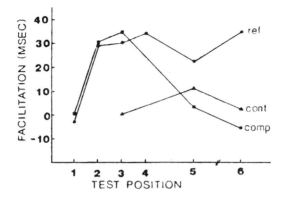

Figure 9.4
The average amount of priming for different test words in different positions in the last sentence of a discourse. Position 2 is 250 ms before the anaphoric element; positions 3, 4, and 5 are 500, 750, and 1250 ms after this element; and position 6 is after the sentence. The time of course of priming for the referent of the anaphora (*ref*), a companion word (*comp*), and a control (*cont*) is shown. (Reproduced with permission from Dell et al., 1985, p. 128.)

the sentence and presented in capital letters—after one of the positions indicated in passage (21). Subjects were to indicate whether this word had previously appeared in the passage. The same words as were used above were used again. Reaction time benefits for the "repeated" word (*burglar*) and the word in the same clause (*garage*) are shown at the various points of probe presentation in figure 9.4. This figure shows that there is an immediate benefit for both the repeated word and for the word from its clause, as soon as the definite NP is uttered. However, the advantage for the word from the same clause drops off rapidly. If we take the time course of the advantage for *the word from the clause* as an indication of the temporal course of activation of some aspect of discourse information (in this case, the information regarding the proposition containing the repeated word), we may (tentatively) conclude that this information both rises and decays quite rapidly.

Thus, experimental evidence, though incomplete, suggests that some aspects of discourse structure are activated very quickly and that they, in turn, influence some aspects of word and sentence processing. It also appears that some discourse-relevant information sees its level of activation fall over a relatively short period of time. The rapid rise of activation of discourse-relevant information is likely to be the basis for our subjective impression that we integrate new material into a discourse "on-line"—as it is being presented. The possibility that this information decays over a few sentences is in keeping with our sense that older information is not as active as that which is currently being presented. However, we easily return to previous portions of a discourse, even those separated from the present utterance, when the need for such returns is indicated in a discourse. How this is accomplished, and how different aspects of discourse structure are rapidly created on-line, remain topics for further research.

Another issue that has been addressed in the psycholinguistic literature that is closely tied to the question of how rapidly discourse structures are built is the nature of the representations that are utilized in processing discourse. Exactly how are items and propositions represented in a discourse? Are the kinds of representations depicted in figuress 9.1 and 9.2 all maintained in speakers' and listeners' minds while a discourse is going on, or only some of these representations? Are these the only kinds of representations maintained in their minds? I cannot review these important and interesting psycholinguistic issues here in a truly adequate fashion, but I shall touch on several aspects of this question to give the reader a sense of the problem and of some work that bears on it.

Let us begin by considering the first of these questions: How are items represented in a discourse? If we represent the items in a discourse semantically, we can run into the following problem (Johnson-Laird, 1983): the more a person knows about an item, the more information he will have to represent. Assuming that representing information takes up mental "space," this would imply that the more a person knows about the items in a discourse, the more costly it is for him to represent the discourse and the harder it is for him to process it. A related problem, much discussed by philosophers, is how to represent items that are qualified by indefinite and universal quantifiers. Suppose we hear a sentence such as (22) or (23):

(22)   Jennifer wants a puppy for her birthday.

(23)   All politicians are dishonest.

We might represent *Jennifer* as some set of features characteristic of Jennifer. But we cannot represent *a puppy* or *all politicians* this way: we don't know what the specific characteristics of the puppy Jennifer wants are, and we certainly cannot include in a discourse representation features of all the politicians on earth.

I cannot review the enormous literature on these issues here, but will outline one possible solution to these problems. This solution is to assume that only partial information about each object is placed in a discourse representation. For instance, in a discourse like (24), the information that cats have fur is more readily available to a reader than that cats have claws, whereas the opposite is true in (25). This suggests that different properties of objects may be represented in different discourses.

(24)   Mary is very fond of cats. She enjoys having them sit on her lap while she pets them.

(25)   Cats are very good hunters. I have seen one kill a mouse with a single blow to the neck.

Another type of answer to this question has been to entertain the possibility that semantic representations of words are not the only types of representations carried along in processing a discourse. Perhaps listeners (and speakers) maintain information in another code, from which the semantic properties of objects and propositions can be recovered. One candidate for such a code is the phonological form of a word.

Several lines of research suggest that this code is used in discourse processing. Several results indicate that the verbatim form of one or two sentences (or clauses in a complex or compound sentence) can be recalled immediately after a sentence is presented (Marslen-Wilson and Tyler, 1976; Jarvella, 1970, 1971). This suggests that this portion of a discourse may be maintained in phonological form in short-term memory. Murphy (1985a,b) studied the role of sentence form in determining ease of understanding of sentences containing either VP ellipsis or the phrase *do it*. He found that both the length and the form of an antecedent affected reading times for sentences containing both these types of anaphora, as long as the antecedent was in the sentence immediately preceding the anaphoric elements (these effects did not occur for more distant antecedents). For instance, reading times were longer for (26) than for (27):

(26) The ball was kicked by Leslie, but Fran
      a) wouldn't.
      b) wouldn't do it.

(27) Leslie kicked the ball, but Fran
      a) wouldn't.
      b) wouldn't do it.

Though these results do not prove that some co-indexation operations refer back to phonological form, they do suggest that some of these operations do refer back to the surface form of an utterance.

We have reviewed a selected number of studies of on-line discourse processing, all of which have dealt with processing at the level of microstructure (or, in Grosz's terminology, within a discourse segment). There are very few studies of how higher-order aspects of discourse structure affect on-line processing (see Townsend, 1983, for one such study). However, there are many studies that deal with the issue of how higher-order discourse structures affect memory for verbal material. The conclusion that emerges very clearly from these studies is that discourse structure has a profound effect on what is remembered.

For instance, Kintsch and Keenan (1973) selected one proposition from a discourse as the one that best describes the topic of the discourse. They called this proposition the "first-order" proposition. They then selected all propositions that shared an item with the first-order proposition, and called them "second-order" propositions; all propositions that shared an item with the second-order propositions were called "third-order" propositions; etc. They found that memory declined in a very direct manner for lower-order propositions. Many other researchers have reported similar results (Perfetti and Goldman, 1974; Kintsch et al., 1975; Mandler and Johnson, 1977; Thorndyke, 1977; Fletcher, 1981). Interestingly, subjects do not only recall the propositions that are actually found in a discourse (Kintsch et al., 1975); they recall at least some of the inferences that are needed to make the discourse coherent as well (Keenan and Kintsch, 1974; McKoon, and Kintsch, 1974; Hildyard and Olson, 1978; Keenan, 1978).

I conclude this section by touching on the question of how discourse is planned by the speaker. We have seen that a very large number of factors all coalesce at the level of discourse. The many features of discourse structure that have been described—the basic intentions of the speaker, the topic of a discourse segment, the topic of individual sentences, whether an item or action is newly introduced into the discourse or has already been part of the discourse, the assumptions the speaker makes about the listener's knowledge of the world, the level of formality of the discourse, etc.—affect the activation of elements of the language processing-system. They enter into the encoding process to influence the choice of vocabulary elements, aspects of syntactic form, and features of intonational contours. Speech production models such as that proposed by Garrett (1976, 1980; see chapter 8), group all these different aspects of discourse into a single component of the production process—the creation of the message-level representation. Presumably, many of these different aspects of discourse are planned separately, but very little is known about the components of these very abstract planning processes. Some theorists (e.g., Fodor, 1983) have suggested that, at this level of abstraction, there is no modularity to the language-processing system, that all these factors interact freely. Other theorists disagree (e.g., Shallice, 1988). Not enough is known about these processes to have a reasonable basis for adjudicating this debate. The reader is referred to Frederikson et al (1990) for one model that begins to identify the subprocesses involved in planning at the discourse level.

   Finally, the perennial question arises of how far in advance different aspects of discourse are planned (see chapters 4 and 8 for discussion regarding look-ahead in planning word sounds and sentence forms). Though it seems intuitively clear that speakers have some idea of their subject quite far in advance of much of their actual output, whether any detailed representation of discourse structure evolves much in advance of activating lexical items, syntactic forms, and intonational contours, is not clear. For an argument in favor of a incremental production process in which discourse representations trigger lexical, syntactic, and prosodic forms with virtually no look-ahead, see Levelt (1989).

DISORDERS AFFECTING THE PRODUCTION AND COMPREHENSION OF DISCOURSE-LEVEL STRUCTURES

Patients frequently have difficulty with the production or comprehension of the discourse level of language. If the disturbances affecting words, word formation, and sentences are any indication of how disturbances of discourse occur, we would expect these problems could fractionate along at least two major lines. They could occur in either comprehension or production, and they could occur in either the auditory-oral or written modalities. We might also expect there to be separate disturbances of memory for discourse, even if comprehension of discourse is intact. Indeed, if the disturbances affecting words, word formation, and sentences are a guide to the nature of disturbances of discourse, we might expect to see a much more specific fractionation of these disturbances along linguistic lines. For instance, it is possible that some patients only have trouble with finding the antecedents of pronouns, and others only with making certain types of inferences. Disturbances affecting discourse could also could occur with or without other language disturbances (i.e., with or without an aphasia). Many of these possible disturbances have been attested to in the existing literature. Because of the importance of separating disturbances of discourse from those of word- and sentence-level processing, my review of disturbances of discourse falls under two main headings: those that occur in patients with and without other aphasic language disturbances.

Discourse Comprehension and Production in Nonaphasic Patients

Recent studies have documented disturbances affecting the comprehension of discourse in patients without other language impairments. The most extensive studies of this type have been carried out in right-handed patients with right hemisphere lesions (mostly strokes). These patients have been shown to fail to draw certain types of inferences from discourse.

Perhaps the best-known of these studies are those that indicate that right hemisphere–lesioned patients have difficulty in appreciating certain aspects of jokes. Brownell and his colleagues (Brownell et al., 1983; Brownell and Gardner, 1988) claimed that the humor in a joke is due to the punchline of the joke being coherent with the initial material in the joke, but surprising given that material. Brownell et al. (1983) tested the abilities of 12 patients with right hemisphere lesion to choose the punchlines of jokes. After reading and hearing the opening lines of a joke, the patients had to select a humorous continuation from three possibilities: the real punchline, a nonsequitur, and a nonhumorous coherent ending. A typical stimulus is presented in (28):

(28)   The quack was selling a potion which he claimed would make men live to a great age. He claimed he himself was hale and hearty and over 300 years old.

"Is he really as old as that?" asked a listener of the youthful assistant.

"I can't say," said the assistant.

Correct punchline: "I've only worked with him for 100 years."

Non sequitur: "There are over 300 days in the year."

Coherent nonhumorous ending: "I don't know how old he is."

Right hemisphere–lesioned patients made more errors than normal controls. Critically, they chose nonsequitur endings more often than normal controls, indicating that they knew that the ending of a joke should be surprising, but had less ability than normals to make it coherent with the first part of a joke.

This result was replicated in a second study (Birhle et al., 1986) using both verbal materials and cartoon sequences to present the first part of a joke. In these studies, a fourth ending was also supplied. This fourth choice was a humorous nonsequitur—a statement that was not coherent with the text, but which was humorous because it contained an element of slapstick or surprise in and of itself. Ten right hemisphere–lesioned patients again made more errors than normals, and chose these humorous nonsequiturs more often than normals. (Seven others did very well.) This pattern confirmed that right hemisphere–damaged patients had trouble recognizing the coherence of a statement with respect to previously presented materials. Interestingly, it also indicated that aphasic patients had less trouble with this aspect of comprehension.

A more direct study of right hemisphere–damaged patients' abilities to make inferences on the basis of a discourse—one that is not complicated by the issue of humor or surprise—was reported by Brownell et al. (1986). They presented discourses in which an inference that might be drawn from a single sentence was changed because of the remaining discourse. For instance, they argue that, in isolation, sentence (29) suggests that Jane was late for an appointment, and sentence (30) suggests that a vehicle was in an accident:

(29)   Jane hurried into the dentist's office.

(30)   The windshield was shattered.

These researchers embedded these sentences in discourses that made it clear that these implications were incorrect. In half the discourses, the sentence that modified these implications occurred before the critical sentence, as in (31). In half the discourses, it occurred after the critical sentence, as in (32):

(31)   Johnny missed the wild pitch. The windshield was shattered.

(32)   Jane hurried into the dentist's office. She saw her purse on the table in the waiting room.

In (31), the first sentence leads the listener to conclude that a ball broke the windshield. In (32), the second sentence leads the listener to conclude that Jane had been in the office before and forgotten her purse, and that the reason for her hurrying was that she wished to recover it as soon as possible.

Subjects were presented these passages in both written and oral form, and then asked to state whether four other sentences were true or false. Two questions were directed at statements in the discourse itself. The remaining two tested inferences. One was the statement that would be drawn from the critical sentence in isolation (that Jane was late for an appointment; that a vehicle had been in an accident). The other inferential statement was the implication that would be drawn from the discourse as a whole (that Jane had forgotten her purse in the office; that the wild pitch had broken the windshield). Eight right hemisphere–damaged patients showed a very selective impairment on this task, compared with normal control subjects. In passages like (32), in which the critical sentence came first, they were more likely to accept the incorrect inference (that Jane was late for an appointment) and less likely to accept the correct inference (that she had forgotten her purse) than normal controls. However, they did not show comparable impairments in verifying facts from the discourses or in verifying inferences when the critical information came second. This pattern suggested to these investigators that patients with right hemisphere damage can draw inferences from sentences and discourse, but cannot revise them when new information comes up in a discourse.

Patients with short-term memory impairments may also have difficulties revising representations of discourse structure that they have constructed. Vallar and Baddeley (1987) presented data on auditory comprehension in a patient, P.V., with a severe limitation of verbal short-term memory. P.V. was excellent in syntactic comprehension, in verification of lexical semantic anomalies, and in grammaticality judgments in short sentences. She was near perfect on grammaticality judgments in longer sentences in which the error-producing segments were separated by more words than her span. She was able to recall information and make inferences in passages of several sentences. P.V. made a few errors in detecting anomalies in sentences when different error types (number and gender agreement, word order inversion, semantic) were presented in mixed lists. She did worse in detection of number and gender anomalies when they were separated by several sentences in a passage, though her error rates were close to normal. She made no errors on permuted word anomalies in these passages.

P.V.'s performance in detecting anomalies based upon gender and number in discourse passages is exemplified in the following passage:

(33)   The businessman from Milan was traveling in his luxurious car. The car was very speedy and silent. Fortunately, that day the motorway was empty.
   a)   He had to arrive in Rome . . .
   b)   They had to arrive in Rome . . .

The continuation in b) is infelicitous because the antecedent of the pronoun *they* has not been previously mentioned in the discourse. Normal subjects judged such passages as anomalous; P.V. accepted these passages. This performance might reflect a limitation in her ability to recognize infelicitous discourse due to pronominal reference. Such a limitation would have a general similarity to right hemisphere–damaged patients' difficulties with revising inferences. In both cases, the patients tolerate and cannot revise discourse-level anomalies (either in co-indexation or in inferences).

There is some indication that particular discourse processes may be quite selectively impaired in some populations. For instance, Lesser (1986) presented nine right brain–damaged subjects stories consisting of five sentences, in which the propositions were related through spatial, temporal, or class-inclusion ("categorical") factors. Subjects were given the sentences in the stories in random order and had to arrange them to tell a coherent story. The right hemisphere–damaged patients performed less well than controls, and did worst on those discourses that were linked by spatial factors. This order of difficulty was not found in a similar sentence arrangement task given to ten right hemisphere–damaged patients by Delis et al. (1983). In that study, the right hemipshere–damaged patients had more trouble with the passages in which sentences were related on categorical grounds than those in which the sentences were related by spatial factors. It may be that different patients have greater problems with different elements making for coherence.

Other researchers have found deficits in the ability of some nonaphasic patients to produce aspects of discourse. Joanette and Goulet and colleagues (1990; Joanette et al., 1986) described the results of a study of 36 right hemisphere–damaged patients' and 20 normal controls' abilities to describe a story depicted through a series of eight line drawings. They analyzed the patients' responses in terms of the linguistic devices that were used, the cohesion and coherence of the discourses that were produced, and the nature of the story schemata that were produced. Ten aspects of linguistic form were measured: the percentages of nouns, verbs, adjectives, and adverbs compared to total words; the verb-noun, adjective-noun, and pronoun-concept ratios; the use of lexical items for the main concepts in the story; the number of different lexical items used; and the number of subordinate clauses produced. The right hemisphere–damaged patients performed similarly to normal controls on all these measures except for producing fewer adjectives overall and a larger number of different words to refer to the concepts depicted in the sequence of drawings. Similarly, the right brain–damaged subjects produced discourses that were similar in terms of their coherence and cohesion to those of normals, as measured in terms of the adherence of the discourses to four rules governing cohesion developed by Charolles (1978).

However, right brain–damaged patients differed from controls in their production of aspects of story schemata. The researchers assigned utterances to propositions, each consisting of a predicate and one or more arguments. A simple proposition was considered to be one in which the arguments were not themselves propositions; complex propositions were ones in which at least one argument was a proposition. These propositions were organized into a story schema, consisting of an introduction, a complication, and a resolution. The right hemisphere–damaged patients produced discourses that contained these three parts of a story. However, they produced fewer propositions, fewer complex propositions, and fewer frequently produced propositions than normal controls. They also tended to produce fewer propositions pertaining to the complication of the story. This is consistent with these patients' tendency to omit adjectives, and suggests that they tend not to elaborate upon the details of a discourse.

It does not appear that these disturbances in comprehension and production of discourse-level structures are due to a primary loss of right hemisphere–damaged patients' knowledge of the basic organization of actions and events, that is, to a loss of knowledge regarding "scripts." Scripts are abstract descriptions of events, such as that eating at a restaurant involves ordering food, eating, paying the bill, etc. The evidence for the integrity of right hemisphere–damaged patients' knowledge of at least the basic aspects of scripts come from several sources. Roman et al. (1987) explicitly evaluated six right hemisphere–lesioned stroke victims' knowledge of the basic aspects of scripts pertaining to changing a tire and dining in a restaurant. They found that, in both free production and three constrained tasks (judging whether a statement pertained to the script; ordering statements in order of importance in the script; and ordering statements temporally within the script), the patients did quite well. The problem some nonaphasic patients appear to have is mapping this knowledge onto more complex linguistic forms and sequences of sentences—either in comprehension, or production, or both.

Overall, the problems in comprehending and producing discourse we have described in these nonaphasic patients are relatively mild. On the comprehension side, right hemisphere–damaged patients can make inferences from discourses, as long as these inferences follow directly from the sequence of propositions in the discourse. They retain the ability to produce discourses with the normal components of a story grammar. Patients with short-term memory limitations also appear to process aspects of discourse such as the assignment of antecedents to a pronoun, though they also may have trouble when a discourse is infelicitous. Short-term memory patients also appear to produce well-formed, coherent discourses (Shallice and Butterworth, 1977).

Discourse Comprehension and Production in Aphasic Patients

We have seen that theories of the structure of discourse all begin with a representation of the items and propositions in a discourse.

Patients with disturbances affecting the word and sentence level of language processing would therefore be expected to have impairments of processing at the level of discourse. We might expect that a challenge for a researcher or clinician is to determine which aspects of a disturbance of discourse comprehension or production are due to disturbances of word and sentence processing, and which are due to primary impairments of processing at the discourse level. However, the expectation that aphasic patients will have considerable trouble with discourse processing appears to be mistaken. Though aphasic patients do have some trouble with discourse structures, the ability to process discourse is often preserved to a surprising degree in aphasic patients.

Several studies come to this conclusion with respect to the comprehension of aspects of discourse structure. In one of the first of these, Stachowiak and collaborators (1977) read short texts to 19 aphasic subjects, and an equal number of right hemisphere–damaged patients and normal control subjects. Each story ended with an idiom. For instance, a story about a man who took on too much work ended with the German sentence *Da hat er sich seine schöne Suppe eingebrockt*, literally meaning "He then crumbled some pieces of bread into his soup," but interpreted in its figurative meaning as "He got himself into a nice mess." In half the stories, the literal and figurative meanings of this sentence were closely related; in half, they were not (as in the case of *Da hat er sich seine schöne Suppe eingebrockt*). Subjects were to match the last sentence in the text with one of five pictures, depicting the literal meaning of the sentence, the figurative meaning of the sentence, or a lexical foil (an inappropriate action by a character in the story, or a person not mentioned in the story). Overall, the aphasic subjects performed at the same level as both the right hemisphere–damaged patients and the normal controls. All groups also chose more literal pictures when the literal and figurative meanings of the sentence were closely related. This basic patten of results was found in all types of aphasics.

Brookshire and Nicholas (1984) reported a similar finding regarding the retention of main ideas and details in discourses on the part of aphasic patients. Six narratives were read to subjects (15 aphasic patients, 5 right hemisphere–damaged patients, 5 normal controls). Following the presentation of the narrative, subjects were read pairs of statements, one of which was true of the narrative and one of which was false. The statements referred to either main ideas or details. Main ideas were better verified than details in all groups. The effect of group was marginally significant ($P = .08$), indicating a weak tendency for aphasic patients to perform less well than the other two groups. This tendency was due to "fluent" and "mixed" aphasic patients performing less well than right hemisphere–damaged patients and controls (as well as less well than "nonfluent" aphasic patients), but the authors emphasize that there was considerable overlap in performances across the various types of aphasia.

Wegner, Brookshire, and Nicholas (1984) extended this result. These researchers presented stories to subjects that were either coherent or incoherent. Incoherent stories had no overall topic, but contained sentences that maintained reference, as in (34):

(34)   Joe and Bill were avid golfers. They golfed every Wednesday because it was Joe's day off from the restaurant where he worked. The owner of the restaurant was a famous doctor . . .

Subjects were tested, as in the Brookshire and Nicholas experiment, for verification of main ideas and details from these two types of stories. Ten aphasic patients performed less well than ten control subjects. There was no effect of coherence, but main ideas were better recalled than details. The interaction of group by salience was significant: aphasic patients performed worse than controls in verifying details than they did in verifying main ideas. In addition, there was a significant three-way interaction (group by condition by salience). The aphasic patients did worse in verifying details in coherent paragraphs, while the controls had their greatest problem with details in the incoherent paragraphs. The authors suggest that details may have been lost by the aphasic patients in the coherent paragraphs because these paragraphs contained many semantically related items that the aphasic patients could not keep separate. Another possibility is that aphasic patients constructed a discourse representation and kept main ideas preferentially in mind whenever they could be related to the topic of a discourse, forgetting supporting details once the topic was clearly established.

Finally, Huber and Gleber (1982) reported that aphasic patients, right hemisphere–damaged patients, and normal controls (18 subjects per group) performed similarly in certain respects on both a sentence-ordering and a picture-ordering task. Subjects were given six sentences or drawings in random order and requested to arrange them to tell a story. Sentence sets were either "high cohesion" or "low cohesion." High-cohesion sentence sets contained connective phrases (e.g., "in order to") and descriptions of motivations and emotional states (e.g., "This made the gentleman feel good") that served to link propositions; low-coherence sets simply reported actions. Aphasic patients were more impaired than controls in arranging sentences, and right hemisphere–damaged patients had more trouble with arranging pictures. However, none of the groups found it more difficult to arrange the low cohesion sentence sets than the high-cohesion sets. The authors conclude that all these groups of subjects construct discourse-level representations on the basis of propositional content, and do not rely on "microstructural" features of sentences to build such structures.

Aphasic patients also appear to be similar to normal subjects in that they have more trouble with more complicated discourses. Caplan and Evans (1990) studied the abilities of 16 aphasic patients' to answer questions pertaining to stories. Two narratives and two folk tales were composed. The folk tales had more complicated structures than the narratives because they included more events. A set of 18 true/false probes was designed for each of the stories to assess comprehension. There were three categories of probes: (1) Event frame probes were designed to assess an individual's ability to retain the sequential order of events in a story. Probes were statements involving event sequences in the stories. (2) Problem frame probes were designed to assess a person's ability to make inferences based on the problems included in each story that were considered necessary in order for a person to have fully understood the story. These probes tested the ability of patients to form inferences related to the topic and coherence of the macrostructure of the discourse. (3) Verbatim probes contained direct statements from the story texts. The folk tale problem frame probes were significantly more difficult to verify than the narrative story problem frame probes. The familiar content and simpler structure of narratives appeared to result in making it easier for aphasic (and nonaphasic) patients to respond to problem inference probes. Comparison of other studies leads to the same conclusion. Brookshire and Nicholas (1984) and Wegner et al. (1984) found no difference between these different types of information in aphasics patients' retelling of short narratives that had simple problem frames, while Ulatowska and her colleagues (1981b, 1983), using a modified fable as one of their story stimuli, found that their aphasic subjects, when asked to recall and summarize the presented discourse, produced few propositions which evaluated story events and formed conclusions and judgments. All these results suggest that aphasic patients are better able to draw inferences in simple discourses than in complex ones (or, perhaps, in certain types of discourses, such as narratives, than others, such as folk tales). This is also true of normal subjects.

Is there any relationship between aphasic patients' abilities to comprehend words and sentences and their ability to comprehend aspects of discourse? In the studies just described, the authors independently assessed aspects of the aphasic patients' comprehension of words and sentences. Almost no correlation was found between patients' performances on the word and sentence comprehension measures and their performances on the tasks that were sensitive to discourse structure in four of the studies described above. (Stachowiak et al., 1977; Brookshire and Nicholas, 1984; Wegner et al., 1984; Huber and Gleber, 1982). However, there was a relationship between syntactic comprehension and story comprehension in the Caplan and Evans (1990) study. These researchers systematically varied the syntactic structure of the sentences in the discourses that were presented. Though there was no effect of syntactic complexity on patients' story comprehension performance, the aphasic subjects' total score on a syntactic comprehension test was significantly correlated with their total story comprehension test score. These results indicate that, in common discourse structures containing semantically and discourse-constrained sentences, the syntactic complexity of the sentences in the discourse does not have an independent effect upon aphasic patients' abilties to answer questions about the content of a passage, regardless of a patient's ability to comprehend sentences by a syntactic route. However, sentence and discourse comprehension may share some processing resources, and patients' reductions in this resource system may partially determine the magnitude of their failure on both tasks.

These studies indicate that aphasic patients have some impairments, relative to control subjects, in tasks that require comprehending and retaining aspects of discourse structure. However, what is striking about the studies is how well these subjects performed, and, especially, how much evidence there is that they extract main ideas and topics from discourses (and even from sets of sentences that are in random order). How might this happen? Stachowiak et al. (1977) and Waller and Darley (1978) proposed that aphasic patients could comprehend spoken discourse through a process of contextualization that involves recruiting internal knowledge structures that guide a listener's semantic construction of a discourse. This idea is supported by a study of Armus, Brookshire, and Nicholas (1989) that provided evidence for the integrity of knowledge of scripts in aphasic patients. Twelve aphasic patients performed as well as control subjects in discriminating events that would occur in a script from those that would not be expected to be part of a given script, and in ordering events in scripts. The patients performed almost as well as the controls in choosing the most central propositions in scripts. It thus appears that knowledge of common events—scripts—can be preserved in aphasic patients. Contextualization may be possible in aphasic patients, even on the basis of very little lexical and propositional information, and may be able to compensate for disorders in basic linguistic abilities.

If discourse structures are created by aphasic patients, perhaps on the basis of script knowledge being activated by a limited number of lexical items from which propositional information is inferred, how fast does this process go on? Does it approach the speed of normal discourse-level processing? There are only a few on-line studies of discourse processing in aphasic patients. They suggest that discourse-level processing does go on very quickly and possibly normally (in some respects at least) in some aphasic patients.

For instance, Tyler (1985) studied word monitoring in a patient with Broca's aphasia. She found that word-monitoring latencies were sensitive to violations of semantic and syntactic well-formedness, just as in a group of normal control subjects. Among the violations of semantic well-formedness were pragmatic violations, such as (35a). These were contrasted with acceptable sentences, such as b), and other violations, such as those of subcategorization as in c):

(35a) The singer buried the guitar.
   b) The singer picked up the guitar.
   c) The singer slept the guitar.

Latencies for recognition of *guitar* in (35a) were increased to a similar degree compared to baseline latencies in b) for the aphasic patient and the control subjects. This contrasted with the increase in latencies for monitoring in condition c), which were much longer in the aphasic patient than the control group (relative to baseline). This indicates that the patient was processing pragmatic information (that people don't usually bury guitars) rapidly enough to influence word on-line recognition, as normal subjects did. The greater increase in reaction times for the syntactic anomalies suggests the patient was very sensitive to these anomalies; the fact that he was not overly affected by pragmatic anomalies suggests that he did not have more trouble than normals in recognizing these anomalies and processing sentences that contained them.[3]

Finally, let us turn to discourse production in patients with disturbances of word and sentence production. Studying discourse production in aphasic patients presents the researcher with the challenge of differentiating between disturbances of discourse production and patients' difficulties in producing words and sentences. These problems were highlighted in a study by Berko Gleason and her colleagues (1980). They had their subjects (10 aphasic patients and 5 controls) look at a series of three line drawings, listen to a description of the story the drawings represented, and then tell that story. Some of the abnormalities in production made by the aphasic patients appear to be secondary to disturbances at the word and sentence level. These errors were expected on the basis of the clinical classification of the patients. For instance, the patients with Broca's aphasia produced less speech, fewer verbs, and fewer syntactic forms than normals; the patients with Wernicke's aphasia produced fewer nouns than the normal subjects. However, there were also abnormal aspects of the speech of these patients that appear to be related to discourse considerations. For instance, Wernicke's aphasic patients used many more deictic pronouns (pronouns that "point" to an item in the environment, such as *this* and *that*) than normals. All patients used more third person pronouns for which an antecedent could not be established than normal subjects did. Both these features of the speech production of these patients appear to be due to efforts to achieve reference and to maintain continuity of reference despite impairments in accessing and producing lexical forms; that is, they may reflect compensations for a primary production impairment. Beyond these disturbances, there were abnormalities that appear to be due to limitations in the discourse planning process. For instance, all the patients produced fewer major themes for the stories than did the normal subjects.

Perhaps the most extensive studies of discourse production in aphasia have been reported by Ulatowska and her colleagues. They carried out a series of studies using story recall protocols in several mild and moderately impaired aphasic subjects and one severely impaired aphasic. In these studies, various types of discourse were presented for later recall (Ulatowska et al., 1981, Ulatowska 1983a,b; Freedman-Stern et al., 1984). The authors analyzed their data with reference to aspects of narrative superstructure (Van Dijk, 1977; Van Dijk and Kintsch, 1983; see above). Narrative superstructure categories were defined to include abstract, setting, complication, evaluation, result or resolution, and a code or moral (Ulatowska et al., 1981). In all of their experiments, the authors claimed that the aphasic subjects exhibited well-developed narrative superstructures. They could retell the stories and summarize them, including all the essential elements of the superstructure "explicitly, implicitly or probably," as judged by the experimenters (Ulatowska et al., 1983a). They claimed that their results supported the notion that aphasic patients show a preservation of discourse structure with a selective reduction of information involving elaborative material. As was the case for comprehension of aspects of discourse form, performance on sentence comprehension tests did not predict how the aphasic patients performed on the discourse tasks. The authors concluded that aphasic patients can produce discourse structures despite quite disturbed linguistic systems as tested by conventional procedures. However, it was observed in examining the written discourse of one severely aphasic subject that, when the discourse required the use of complex sentence structures, his impaired syntactic ability adversely affected his success on the test. The authors concluded that severely impaired language functions can lead to collapse of discourse structure (Freedman-Stern et al., 1984).

A more controlled study of the ability of aphasic patients to produce aspects of sentence form on the basis of discourse factors was carried out by Bates, Hamby, and Zurif (1983). These authors presented patients with sequences of three pictures, in which the second and third pictures contained some new and some previously presented material. For instance, a series of pictures might show a woman giving flowers to a child, the woman giving the child candy, and the woman giving the child a toy. Patients with Broca's aphasia were requested to describe the series of pictures. The authors were interested in whether these patients would use linguistic devices to signal new and given information appropriately. For instance, in the description of the series of pictures just given, new information is placed last in the second and third clause (where it would attract intonational stress in spoken language) and is indicated by the use of the indefinite article (*a*) instead of the definite article (*the*), while old (given) information is indicated by the use of the definite article (*the*) instead of the indefinite article (*a*). Despite significant disturbances in production of lexical items, including function words, the patients in this study were able to use these syntactic devices to encode given and new information in the second and third pictures in these series. In addition, they used devices such as pronominalization (the words *she* and *her* to refer to the woman and the child) and explicit connectives (e.g., *and then*) that created cohesion and coherence at the microstructural level of discourse.

These studies have been carried out mostly in patients with acquired exogenous neurological disease, usually left hemisphere strokes. Patients with other neurological conditions also have disturbances of production of discourse along with impairments of producing other linguistic elements. Chief amoung these patients are those with Alzheimer's disease. We have seen in chapter 4 that patients with this condition have semantic disturbances that frequently lead to anomia. However, these disturbances have been separated out from disturbances at the level of production of discourse. Ulatowska, Allard, and Chapman (1991) reported that Alzheimer's patients produced less information than normal control subjects on the discourse production tasks that she used with aphasic patients. Information judged to be essential for the coherence of discourse was frequently absent, and information judged to be tangential or irrelevant was frequently produced. Like the aphasic patients of Berko-Gleason et al., the patients with Alzheimer's disease used a greater number of pronouns than normals; this may reflect their anomia, as we suggested may have been the case in the aphasic group. Other studies confirm the reduction in informativeness of discourse in patients with Alzheimer's disease (e.g., Ripich and Terrell, 1988).

The available studies of discourse processing in patients with other language impairments all argue that the ability to understand and produce important aspects of discourse can be relatively preserved in aphasia. They show that aphasic patients frequently recall and encode macrostructure information and are able to utilize conventional superstructures, such as a narrative superstructure, to guide the comprehension and retrieval of discourse. However, as language impairments become more severe, aphasic patients begin to lose the ability to produce coherent and cohesive discourse, and to retain details of coherent discourse.

SUMMARY

The ability to abstract the major themes of connected discourse appears to be relatively preserved in many brain-damaged patients. Even patients with major disturbances affecting other levels of language appear to retain this ability in some measure. On the other hand, details of discourse are often not retained and not produced, even in patients without other language impairments. Recovery from anomalies in discourse is limited in many patients. Most patients retain basic knowledge of the structure of common events (scripts), and processing of discourse structures may in large part consist of mapping elements in these scripts onto whatever linguistic forms are comprehended and available for production. This mapping does not achieve the full range of linguistically based communication in many patients, although it does allow the most important aspects of discourse to be conveyed and understood.

NOTES

1. At times, the intentions of speakers and listeners become more complex, and include the intention to deceive or mislead. I will not deal with these more complicated intentional states here.

2. Many researchers have argued that the speed of language processing is tied to its structure (e.g. Fodor's (1983) theory of modularity relates those two stems). This view is based on the fact that, though the language code pairs forms and meanings in complex ways, this pairing is "direct" in the sense described earlier in this chapter: basic aspects of literal meaning are determinable by individual linguistic forms and combinations of these forms, without the additional intervention of cognitive processes, such as reasoning or searching through long-term or semantic memory. As we have seen, different processors, each dedicated to the activation of particular linguistic representations and each extremely rapid, are thought to operate in close communication to achieve rapid processing of language. If the "direct" nature of the mapping from form to meaning is essential for language processing to proceed at the speed it does, one would expect that discourse processing, which involves other cognitive processes, would be much slower than other aspects of language processing. However, this is not the case. Despite its partial reliance on inferential and other cognitive processes, at least some aspects of discourse processing appear to take place just as rapidly as other language-processing operations.

3. On the other hand, there is some evidence that some patients do not show effects of discourse on on-line processing, where such effects might be expected. For instance, Swinney, Zurif, and Nicol (1988) reported on the results of a cross-modal lexical priming task for associates of ambiguous words in previously disambiguating contexts in eight aphasic patients. We saw above that, in this task, both the meanings of a lexically ambiguous word like *bug* are activated when the word is heard, and previous context selects out a preferred meaning a few hundred milliseconds after the word has been presented. Four patients with Wernicke's aphasia showed this pattern. However, four patients with Broca's aphasia showed increased activation of only the most common meaning of an ambiguous word at the point where the word was presented. If the contextually preferred reading was less common than the contextually unpreferred reading, it was not activated at this point. This indicates two things: that these patients have a disturbance of lexical semantic access (they do not access all meanings of ambiguous words when such words are presented) and that context does not affect the lexical semantic access process early in some aphasic patients. It remains to be seen whether context has the normal effect on lexical semantic activation data at a later point in the presentation of a sentence to these patients.

10 Brief Notes on Issues Relating to Diagnosis and Treatment of Language Disorders

Though this book is not intended to be a clinical manual, this final chapter is devoted to a brief discussion of a number of issues that arise in the clinical domain. These are: a psycholinguistic approach to diagnosis of language disorders; the classification of language disorders; the neurological basis of language disorders, especially as it relates to localization of language functions; and psycholinguistic approaches to therapeutics. I hope the reader will find this discussion an appropriate ending to this book, and a beginning to the application of the concepts and techniques described in this book to clinical problems.

A PSYCHOLINGUISTIC APPROACH TO THE ASSESSMENT OF LANGUAGE DISORDERS

The goal of a psycholinguistic assessment of a patient is to specify the types of linguistic representations (simple words, complex words, sentences, discourse) that are processed abnormally in each of the four major language-related tasks (speech, auditory comprehension, reading, writing). It should also attempt to identify selective impairments affecting each type of representation in each of these tasks, and the overall level of functioning of the patient with respect to each linguistic representation in each task. This effort will lead to a description of the patient's language disorder in relation to the major components of the language-processing system. Finally, a psycholinguistic approach to diagnosing patients with language disorders will identify compensations the patient makes to these impairments.

To achieve this goal, the clinician must have a reasonable understanding of the language-processing system and its disorders. I have tried to provide a basis for understanding this system and its disorders in this book. In addition, the clinician must have a means of testing patients that can identify disorders of components of the system.

The obvious place to turn for assessment tools is existing aphasia batteries. However, for the most part, these batteries do not provide the basis for an analysis of patients' deficits in terms of language-processing components. We can illustrate the shortcomings of existing batteries by considering one part of the aphasia battery that is probably the most widely used in the English-speaking world, the Boston Diagnostic Aphasia Examination (BDAE; Goodglass and Kaplan, 1972, 1982). I have not selected the BDAE for this criticism because it is a particularly poor test. On the contrary, it is probably one of the better general English-language aphasia tests. Other general language assessment tests, such as the Western Aphasia Battery (WAB) (Kertesz and Poole, 1974; Kertesz, 1979) or the Porch Index of Communicative Ability (PICA) (Porch, 1971), tend to test even fewer language functions than the BDAE.

Let us consider how word comprehension, a critical part of language functioning, is tested on the BDAE. A single word is spoken to a subject, who then must choose a matching picture from a set of alternatives. Words are taken from different categories (letters, numbers, geometric shapes, body parts, and common objects), and the pictures are all presented together in several large displays.

There are quite a number of drawbacks to this method of testing auditory single word comprehension. Anyone who has gone through the material in chapters 2 and 3 of this book will immediately see what these are. First, the BDAE evaluates word comprehension only through word-picture matching. It is possible for a patient to perform abnormally because of a visual agnosia that leads to misidentification of the pictures. The BDAE does not rule out this locus of impairment in the word-picture matching task. The patient must select pictures from a large disorganized array, and may be unable to search through the array properly. A variety of language-processing deficits may also underlie failure on a word-picture matching test. A patient may have a problem with phonemic discrimination or other aspects of auditory processing, or may have lost access to the permanent representation of a word in his vocabulary. A patient who does achieve lexical access—i.e., who recognizes an auditory stimulus as a legitimate word of English—may nonetheless have lost access to the meaning of that word. This, in turn, may be because the access mechanism is not working properly for the word or because the permanent representation of the word's meaning has degenerated. In either of these cases, impairments in understanding the meaning of words can be partial. The BDAE gives no indication of which of these stages of processing are affected in a patient who does poorly on the single word auditory comprehension measure. Finally, the selection of words that are tested is not representative of the most common words of English. A substantial number of the categories sampled, such as letters and numbers, do not involve real-world categories, but formally defined, man-made constructs. Another category that does refer to concrete objects—body parts—requires a very special form of internal representation confined to a personal body schema. There are only six items that evaluate the patient's ability to extract the meaning of common objects from a spoken word. The fact that the stimuli in this test are highly atypical of words in general limits the value of the test in establishing the generality of a patient's deficit.

There are many other, more technical, problems with this test on the BDAE. For instance, a partial score is given if a patient produces the correct response after a 2-second period has passed; there is no reason why that time frame has been chosen rather than another. Timing responses is a very valuable way of looking for the integrity of a function, as we have indicated throughout this book. However, if time measurements are to be used in the assessment of a patient's performance, proper documentation of reaction times in comparison to normal performance will be needed.

In defense of the BDAE and similar tests, we should recognize that none of them was designed to provide a psycholinguistic assessment of language. If these tests accomplish other worthwhile goals, these tests are valuable for other purposes, if not for assessing language disorders from a psycholinguistic point of view. Most general aphasia batteries currently available achieve three things: (1) they establish that there is a language impairment in a patient; (2) they indicate what language-related tasks (speech, auditory comprehension, reading, writing) are affected; (3) they give the clinician some idea of what responses the patient makes in these tasks. Some of the properties of these tests contribute to these achievements. For instance, the items to be tested in the single word auditory comprehension subtest of the BDAE are ones that are frequently disturbed in aphasia (Goodglass and Baker, 1976). Their inclusion on the BDAE helps this test discriminate between the performance of normal and brain-damaged subjects, even if these items are not representative of words in general and the usefulness of the test in determining the extent and nature of a patient's word comprehension disturbance is limited.

Another goal of some aphasia batteries is to help in neurological diagnosis. Some aphasia batteries, such as the BDAE and its derivatives (e.g., the WAB), were closely tied to a neurological theory of language impairments and derive a good part of their justification from their ability to classify aphasic patients into categories derived from this neurological theory. I indicate below that I think this theory is seriously flawed, and that the goal of language assessment should not be to classify patients into the groups identified in this approach.

If the clinician cannot rely on existing general purpose aphasia batteries to assess language psycholinguistically, are there any other means available to accomplish this task? One possibility is to use different parts of different more specific tests (the Wepman [Wepman, 1958], the Peabody Picture Vocabulary Test [Dunn, 1965], the Boston Naming Test [Kaplan, Goodglass and Weintraub, 1977], the Token Test [DeRenzi and Vignolo, 1962], etc.) to assess different aspects of language processing. This approach may help, but it too is far from totally satisfactory. As is true of the more general language assessment batteries, these more specific tests also do not deal adequately with many of the variables that the research we have reviewed in previous chapters indicates are important. For instance, the Token Test is often used as a test of syntactic comprehension. However, the test does not distinguish between a problem a patient may have in syntactic comprehension and one he may have in utilizing the products of comprehension to plan actions.

I do not wish to imply that all of these tests are completely unrevealing with respect to the language-processing problems of a patient. It is possible to cobble together a series of tests that begin to provide the basis for a picture of which language-processing components are affected in a given patient. But existing tests are very hard to use for this purpose. They only occasionally allow the clinician to identify the language-processing components that are affected in a patient, and they never provide a systematic exploration of the nature of disturbances within a component. In addition, existing tests do not assess some important areas of language processing at all, such as comprehension and production of morphological structure.

The last resort is to create one's own tests. My colleague, Dan Bub, and I have, in fact, created a psycholinguistically oriented language assessment battery—the Psycholinguistic Assessment of Language (PAL)—which we use to identify the major deficits in language processing at the level of simple words, morphologically complex words, and sentences (Caplan and Bub, 1990). I present an outline of this battery here as a guide to what types of materials a clinician might use in assessing language-impaired patients along linguistic and psycholinguistic lines. I most emphatically do not want to claim that this is the only way, or the best conceivable way, to assess language disorders psycholinguistically. There are many other ways of assessing these functions; indeed, virtually any test in this battery could be replaced by another properly selected test and the result would still be an appropriate and useful assessment tool. I am only presenting this overview of the PAL to provide a concrete example of an approach to patient assessment that incorporates the perspective adopted in this book.

THE PSYCHOLINGUISTIC ASSESSMENT OF LANGUAGE

The PAL consists of 27 subtests. Each subtest contains items with different structural or categorical features, to assess the specificity of a deficit for particular stimulus types at each level of processing. Each subtest also contains items that vary in difficulty, to provide a measure of the extent to which a particular component is disturbed. In order to evaluate the integrity of a component of the language-processing system, it is necessary to compare a patient's performance on several tests (see discussion below).

Because many of the tests in the battery involve matching language stimuli to pictures or producing language responses on the basis of pictorial stimuli, before the battery is used a screening test for the ability to identify pictures of objects is administered. This test uses a pictorial forced-choice attribute-verification task to ascertain whether a patient can extract semantic information from a picture. In this task, a patient must choose which of two properties is true of an object depicted in a picture (e.g., a picture of a deer is shown, and the subject must answer the question "Does it eat grass or animals?") Patients who show abnormalities that interfere with their abilities to extract semantic information from pictures would only be examined on tests of the battery that do not make use of pictures.

The battery proper contains the following materials. The reader will appreciate that these materials incorporate many of the variables that affect patient performance that we discussed in chapters 2 through 8. At present, it does not assess processing at the level of discourse.

Auditory Comprehenion

The Single Word Level

Three processing components involved in single word input processing are assessed: (1) acoustic-phonetic processing, (2) lexical access, (3) and semantic access. The tests relevant to these components are the following.

Test 1: Phoneme Discrimination. The ability to discriminate phonemes is tested by a same-different task with 40 pairs of monosyllabic nonwords (20 different and 20 identical trials). Different stimuli differ in a single consonantal phoneme with respect to place of articulation, manner of articulation, or voicing. The changed phoneme can occur in stimulus-initial or stimulus-final position, either as a single consonant or as a member of a cluster. Consonants were chosen as the segments to be changed because they have been used more frequently than vowels in research on phonemic discrimination in aphasia. The subject must say whether the two items are identical or different.

Test 2: Auditory Lexical Decision. Auditory lexical access is assessed using a lexical decision task for words and specifically constructed nonwords. The words consist of 40 concrete nouns. They vary in frequency (>40/million or <5/million) and length (one syllable vs. three or more syllables). Half the foils are constructed by changing a single distinctive feature in a single phoneme in different syllabic positions in comparable words. The other 20 foils are created by changing the form of words matched to the positive targets so as to resemble possible words (e.g., *harpsiform* from *harpsicord*); these stimuli were included because having only phonological foils sounded odd in pilot trials with normals. A yes/no (word/nonword) decision is required.

Single Word Auditory Comprehension. We use three means of assessing single word comprehension: (1) a word-picture matching test, (2) a forced-choice attribute-verification procedure, and (3) a relatedness judgment test for abstract words. These three tasks assess a subject's ability to map a word onto a picture and to recognize verbally presented features and synonyms of a word. Across the set of tests, animacy and abstractness are varied. To test for a subject's consistency across different presentations of a given item, there is selective repetition of some words on the forced-choice attribute-verification task and the word-picture selection task (and also on the picture naming and written tasks described below).

Test 3: Word-Picture Matching. In this task, 32 concrete nouns are presented auditorily and the subject must select one of two pictures as the match to the word. Foils are both semantically and visually similar to the targets (e.g., *deer* as target and *moose* as foil). Targets are of either high or low frequency, and are either short (monosyllabic) or long (tri- or quadrisyllabic). They include examples from the categories of animals, fruits and vegetables, and tools. The subject must select the correct picture.

Test 4: Forced-Choice Attribute-Verification Procedure. In this task, sixteen concrete nouns are presented auditorily, and three questions are asked regarding each noun. The questions require either a yes/no answer or the selection of one of two features (e.g., *Does a horse have fur or a hide?*). Three questions relate to physical and three to functional attributes. Nouns are from the categories of animals, fruits and vegetables, and tools, and vary in familiarity.

Test 5: Relatedness Judgment Test for Abstract Words. A target word and two subsequent words are presented auditorily. The subject must select the word most closely related to the target (e.g., *strive—learn/try*). All targets are mono- and bisyllabic, but otherwise vary in frequency and syntactic category.

The Word Formation Level

The following subtests assess recognition and comprehension of affixed words.

Test 6: Auditory Lexical Decision for Affixed Words. Recognition of derived words is assessed through a lexical decision task that tests a patient's ability to recognize derived words as well formed. Positive stimuli consist of high-frequency stems and affixes that are combined to form low-frequency morphologically complex words. Both derivational affixation and inflectional affixation are used. Within derivational affixation, both word-boundary and formative-boundary affixes are used. The positive stimuli thus consist of 24 words—8 with word-boundary derivational affixes (e.g., *heaviness*), 8 with word-boundary inflectional affixes (e.g., *draws*), and 8 with formative-boundary affixes (e.g., *deceptive*)—and an equivalent number of foils consisting of nonexistent derived forms (e.g., *detentive*). The stimuli are presented auditorily to the subject who must indicate whether each is a word or not.

Auditory Comprehension of Affixed Words. The battery tests for comprehension of the meaning conveyed by affixes—e.g., aspect, tense, and number—on a word-picture matching test and a relatedness judgment task.

Test 7: Word-Picture Matching for Affixed Words. Derived words are presented with a picture that conveys each word's meaning and a foil that reflects a different affix (e.g., the word *restless* is presented with a picture-pair showing a person who is restless [pacing] and one who is resting [sitting down relaxing]). Twenty words are presented auditorily, and the subject must select the appropriate picture. Words vary with respect to the nature of the affixation (derivational, inlectional).

Test 8: Relatedness Judgment for Affixed Words. A relatedness judgment task, similar to that used with abstract words, is used to assess patients' abilities to comprehend the meanings of affixes. A target affixed word is presented auditorily along with two affixed versions of another root (e.g., the target word *chosen* presented with the word-pair *selection* and *selected*), and the subject must indicate which of the pair goes best with the target.

The Sentence Level

The battery assesses the various sentence comprehension processes discussed in chapter 7. The first—lexico-inferential processing—is the process whereby a subject infers aspects of propositional semantics, such as thematic roles, from lexical semantic knowledge and pragmatic information. This component of the comprehension system is tested by presenting sentences that are constrained by plausibility factors. The second process—parsing and syntactic comprehension—applies when lexical and pragmatic constraints do not suffice to yield an unambiguous interpretation, i.e., when sentences are semantically reversible, and involves the utilization of syntactic structure to determine propositional meaning. It is tested by presenting syntactically complex semantically reversible sentences. The use of syntactic heuristics to understand sentences is tested by presenting semantically reversible sentences that can be understood through the application of simple comprehension strategies, such as interpreting noun-verb-noun (N-V-N) sequences as agent-verb-theme.

Test 9a: Constrained Sentence Comprehension.

A sentence-picture matching test is used. Pictures consist of the correct interpretation and a foil that varies with respect to one of the words in the sentence (e.g., target: *The car was waxed by the man;* foil: *The car was washed by the man*). Twenty semantically irreversible sentences varying as to voice (active and passive) and nature of foil (verb, preposition, particle) are presented auditorily. The foils are drawn from syntactic categories that are best tested in sentences—verbs, prepositions, and verbal particles. This test thus supplements the tests of single word comprehension (tests 3–5), which focus on nouns and adjectives. The subject must select the appropriate picture.

Test 9b: Syntactic Comprehension.

Twenty semantically reversible sentences with four syntactic structures—active, passive, dative-passive, subject-object relative—are presented in a sentence-picture matching test with correct pictures and syntactically incorrect foils (e.g., target: *The man was pushed by the woman;* foil: *The man pushed the woman*). Sentences are presented auditorily and the subject must select the appropriate picture.

Oral Production

The Single Word Level
Oral production of single words is divided into two components: accessing lexical phonological forms from the meanings of words, and planning phonological output. The tasks relevant to these components are as follows.

Test 10: Picture Homophone Matching. A picture homophone matching task is used to assess a subject's ability to access lexical phonological representations from word meaning, despite any possible disruption of the ability to produce these representations orally. Thirty-two picture-pairs are presented; half are homophones (*bat/bat*) and half differ by a single distinctive feature (*cat/can*). The subject must indicate whether the names of the pictures are homophones.

Test 11: Word and Nonword Repetition. As discued in chapter 4, repetition can be carried out by various mechanisms. It is possible to understand a word and repeat it by reaccessing it from its semantic meaning. It is also possible to repeat a word by recognizing it as a word (i.e., activating a representation in the phonological input lexicon) and using that representation to activate a word in the phonological output lexicon, without understanding it. Finally repetition of both words and nonwords can be accomplished by identifying phonemes and other sound elements and using them to activate units in an output buffer. The battery tests repetition of both words and nonwords. Twenty words—all common concrete nouns that vary in frequency and length—are presented auditorily, and the subject must repeat them. Repetition of nonwords tests the ability to produce phonological structures that have no lexical identity. Twenty nonwords—derived by changing multiple distinctive features in words comparable to the word stimuli—are presented auditorily, and the subject must repeat them.

In the repetition tasks, responses are to be classified into one of a number of major categories: correct responses (i.e., those made by a normal age-matched population), phonetic (dysarthric and dyspraxic) errors, phonological errors (phonemic paraphasias and neologisms), semantically related errors (semantic paraphasias and circumlocutions), unclassifiable errors, and failures to respond. The number of erroneous responses of each type is measured.

Test 12: Picture Naming. This task tests both the ability to access a lexical phonological representation from semantics and the ability to plan and execute the production of the phonological representation thus accessed. Thirty-two line drawings of objects are presented for naming. The objects are the foils in the auditory word-picture matching test described above. The names are all common nouns, which vary as to semantic category, length, and frequency, as described above in the word-picture matching test. Errors are classified as phonetic, phonological, semantic, unclassifiable, and nonresponses. The number of erroneous responses of each type is measured. If a patient does not respond, he is asked to give the first sound of the word and the number of syllables in the word, as evidence of his having accessed some aspect of the word's phonological form.

The Word Formation Level
The goal of this section of the battery is to see whether a patient can produce appropriate morphologically complex forms on the basis of conceptual representations.

Test 13: Affixed Word Production. A sentence completion task using a prespecified lexical item tests subjects' abilities to produce appropriate morphological forms (e.g., COURAGE: If a man has a great deal of courage, we say he is ____). Derivational affixes (both level I and level II) and inflectional affixes are tested. The base form is presented first, and then the sentence. The subject must complete the sentence with a morphological variant of the root (e.g., *courageous* in the example above). Thirty items are used in the test. Responses are scored correct if the production of the root and suffix are identifiable and correct. (Phonological and dysarthric errors are identified at the lexical level. It is expected that they will continue to be seen at these higher levels if they are present at the word level.)

The Sentence Level
The goal of the tasks described in this section is to determine a subject's ability to assign thematic roles and to use active, passive, and embedded sentences as the syntactic structures whereby these

semantic meanings are expressed in oral speech. These goals require a highly constrained task, in the same way as the production of affixed words requires such a task.

Test 14: Sentence Production.   Pictures depicting actions are presented. The subject is told he must describe what is going on in the picture, mentioning the items designated by arrows and using a single sentence (he is told specifically that the word *and* cannot be used). Five syntactic structures conveying thematic roles and attribution of modification are targeted: actives (*The boy pushes the girl*); datives (*The boy gives the rattle to the baby*); passives (*The boy is pushed by the girl*); dative passives (*The rattle was given to the baby by the woman*); and subject-object relatives (*The girl pushing a cart is opening the door*).

To constrain production to arrive at these targets, the subject is instructed to: (1) mention all the items that are designated, (2) begin with an item indicated by a dot next to the arrow, and (3) use the verb(s) provided by the examiner. For instance, a picture depicting a truck pushing a car is presented, and the subject's task is to describe the picture mentioning the car before the truck and using the verb *push*. These constraints induce the subject to use a passive form.

Scoring of responses attributes credit for (1) producing the correct lexical items, (2) assigning the correct thematic role to each lexical item, and (3) using the correct aspects of sentence structure. Thus, a simple active sentence (e.g., *The boy pushed the girl*) can produce a score of four points (the two nouns produced correctly, and the two thematic roles—agent and theme—assigned to each of them correctly), whereas a dative passive (e.g., *The rattle was given to the baby by the woman*) can produce a score of nine points (three nouns, three correct thematic roles, three syntactic markers—the passive form, the preposition *by* and the preposition *to*).

Written Comprehension

The Single Word Level
Words may be spelled regularly (e.g., *cat*) or irregularly (e.g., *island*). It is possible for a reader to sound out regularly spelled words, but irregularly spelled words must be recognized on the basis of their whole word forms. In terms of the model presented in chapter 5, regularly spelled words may be recognized by converting sublexical

orthographic units to their corresponding, predictable phonological units, while irregularly spelled words are recognized by accessing orthographic lexical forms in a mental written-language dictionary (the "orthographic input lexicon"). The battery tests both the ability to convert sublexical orthographic units to phonological units and to activate entries in the orthographic input lexicon.

Test 15: Written Lexical Decision. Lexical access from print is tested by a written lexical decision task. Word stimuli consist of 32 common nouns that vary in frequency, abstractness, length, and orthographic-phonological regularity. An equal number of nonwords are created by changing one letter in words appropriately matched to the target set. Stimuli are presented visually and a yes/no (word/nonword) decision is required.

Test 16: Word-Picture Matching. The words for the foils in the auditory word-picture matching test are presented visually in a written word-picture matching test, with the same pairs of pictures used previously.

Test 17: Forced-Choice Attribute-Verification. The stimuli and questions used in the auditory version of this task are presented visually.

Test 18: Relatedness Judgment Test for Abstract Words. The materials used in this task in the auditory modality are presented visually.

Transcoding of Written to Spoken Forms. As with repetition, words may be read by understanding them and reaccessing their sounds on the basis of their meanings, by relating the written form of the word to its pronunciation as a whole, or sounding out a word based on correspondences between spelling units and sounds (grapheme-phoneme correspondences).

Test 19: Oral Reading. Thirty-two words, varied as to frequency, length, spelling-sound regularity, and abstractness are presented in written form. An equivalent number of nonwords derived from matched words by changing one letter are also presented. The subject must read each stimulus aloud. Responses are characterized as correct, semantic paralexias, morphological paralexias, visual errors, regularizations, and lexicalizations.

The Word Formation Level

Test 20: Lexical Decision for Written Affixed Words.   A lexical decision task is used with a written version of the stimuli described above for auditory presentation. Presentation is as in the written lexical access test with single words.

Tests 21 and 22: Comprehension of Written Affixed Words.   The materials described above to assess this function in the auditory modality are used with written materials. In the word-picture matching test (test 21), the affixed word is presented in written form along with the target picture and the foil described above. In the relatedness judgment task (test 22), both the target and the two items from which the subject must choose are presented in visual form. In both tests, the subject must indicate which of the two possible choices is best.

The Sentence Level
The two tests used for auditory sentence comprehension are used in written form.

Test 23: (a) Constrained Written Sentence Comprehension and (b) Written Syntactic Comprehension.   Written versions of test 9 are presented.

Written Production

The Single Word Output Level
Single word written production is assessed in two ways: the production of written forms from semantics (writing the names of pictures) and the production of written forms from phonological forms (writing to dictation). In the latter case, words may be written based on their whole word forms or on correspondences between sounds and spelling units (phoneme-grapheme correspondences).

Test 24: Written Naming.   The pictures used as foils in the written word-picture matching test are used as targets. These 32 stimuli are all concrete common nouns that vary as to frequency and length. Written responses are classified as correct, legibility problems, orthographic (spelling) errors, semantic errors, and unclassifiable responses. The number of errors of each type is measured.

Test 25: Writing to Dictation.   Twenty words varying in sound-to-spelling regularity (e.g., *tent* vs. *lamb*) and 20 nonwords are presented to the subject, who must write them from dictation. Words are all of moderate frequency and from one to three syllables in length. The 20 nonwords are constructed by changing one letter in words matched to the positive stimulus set. Responses are classified as above as correct, legibility problems, regularizations (for words), lexicalizations (for nonwords), other orthographic (spelling) errors, semantic errors, and unclassifiable responses. The number of errors is measured for regular words, irregular words, and nonwords.

The Word Formation Level

Test 26: Written Affixed Word Production.   The materials used to assess this function with oral production are used with written presentation, and the output is required to be in writing. Responses are scored correct if the production of the correct root and suffix are identifiable. (Spelling and other errors are identified at the lexical level.)

The Sentence Level

Test 27: Written Sentence Production.   The test used for oral sentence production is given with a written output being required. The responses are not judged for orthographic errors, which have been assessed previously, but only for lexical production and the aspects of sentence meaning and form being tested here.

THE PSYCHOLINGUISTIC ASSESSMENT OF LANGUAGE: IDENTIFICATION OF DEFICITS IN LANGUAGE-PROCESSING COMPONENTS

The PAL provides a database that allows the examiner to assess the integrity of the major components of the language processing system. (Again, other structured sets of tests could accomplish the same goal.) Patients who do significantly less well than normal age-matched subjects with similar educational and socioeconomic backgrounds on a subtest of the PAL can be assumed to have some problem that prevents them from accomplishing that subtest. The analysis of the results obtained with PAL (or a comparable set of tests) is directed toward ascertaining how the pattern of tests on which a patient does well and poorly can be understood in terms of the integrity and impairment of the major language-processing components.

To undertake this analysis, the examiner must first determine that major nonlinguistic factors are not affecting performance. The subject must be paying attention, making a serious effort on the task, and able to accomplish the actions needed for a subtest of the battery. Observation of the patient in the clinical setting, as well as more formal neuropsychological evaluations can help rule out these types of disturbances as the basis for a patient's abnormal performance. In general, it is also likely that a patient who cannot accomplish a handful of tests on a battery such as the PAL, but who performs normally on many others, has a specific problem with these tests, not a general problem with attention, or other general cognitive furctions.

If the examiner is confident that major nonlinguistic factors are not affecting performance, the pattern of performance on a series of tests gives an indication of what language-processing components are affected. The examiner can attribute a *primary* deficit in a particular processing component to a patient if (and only if): (1) his performance on the test(s) that requires that component is abnormal, and (2) the linguistic input to that component is intact (as judged by performance on other subtests). Thus, for instance, the auditory lexical access component may be considered to be the locus of an independent deficit if (and only if): (1) performance on the auditory lexical decision test is abnormal and (2) performance on the phonemic discrimination test is normal. It is inappropriate to conclude that a patient has a *primary* deficit in recognizing words if he cannot discriminate phonemes. The examiner can make the diagnosis of a *secondary* deficit in a language-processing component when both performance on the test(s) that requires that component and performance on the subtests that assess processing of linguistic structures needed for the operation of the deficit component are abnormal. For instance, the auditory lexical access component can be considered to be the locus of a deficit that is secondary to a disturbance of acoustic-phonetic processing if: (1) performance on the auditory lexical decision test is abnormal and (2) performance on the phonemic discrimination test is also abnormal.

In general, a patient's performance must be compared across several subtests to come to a decision as to which component of the language-processing system is impaired. In tables 10.1, 10.2, 10.3, we present the basic pattern of performance on the subtests of the PAL battery that can be taken as evidence for a primary deficit in each of the language-processing components that have been described. (The deficits that we recognize in processing written language above the single word level are the same as those that we recognized for the auditory-oral modality, and are not listed in a separate table.)

This approach to attributing deficits in specific language-processing components to a patient must be qualified by the recognition that a patient may fail on a subtest because of a highly specific cognitive disturbance that is external to the linguistic processing demands of that subtest but that does not show up in other tasks clearly. For instance, failure on the homophone matching test (test 10) may be due to an inability to *compare* two phonological representations, not to a failure to *activate* them. The possibility that failure of a patient on a subtest is due to these types of cognitive factors can be addressed in several ways. First, careful observation of each patient during testing can identify factors such as fatigue that can arise at one point in testing and thus lead to impaired performance on a given subtest. Second, comparisons across tests can serve to rule out several reasons for failure. For instance, a patient who fails on the lexical decision test for affixed words but performs well on the lexical decision test for simple words cannot have a general problem with nonlinguistic aspects of lexical decision tests (such as making decisions). As indicated in tables 10.1, and 10.2, and 10.3, comparison across tests can also provide converging evidence regarding the deficit underlying poor performance on selected tests. For instance, in the example of homophone matching given directly above, a patient's performance on the tests of picture naming and word and nonword repetition can provide converging evidence regarding his or her ability to access phonology from semantics. An inability to produce words coupled with an intact ability to repeat them would be consistent with an inability to access phonology

Table 10.1
Deficits in Auditory Comprehension, Defined by Performances on the PAL
Battery*

Deficient Component	Pattern of Performance on Subtests
A. *Word level*	
1. *Acoustic-phonetic processing*	*Abnormal performance on the phonemic discrimination test*
2. *Auditory lexical access*	Normal performance on the phonemic discrimination test *Abnormal performance on the lexical decision task with words*
3. *Lexical semantic access*	Normal performance on the phonemic discrimination test Normal performance on the lexical decision task with words *Abnormal performance on any lexical comprehension test*
B. *Affixed word level*	
1. *Morphological analysis*	Normal lexical access *Abnormal performance on lexical decision for affixed words*
2. *Morphological comprehension*	Intact single word input processing Normal lexical decision for affixed words *Abnormal performance on any test of affixed word comprehension*
C. *Sentence level*	
1. *Lexico-inferential comprehension*	Normal lexical semantic access and morphological comprehension *Abnormal performance on constrained sentence comprehension*
2. *Parsing and syntactic comprehension*	Normal lexical semantic comprehension Normal lexical semantic access and morphological comprehension Normal performance on constrained sentence comprehension *Abnormal performance on comprehension of semantically unconstrained syntactically complex sentences*

*Subtests on which the subject must perform normally are indicated in
plain type. Subtests on which abnormal performance is a criterion for the
assignment of a particular deficit are italicized.

Table 10.2
Deficits in Oral Production, Defined by Performances on the Battery*

Deficient Component	Pattern of Performance on Subtest
A. Word level	
1. Accessing lexical phonological forms (from semantics)	Normal performance on picture comprehension screen *Abnormal performance on naming task* *Abnormal performance on homophone judgment task*
2. Phonological output planning	Normal performance on picture comprehension screen, homophone judgment, phonemic discrimination, auditory and written lexical decision *Phonemic paraphasias in naming, repetition, and oral reading tasks*
B. Affixed word level	
1. Accessing affixed words (from semantics)	Naming and repetition adequate for the patients' oral production of words to be recognized *Abnormal performance on affixed word production*
C. Sentence level	
1. Expression of thematic roles	Normal word production in isolation Normal performance on affixed word production *Failure to produce word sequences that convey correct thematic roles on sentence production task*
2. Construction of syntactic structures	Normal word production in isolation Normal performace on affixed word production *Failure to produce complex structures (e.g., passives) on sentence production task*
3. Insertion of function words into syntactic structures	Normal word production in isolation Normal performance on affixed word production *Agrammatism/ paragrammatism on sentence production task*
4. Insertion of content words into syntactic structures	Normal word production in isolation Normal performance on affixed word production *Anomia/phonemic paraphasias in content words on sentence production task*

* Subtests on which the subject must perform normally are indicated in plain type. Subtests on which abnormal performance is a criterion for the assignment of a particular deficit are italicized.

Table 10.3
Deficits in Written Single Word Processing, Defined by Performances on the Battery

Deficient Component	Pattern of Performance on Subtest
Comprehension of written words	
1. *Written lexical access*	*Abnormal performance on the written lexical decision task*
2. *Written lexical semantic access*	Normal performance on the written lexical decision task
	Abnormal performance on any written lexical comprehension task
Production of written words	
1. *Accessing lexical orthography from semantics*	Normal performance on picture comprehension screen
	Normal writing of words to dictation
	Abnormal performance on written picture naming task
2. *Accessing lexical orthography from lexical phonology*	Normal auditory lexical access
	Normal writing of nonwords to dictation
	Abnormal (regularized) writing of irregular words to dictation
3. *Accessing sublexical orthography from sublexical phonology*	Normal phoneme discrimination
	Normal writing of words to dictation
	Abnormal writing of nonwords to dictation
Reading single words	
1. *Accessing lexical phonology from lexical orthography*	Normal written lexical access
	Normal regular word reading and nonword reading
	Abnormal (regularized) reading of irregular words
2. *Accessing sublexical phonology from sublexical orthography*	Normal oral naming
	Normal word reading
	Abnormal nonword reading

* Subtests on which the subject must perform normally are indicated in plain type. Subtests on which abnormal performance is a criterion for the assignment of a particular deficit are italicized.

from semantics, also suggested by failure on homophone matching. Third, a patient's performance on these language tests can be compared with his performance on other neuropsychological tests. This should serve to help decide whether some abnormal performances are due to extralinguistic factors, such as difficulty making comparisons or decisions.

Another problem that occasionally arises in interpreting the results of a battery such as the PAL is that unexpected patterns of performance occur. For instance, a patient may do well on all the tests pertaining to single word comprehension—phoneme discrimination, auditory lexical decision, all the word comprehension tasks—and also on the naming test, but still be poor at repetition of words. At first blush, this would seem impossible. If the subtests are good measures of processing, they are indicating that the patient can discriminate the sounds of words, recognize words, understand words, and produce spoken words from semantic representations. He should be able to repeat, at least by understanding a word and activating its form from its meaning. Why can't he?

One possibility is that the entire model of how single word repetition takes place is wrong. Perhaps words are repeated through some form of mimicry of their nonlinguistic acoustic properties, and the ability to analyze or produce these nonlinguistic features of an auditory stimulus is affected in the patient. This sort of explanation of how repetition takes place and why it might fail in a patient seems extremely unlikely, especially given the data presented in chapter 4 about repetition and its disorders. Another possibility is that the patient cannot chain together all the steps involved in repetition, even if he or she can accomplish each step by itself. This has been suggested as the basis for certain repetition disorders (see chapter 4). Such a disturbance may be related to certain kinds of limitations of auditory-verbal short-term memory (Shallice and Warrington, 1977). A third possibility is that there is a special processor devoted to repetition that is independent of those that are involved in word comprehension and word production (see chapter 4). A patient may be trying to use this special processor and it may be damaged; for some reason (related to how the patient unconsciously determines which processing components are used in any psycholinguistic task), the patient may not be using the alternative routes to repetition based upon single word comprehension and production. The point is that what at first seems to be an inexplicable pattern of results may be interpretable.

Exploring the possibilities just enumerated will require further testing. The occurrence of a puzzling pattern of performance is just one circumstance in which a clinician may decide that it is necessary to add to the tests in a battery such as the PAL. The clinician may feel it is important to test comprehension of types of linguistic elements that are not well represented in this battery, such as a range of function words. In most patients it is important to test comprehension and production of discourse. Different clinical circumstances will require different levels of depth and breadth of patient deficit analysis.

The approach to patient diagnosis we have outlined is not a simple one to apply. As I indicated above, it requires the clinician to be familiar with basic aspects of language structure and psycholinguistic processing, and to master the administration and interpretation of a set of psycholinguistically oriented tests of language functions. In some cases, it may require the clinician to think in novel ways about what is wrong with a patient, as in the example of a patient who understands and produces words but has difficulty repeating them. Given the demands—intellectual and time-related—of a psycholinguistically oriented approach to patient assessment, we must ask whether this approach is realistic. Can the PAL—or its equivalent—be administered in a reasonable period of time? Will the effort to interpret patients' performances as deficits in specific language-processing components prove worthwhile in identifying patients with language disorders and in designing therapy?

Clearly, this approach is too new for anyone to be sure of the answers to these questions. The answers may well depend upon the goals of an assessment of language in a patient. If the goal of a language assessment is simply to say whether a patient is language-impaired, as is the case in many neuropsychological assessments in acute care settings, this battery or an equivalent approach is probably unnecessary. A language assessment battery need only have discriminating value to serve this type of diagnostic function. However, if the clinician must plan and undertake therapy for a patient who is shown to have a language problem, a psycholinguistic assessment can be extremely useful in guiding the choice of therapeutic materials. It gives the clinician a basis upon which to focus on one or another aspect of language processing, and upon which to choose particular types of linguistic stimuli for use.

In many settings, clinicians who are charged with treating as well as diagnosing language disorders have limited contact time with their patients. In the United States, for instance, clinical practice now frequently limits patients' stays to a few days in acute care hospitals after illnesses such as stroke. Clinicians in these settings frequently rely on a very short assessment—often taking an hour or less—and then begin therapy. Is the psycholinguistic approach possible for this type of clinical need?

The answer to this question is clearly affirmative. The battery I have outlined above can be considerably truncated. For instance, all the written language subtests can simply be eliminated, reducing administration time to half. Only one test of comprehension can be administered for simple and complex words, rather than the two or three provided. The homophone matching test can be eliminated. Only half of the stimuli in each of the remaining subtests can be presented. This barebones battery usually takes less than an hour to administer. Though it cannot provide as much information as the full battery, what information it does provide is a systematic guide to important psycholinguistically defined deficits that are frequently seen in the acute neurological patient.

This battery, and the psycholinguistic approach to language impairments in general, is not limited to use with neurological patients, let alone patients with selected neurological disease such as stroke. It provides a representative and rational basis for assessing important aspects of language function in anyone—child or adult, brain-damaged or neurologically intact, demented or schizophrenic, etc. I have only emphasized neurological patients in this book because psycholinguistically defined language-processing disorders have been most clearly demonstrated in these patients.

What is most important, in my view, is not that the clinician find a way to administer the PAL or any other particular language assessment battery in a given clinical setting. What is most important is that the clinician carefully examine the purpose of his or her diagnostic activities, and choose tests that are appropriate for those purposes. If these include an analysis of what has gone wrong with the patient's language, a psycholinguistic approach to diagnosis is likely to be useful.

CLASSIFICATION OF PATIENTS WITH LANGUAGE DISORDERS

Speech-language pathologists and neuropsychologists often classify patients into groups. In most contemporary clinical settings, this classificatory process is one basis for an interaction between speech-language pathologists and neuropsychologists, on the one hand, and members of the medical profession, whose charge is to diagnose and deal with the organic aspects of disease, on the other. A set of clinical classes of aphasia has grown up over the last 125 years or so that largely satisfies the need for this interdisciplinary communication regarding the nature of a patient's language disorder (as well as some intradisciplinary communication). I have frequently referred to this system of patient classification in this book, speaking of clinical aphasic syndromes such as Broca's aphasia, Wernicke's aphasia, conduction aphasia, etc. This clinical approach to classification differs significantly from an approach to patient classification based on the psycholinguistic approach to individual patient diagnostics. Given the widespread use of the clinical approach to classification of aphasic patients, it is important to understand the differences between it and the psycholinguistic approach.

Early researchers into aphasia made the claim that a handful of constellations of symptoms were reflections of isolated impairments of the language-processing system. For instance, Broca's aphasia was considered to reflect an isolated disturbance of the speech production system; Wernicke's aphasia was said to reflect a disturbance in a storehouse for the auditory form of words used in both auditory comprehension and speech production (translated into modern terms, this would be phrased as a disturbance of a single phonological lexicon); and other traditional aphasic syndromes received similar theoretical analyses. These syndromes are listed in table 10.4.

The research we have reviewed in this book leads to the conclusion that these syndromes have two serious limitations as reflections of impairments to single language-processing components. These limitations are related to how the syndromes are defined in theoretical and operational terms.

The problem with how the classic aphasic syndromes are defined, in theoretical terms, is that their definitions often specify disturbances of more than a single language-processing component. For instance, Benson and Geschwind (1971) describe Broca's aphasia as follows:

> The language output of Broca's aphasia can be described as nonfluent. It is sparse, dysprosodic, and poorly articulated; it is made up of very short phrases and it is produced with effort, particularly in initiation of speech. The output consists primarily of substantive words, i.e., nouns, action verbs, or significant modifiers. The pattern of short phrases lacking prepositions is often termed "telegraphic speech." The substantive quality of the output often enables the Broca's aphasic to communicate ideas despite a gross expressive difficulty.... Repetition of spoken language is always abnormal, but in most cases repetition is somewhat superior to spontaneous output. Similarly, confrontation naming ability is abnormal in Broca's aphasia but may be good relative to the paucity of spontaneous speech.... Writing is always abnormal in Broca's aphasia, usually consisting of scribbling and complicated by misspelling and omission of letters. (pp 7–8)

The abnormalities which determine that a patient has Broca's aphasia are only related to each other at a very general level of description of the language-processing system. For instance, it is not clear how the symptoms of "dysprosodic," "poorly articulated" speech are related to the presence of "nouns, action verbs, or significant modifiers." We would have to accept a very general characterization of language functions that only identifies the four major on-line tasks of language use (speaking, auditory comprehension, reading, and writing) and a few other less usually performed tasks such as repetition, and naming objects and pictures, to view syndromes such as Broca's aphasia as reflections of impairments of a single language-processing component. We cannot use a diagnostic label such as Broca's aphasia to convey information about which levels of the language code are impaired in the speech or writing of a patient.

A consequence of the overly broad nature of the classic syndromes is that, in practice, many syndromes are identified by a check list of symptoms that only co-occur statistically. This does not establish unique criteria for membership in a group. As Benson (1979) indicates, any of the above symptoms may be absent in a case of Broca's aphasia. Schwartz (1984) pointed out that the actual application of these criteria has led to grouping together many patients with no symptoms in common. The reverse is also frequently encountered: patients are often not uniquely classifiable. The criteria for inclusion of patients in different aphasic groups overlap (the presence of

Table 10.4
The Classic Aphasic Syndromes

Syndrome	Clinical Manifestations	Hypothesized Deficit	Classic Lesion Location
Sydromes Attributed to Disturbances of Cortical Centers			
Broca's aphasia	Major disturbance in speech production with sparse, halting speech, often misarticulated, frequently missing function words and bound morphemes	Disturbances in the speech planning and production mechanisms	Primarily posterior aspects of the 3rd frontal convolution and adjacent inferior aspects of the precentral gyrus
Wernicke's aphasia	Major disturbance in auditory comprehension, fluent speech with disturbances of the sounds and structures of words (phonemic, morphological, and semantic paraphasias)	Disturbances of permanent representations of the sound structures of words	Posterior half of the 1st temporal gyrus and possibly adjacent cortex
Anomic aphasia	Disturbance in the production of single words, most marked for common nouns with variable comprehension problems	Disturbances of the concepts or the sound patterns of words, or both	Inferior pariental lobe or connections between parietal lobe and temporal lobe
Global aphasia	Major disturbance in all language functions	Disruption of all language-processing components	Large portion of the perisylvian association cortex
Syndromes Attributed to Disruptions of Connections Between Centers			
Conduction aphasia	Disturbance of repetition and spontaneous speech (phonemic paraphasias)	Disconnection between the sound patterns of words and the speech production mechanism	Lesion in the arcuate fasciculus or corticocortical connections between temporal and frontal lobes

Transcortical aphasia	Disturbance of spontaneous speech similar to Broca's aphasia with relatively preserved repetition	Disconnection between conceptual representations of words and sentences and the motor speech production system	White matter tracts deep to Broca's area
Transcortical sensory aphasia	Disturbance in single word comprehension with relatively intact repetition	Disturbance in activation of word meanings despite normal recognition of auditorily presented words	White matter tracts connecting parietal lobe to temporal lobe or in parietal lobe
Isolation or the language zone	Disturbance of both spontaneous speech (similar to Broca's aphasia) and comprehension, with some preservation of repetition	Disconnection between concepts and both representations of word sounds and the speech production mechanism	Cortex just outside the perisylvian association cortex

phonemic paraphasias is noted in several categories; anomia is mentioned in almost all categories), so that a patient who shows only or chiefly these symptoms cannot be uniquely classified. Most applications of the clinical taxonomy result in frequent disagreement as to a patient's classification (Holland, Fromm, and Swindell, 1986) or to a large number of "mixed" or "unclassifiable" cases (Lecours, Lhermitte, and Bryans, 1983).

We should briefly mention the application of statistical methods of grouping patients on the basis of their performances on aphasia batteries such as the BDAE and the WAB, which is sometimes said to support the clinical classification (Goodglass and Kaplan, 1972, 1982; Kertesz, 1979). There are many problems with the statistical treatment of the data obtained through the use of these batteries and with the interpretations offered regarding the statistical results. Statistical clustering analyses have often been carried out on the values derived from both the language and nonlanguage aspects of the "aphasia" batteries, making the resulting patient groups reflections of nonlanguage as well as language impairments. In some studies (e.g., Goodglass and Kaplan 1972, 1982), different factor analyses have produced different factor compositions in different aphasic populations tested by the authors, raising the question of which of the analyses are reliable indications of patient clustering. Statistical analyses have been performed on inappropriate data, such as using factor analyses to analyze categorical data (Kertesz, 1979). The most important point, however, is that analyses of this sort—if carried out properly—could only indicate that certain symptoms co-occur reliably in particular brain-damaged populations. They could not indicate which of the co-occurrences were due to two or more symptoms resulting from a single functional deficit and which were due to the fact that a given neurological insult may affect more than one language-processing component. We have discussed the ways psycholinguistically oriented aphasiologists have attempted to determine whether two abnormal performances are due to impairments in two separate language-processing components or in a single functional component that is used in the two tasks (see chapters 3 through 7 for discussion of this important topic). The statistical analysis of data provided by these batteries is only a small part of these methods. For all these reasons, these statistical approaches provide no reasons to think that the classic syndromes are interpretable in psycholinguistic terms.

The second problem with the classic syndromes is operational, and derives from how they have been identified in clinical practice. We may exemplify this problem by considering Wernicke's aphasia. Patients with Wernicke's aphasia have a major disturbance affecting auditory comprehension. Wernicke's original description attributed this disturbance to an inability to activate the phonological representations of words. However, Wernicke did not show that his patients had this single impairment, rather than impairments to other mechanisms involved in comprehension. To sustain Wernicke's analysis, it would be necessary to show that phonetic decoding mechanisms were intact in his patients (e.g., by showing that they had good performance on phoneme discrimination tasks), and that their comprehension deficits were not due to disturbances affecting word meanings or the process of accessing word meanings (e.g., they should have been able to understand those words that they did recognize). In patients with this pattern of functional capacities, it would also be important to have independent evidence that the phonological lexicon was impaired (e.g., inability to make judgments as to whether utterances are real words or nonwords in lexical decision tasks; the absence of word superiority effects in auditory-oral tasks such as repetition; abnormal performance on gating tasks; see chapter 2). Needless to say, Wernicke did not undertake these studies in his original paper. Indeed, as I pointed out in chapter 2, there is not a single case of Wernicke's aphasia in the published literature on aphasia in which a researcher has undertaken these or similar experiments to show that Wernicke's analysis is correct, despite the fact that his original analysis still forms the basis for an aphasic syndrome described in most textbooks of psychology, neurology, and speech-language pathology!

These two problems—the overly broad nature of many characterizations of aphasic syndromes (as in Broca's aphasia) and the inadequate operational identification of patients with syndromes that have been more narrowly defined (as in Wernicke's aphasia)—both stem from not approaching aphasic phenomena with a sufficiently detailed model of language and the language-processing system and an understanding of how to test for the integrity of the components of this system. Operating at the level of the traditional clinical aphasic syndromes tends to trivialize language, its processing, and its disorders. Because it lumps together many different types of impairments, it tends to lead the clinician to ignore the details of a patient's language impairment. In defense of the traditional approach, it may be said that only recently has the linguistic and psycholinguistic approach to language disorders developed enough to form the basis for a clinician to identify the language-processing components that are disturbed in individual patients at a greater level of detail. Now that we do have such analyses, however, the classic taxonomy of aphasic syndromes has outlived its usefulness, and it is time to replace it with one based on a description of the individual psycholinguistic processing deficits in each patient.

As I have said at many points in this book, such an approach consists of identifying the disturbances in the major components of the language-processing system that are present in each patient. I have illustrated this approach in the discussion of diagnostics above. In this approach to taxonomy a patient is likely to have more than one deficit (e.g., a patient can have a disturbance of the nonlexical reading route, a separate disturbance in auditory comprehension of derived words, and a third disturbance in producing the form of sentences orally). Depending on the level of detail in which aphasic impairments are described, there may be hundreds of primary language-processing impairments. From a practical point of view, however, a very detailed taxonomy based upon specific deficits is unrealistic. For many clinical purposes, the best way to approach a psycholinguistic taxonomy of aphasic impairments is at the level of detail that identifies language-processing components with the sets of related operations responsible for activating the major forms of the language code and their associated meanings in the usual language tasks of speaking, comprehending auditorily presented language, writing, and reading.

NEUROLOGICAL MECHANISMS AND APHASIA

It is well established that the association cortex in the region of the sylvian fissure (usually in the left hemsiphere) is responsible for language capacities. The relationship of portions of this perisylvian association cortex to different components of the language-processing system remains the subject of controversy and research. Holistic models maintain that the entire region, or at least large portions of it, acts as a whole to support all language functions. Localizationist models argue that specific language processes are universally carried out in relatively restricted areas of this region. Neither of these types of models appears to be adequate.

The finding that multiple different individual language deficits arise in patients with small perisylvian lesions provides strong evidence against the complete adequacy of any holistic model. These selective deficits could not arise if all language processing took place in all parts of the language zone and obeyed holist principles, such as those of mass action and equipotentiality enunciated by Lashley (1929, 1950). Mass action refers to the idea that the efficiency of a process is directly related to the amount of neural structure involved in carrying out that process. Equipotentiality refers to the idea that all parts of a given neural area contribute equally to carrying out any process. If these principles applied, and if all language functions depended on all parts of the perisylvian association cortex, small lesions should always affect all language functions to a minor degree, and major isolated deficits should not occur following small lesions.[1]

Since there are many localizationist models, their value has to be assessed on an individual basis. The best-known localizationist model is probably the "Connectionist" model initially developed in the 19th century and rediscovered, revised, and placed on a firmer neuroanatomical basis by Geschwind and his associates (Geschwind, 1965). Since this is such a well-known model of how the brain is organized to process language, and because many existing aphasia batteries are closely tied to this theory, we shall deal with it in some detail.[2]

According to this Connectionist model, depicted in figure 10.1, the permanent representations for the sounds of words (a phonological lexicon, in modern terms) are stored in Wernicke's area, the association cortex of the second temporal gyrus. These auditory representations are accessed following auditory presentation of language stimuli. They, in turn, evoke the concepts associated with words in the "concept center." According to Lichtheim (1885), the concept center is diffusely represented in association cortex; according to Geschwind (1965), a critical part of this process involves the inferior parietal lobe. In spoken language production, concepts access the phonological representations of words in Wernicke's area, which are then transmitted to the motor programming areas for speech in Broca's area, the association cortex of the pars triangularis and opercularis of the third frontal gyrus and possibly that of the

SYNDROMES OF APHASIA

Perisylvian aphasia syndromes	Nonlocalizing aphasic syndromes
Broca's aphasia	Anomic aphasia
Wernicke's aphasia	Global aphasia
Conduction aphasia	Alexia
Borderzone aphasia syndromes	Parietal temporal alexia
Transcortical motor aphasia	Occipital alexia
Aphasia of anterior cerebral	Frontal alexia
artery infarction	Agraphia
Transcortical sensory aphasia	Related syndromes
Mixed transcortical aphasia	Aphemia
Subcortical aphasia syndromes	Pure word deafness
The aphasia of Marie's	Apraxia of speech
quadrilateral space	Nonaphasic misnaming
Thalamic aphasia	
Striatal aphasia	
Aphasia from white matter lesions	

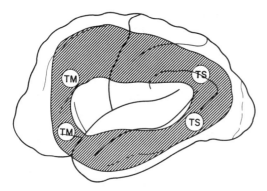

Diagram of approximate boundaries of borderzone area. Pathologic changes are present in the lined area but not in the inner language area in most instances of borderzone aphasia. *TM* = possible sites of transcortical motor aphasia; *TS* = possible sites for transcortical sensory aphasia. Involvement of borderzone area both anteriorly and posteriorly underlies the mixed transcortical aphasia picture.

Figure 10.1

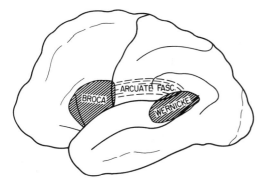

Diagrammatic view of left lateral hemisphere outlining cortical areas commonly associated with Broca's and Wernicke's aphasia plus a schematic illustration of the arcuate fasciculus, site of pathologic changes in some cases of conduction aphasia.

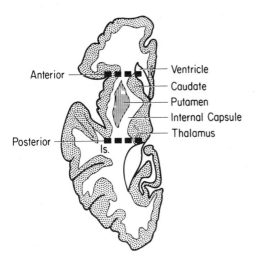

Diagrammatic sketch outlining Marie's quadrilateral space. The *heavy broken lines* indicate the anterior and posterior boundaries of the space. Destruction of tissue posteriorly, particularly involving the temporal isthmus (*Is.*), was considered necessary to produce a true Wernicke's aphasia.

Figure 10.1
The classic aphasic syndromes and their localization. (Modified with permission from Benson, 1979, pp. 63, 77, 90, 95.)

Rolandic operculum. Simultaneously, according to theorists such as Lichtheim (1885), Naeser and Hayward (1978), and Alexander, Naeser, and Palumbo (1987), the concept center or other higher-order center activates Broca's area. The proper execution of the speech act depends upon Broca's area receiving input from both these different cortical areas.

The principal evidence in favor of this model is said to be the occurrence of the classic syndromes we outlined above after lesions of these centers and the connections between them (Wernicke, 1874; Lichtheim, 1885; Geschwind, 1965; Benson and Geschwind, 1971; Benson, 1979; see table 10.4 and figure 10.1). The most serious problem with this evidence is the inadequacy of the functional analysis of patients' deficits as indications of specific processing deficits, which we discussed above. These studies give information about the localization of the classic syndromes only, not individual language-processing components. For reasons discussed above, in almost all studies, the patient groupings corresponding to the classic syndromes do not consist of patients with similar deficits in language-processing components. For instance, in a study by Damasio and Damasio (1980), patients with conduction aphasia were not homogeneous with respect to functions like auditory comprehension. In a study of transcortical sensory aphasia by Kertesz, Sheppard, and MacKenzie (1982), some of the patients had fluent jargon speech output and others had only a few phonemic paraphasias. In general, though there is good evidence that the *classic aphasia syndromes* have predictive value with respect to lesion localization in stroke cases, the *components of language functioning* that are being localized in these studies cannot be ascertained.

Neuroanatomical studies of patients with specific psycholinguistic impairments are limited, and have often reported deficit-lesion correlations incompatible with the standard Connectionist model. For instance, patients with anterior lesions can have disturbances of phoneme identification and discrimination, and patients with temporal lesions can be spared these problems (Blumstein et al., 1977a,b; Basso et al., 1977, see chapter 4). Caplan and his colleagues (Caplan et al., 1985; Caplan, 1986, 1987b) reported that deficits in the use of syntactic structure to determine sentence meaning varied greatly in patients with lesions restricted to any one of the three lobes in the perisylvian area. Data regarding localization from positron emission tomography (PET) scanning in normal subjects also have not supported the Connectionist model. PET studies have found that the inferior parietal lobe—a crucial language area according to all theories—shows no activation in any language test (Peterson et al., 1988; Posner et al., 1988). Studies using electrocortical stimulation during neurosurgical operations have led to a different localizationist model, and have shown considerable individual variation in the localization of language processes (Ojemann, 1983). In all, the database regarding the localization of specific components of the language-processing system is scanty and contradictory. Many results suggest that different areas within the perisylvian cortex are capable of supporting different aspects of language functions in different people. This would imply that identifying a specific processing deficit in a patient would, at most, only lead to a probable localization of the patient's lesion within the perisylvian cortical region.

If language-processing components occupy different parts of the perisylvian cortex in different people, what is the basis for the correlations between the classic syndromes and lesions in specific areas of the perisylvian cortical area? One possible explanation is that the classic syndromes reflect the co-occurrence of variable combinations of language-processing deficits with motor speech impairments. If a patient has many or severe language function deficits, he either has global aphasia (if motor speech mechanisms are affected) or one of the types of classic Wernicke's aphasia (if motor speech mechanisms are not involved). If he has only a few or minor language function deficits, he has one of the types of classic Broca's aphasia (if there are motor speech impairments) or one of the minor "fluent" aphasias, such as anomia, conduction aphasia, transcortical sensory aphasia, etc. (if there are no motor speech impairments). It is entirely possible that the localizing value of the classic syndromes is due to the invariant location of the motor system, while language-processing components are themselves quite variable in their localization in different persons.

We believe that, while neurological factors are obviously important to the speech-language pathologist and neuropsychologist, they should not be overly concerned with the exact localization of a lesion within the association cortex around the sylvian fissure. Anterior lesions in the area will cause impairments of the motoric aspects of speech and writing, because of the fact that they damage the motor cortex and its output fibers, and more posterior lesions in this area will spare motor output. However, the effects of lesions in these parts of the language zone on language processing per se may differ in different persons.

There are neurological issues regarding language disorders other than the question of localization. The nature of aphasic symptoms may give clues to the etiology of a patient's lesion. For instance, it is rare to find jargonaphasia in a patient with a slowly growing tumor, although jargonaphasia does occur reasonably frequently in rapidly growing tumors with necrotic areas and after surgical biopsies and partial resections of many tumors. A relatively pure disturbance of the meaning of words, without major disturbances in the processing of word form, is often associated with slow degenerative dementing processes, such as Alzheimer's disease. Though it is not possible at present to predict lesion type from most aphasic symptoms, present work shows considerable promise regarding the predictive nature of a few specific language disturbances. These types of inferences from the type of language impairment to the etiology, rather than the location, of neurological disease are often of great help to the medical practitioner, and are among the most important potential uses of psycholinguistic analyses of patients' language disturbances.

More is known about the prognosis associated with certain aphasic symptoms, especially when something is known about the neurological lesion that produces the symptoms. Obviously, lesion etiology influences the natural history of a language disorder, with advancing lesions like tumors and degenerative diseases carrying worse prognoses than single-event lesions like stroke and head trauma. It is also established that certain classic aphasic syndromes tend to evolve into others, at least in vascular cases. For instance, patients with Wernicke's aphasia are likely to develop anomia or conduction aphasia over time (Kertesz, Harlock, and Coates, 1979). Here again, what we know about the prognosis and the natural history of aphasic impairments is primarily linked to descriptions of patients in terms of the classic aphasic syndromes, and does not give us much information about the natural history of specific processing deficits. Research into this important question requires psycholinguistically oriented assessment tools, and hopefully such will be forthcoming in the near future.

THE RELEVANCE OF LINGUISTICS AND
PSYCHOLINGUISTICS TO THERAPEUTICS

From the perspective of the practicing speech-language pathologist, the acid test of any approach to describing and classifying patients' language impairments is whether the descriptions lead to effective therapy, and whether the classification is useful in predicting outcome and in deciding what patients will benefit from which therapeutic measures. The psycholinguistic approach to aphasia invites a therapeutic effort based upon an undertanding of each patient's primary deficits. Either specific therapy can be directed at a deficit, or the patient can be trained to use compensatory procedures to circumvent the deficit. The more specific our understanding of a patient's deficits, the more specific therapeutic materials can be. Though the field of psycholinguistically based therapeutics is in its infancy, some early reports are encouraging.

Several studies show that specific deficits can improve when therapy is directed at them. Byng (1988), for instance, reported on her rehabilitation efforts with a patient who had been in speech therapy for over 5 years. B.R.B. had a specific impairment in comprehension of sentences, which Byng (1988) identified through the use of a psycholinguistically oriented test battery. He was able to understand concrete nouns, as measured by both a synonym judgment and a triadic relatedness test. He could not understand sentences in which either of the nouns could accomplish the action of the verb, such as: *The bishop weighs the mayor.* In sentences like this, he frequently chose a picture showing a mayor weighing a bishop, but never one showing a different type of person. B.R.B. also had trouble with reversible locative sentences (e.g., *The hook is above the switch*), and in judging whether sentences were correctly formed when they were missing needed objects or had additional objects (e.g, ** The council opposed to the new road; * The council objected the road*). B.R.B. had no trouble understanding sentences that could only have one possible meaning (e.g., *The boy ate the cake*). Byng concluded that B.R.B. had trouble mapping syntactic structures onto thematic roles (who is doing what to whom in the action conveyed by a sentence; see chapter 7 for a discussion of this sort of deficit). She fashioned materials to train the patient on this task. She presented B.R.B. with pictures indicating the meaning of a preposition, including pictorial information regarding the thematic roles of the nouns that occurred before and after the preposition. She presented these pictures with both abstract drawings and more concrete drawings, indicating thematic roles through color codes. Within a 2-week period, B.R.B. developed the ability to understand reversible locative sentences rapidly and effortlessly. The effect extended to the auditory modality (the training had used written sentences) and to N-V-N sentences. That this effect was due to the specific therapy was shown in two ways: first, B.R.B had been receiving nonspecific therapy for years and had not improved on this aspect of sentence comprehension; and second, when B.R.B. was tested on other language-processing tasks before and after this therapy, his performance on these other tasks did not improve. Other researchers have shown similar results with psycholinguistically based analysis of deficits and therapeutic programs that are focused on patients' specific deficits (Howard, 1985; Kohn, Smith, and Arsenault, 1990). The approach of bypassing an identified deficit using residual processing abilities has also been successfully employed.

Though few in number, these reports are extremely encouraging. If even a small percentage of aphasic patients can be successfully rehabilitated using materials directed at psycholinguistically defined processing deficits, the psycholinguistic approach to diagnostics and therapeutics will be important for the clinician to master.

CONCLUDING COMMENTS

The study of language disorders is increasingly influenced by research on normal language and its processing. These studies have major implications for clinical matters. They have led to changes in how aphasic patients are viewed, to a rejection of current taxonomic practice, and to a serious questioning of basic aspects of theories of neural mechanisms supporting language. These studies suggest new approaches to diagnostics and therapeutics. It is possible for clinicians directly responsible for the assessment and treatment of patients with language disorders to incorporate the psycholinguistic approach into their practice. This chapter has illustrated some of these efforts. Hopefully, familiarization with the kinds of studies reviewed in this book will enable clinicians to expand the range of these clinical applications and evaluate their effects.

NOTES

1. See Shallice (1988) for a discussion of some possible exceptions to this general argument in some PDP systems.

2. Note that the term *Connectionist* applies here to a neurological model that involves localization of language processes. This must not be confused with the modern "connectionist," PDP models which are not localizationist.

References

Alajouanine, T., Ombredane, A., and Durand, M. (1939). *Le syndrome de désintégration phonétique dans l'aphasie.* Paris: Masson.

Albert, M. L., and Bear, D. (1974). Time to understand: A case study of word deafness with reference to the role of time in auditory comprehension. *Brain, 97,* 373–384.

Alexander, M. P., Naeser, M. A., and Palumbo, C. L. (1987). Correlations of subcortical CT lesion sites and aphasia profiles. *Brain, 110,* 961–991.

Allport, D. A., and Funnell, E. (1981). Components of the mental lexicon. *Philosophical Transactions of the Royal Society of London B, 295,* 397–410.

Altmann, G., and Steedman, M. J. (1988). Interaction with context in human syntactic processing. *Cognition, 30,* 191–238.

Anderson, S. R. (1982). Where's morphology. *Linguistic Inquiry, 13,* 571–612.

Armstrong, S. L., Gleitman, L. R., and Gleitman, H. (1983). What some concepts might not be. *Cognition, 13,* 263–308.

Armus, S. R., Brookshire, R. H., and Nicholas, L. E. (1989). Aphasic and non-brain–damaged adults' knowledge of scripts for common situations. *Brain and Language, 36,* 518–528.

Aronoff, M. (1976). *Word formation in generative grammar.* Cambridge, Mass.: MIT Press.

Auerbach, S. H., Allard, T., Naeser, M., Alexander, M. P., and Albert, M. L. (1982). Pure word deafness: Analysis of a case with bilateral lesions and a defect at the pre-phonemic level. *Brain, 105,* 271–300.

Baars, B. J., Motley, M. T., and MacKay, D. (1975). Output editing for lexical status from artificially elicited slips of the tongue. *Journal of Verbal Learning and Verbal Behavior, 14,* 382–391.

Baddeley, A. D. (1966a). The influence of acoustic and semantic similarity on long-term memory for word sequences. *Quarterly Journal of Experimental Psychology, 18,* 302–309.

Baddeley, A. D. (1966b). Short-term memory for word sequences as a function of acoustic, semantic and formal similarity. *Quarterly Journal of Experimental Psychology, 18,* 362–365.

Baddeley, A. D. (1979). Working memory and reading. In P. S. Kolers, M. E. Wrolstad, and H. Bouma (Eds.), *Processing of visible language* New York: Plenum.

Baddeley, A. D., Eldridge, M., and Lewis, V. (1981). The role of subvocalisation in reading. *Quarterly Journal of Experimental Psychology, 33A,* 439–454.

Baddeley, A. D., Lewis, V. J., and Vallar, G. (1984). Exploring the articulatory loop. *Quarterly Journal of Experimental Psychology, 36,* 233–252.

Baddeley, A. D., Thompson, N., and Buchanan, M. (1975). Word length and the structure of short-term memory. *Journal of Verbal Learning and Verbal Behavior, 14,* 575–589.

Baddeley, A. D., Vallar, G., and Wilson, B. (1987). Comprehension and the articulatory loop: Some neuropsychological evidence. In M. Coltheart (Ed.), *Attention and performance XII* (pp. 509–530). Hillsdale, N.J.: Lawrence Erlbaum.

Badecker, W., and Caramazza, A. (1985). On considerations of method and theory governing the use of clinical categories in neurolinguistics and neuropsychology: The case against agrammatism. *Cognition, 20,* 97–125.

Badecker, W., and Caramazza, A. (1986). A final brief in the case against agrammatism. *Cognition, 24,* 277–282.

Badecker, W., and Caramazza, A. (1987). The analysis of morphological errors in a case of acquired dyslexia. *Brain and Language, 32,* 278–305.

Badecker, W., Hillis, A., and Caramazza, A. (1990). Lexical morphology and its role in the writing process: Evidence from a case of acquired dysgraphia. *Cognition, 35,* 205–234.

Baker, E., Blumstein, S. E., and Goodglass, H. (1981). Interaction between phonological and semantic factors in auditory comprehension. *Neuropsychologia, 19,* 1–16.

Banks, W. P., and Flora, J. (1977). Semantic and perceptual processing in symbolic comparison. *Journal of Experimental Psychology: Human Perception and Performance, 3,* 278–290.

Barnard, P. (1985) Interacting cognitive subsystems: A psycholinguistic approach to short-term memory. In A. W. Ellis (Ed.), *Progress in the psychology of language. Vol. 2* (pp. 197–258). London: Lawrence Erlbaum.

Baron, R. W., and Strawson, C. (1976). Use of orthographic and word-specific knowledge in reading words aloud. *Journal of Experimental Psychology: Human Perception and Performance, 2,* 386–393.

Barruzzi, A., and Caplan, D. (1985). *The effects of literacy and brain injury upon syntactic comprehension.* Paper presented at the Body for the Advancement of Brain, Behavioral and Language Enterprises, Niagara Falls.

Barton, M. (1971). Recall of generic properties of words in aphasic patients. *Cortex, 7,* 73–82.

Barton, M., Maruszewski, M., and Urrea, D. (1969). Variation of stimulus context and its effects on word-finding ability in aphasics. *Cortex, 5,* 351–365.

Basso, A., Casati, G., and Vignolo, L. A. (1977). Phonemic identification defect in aphasia. *Cortex, 13,* 85–95.

Bates, E. (1976). *Language and context: The acquisition of pragmatics.* New York: Academic Press.

Bates, E., and MacWhinney, B. (1989). Functionalism and the competition model. In B. MacWhinney, and E. Bates (Eds.), *The cross-linguistic study of sentence processing* (pp. 3–73). Cambridge: Cambridge University Press.

Bates, E., and Wulfeck, B. (1989). Cross-linguistic studies of aphasia. In B. MacWhinney, and E. Bates (Eds.), *The cross-linguistic study of sentence processing* (pp. 328–371). Cambridge: Cambridge University Press.

Bates, E., McNew, S., MacWhinney, B., Devescovi, A., and Smith, S. (1982). Functional constraints on sentence processing. *Cognition, 11,* 245–299.

Bates, E., Hamby, S., and Zurif, E. (1983). The effects of focal brain damage on pragmatic expression. *Canadian Journal of Psychology, 37,* 59–84.

Bates, E., Friederici, A., and Wulfeck, B. (1987). Sentence comprehension in aphasia: A cross-linguistic study. *Brain and Language, 32,* 19–67.

Bauer, D. W., and Stanovich, K. E. (1980). Lexical access and the spelling-to-sound regularity effect. *Memory and Cognition, 8*(5), 424–432.

Baum, S. R., and Blumstein, S. E. (1987). Preliminary observations on the use of duration as a cue to syllable-initial fricative consonant voicing in English. *Journal of Acoustic Society of America, 82*(3), 1073–1077.

Baum, S. R., Blumstein, S. E., Naeser, M. A., and Palumbo, C. (1990). Temporal dimensions of consonant and vowel production: An acoustic and CT scan analysis of aphasic speech., *Brain and Language, 39,* 33–56.

Baxter, D. M., and Warrington, E. K. (1985). Category-specific phonological dysgraphia. *Neuropsychologia, 23,* 653–666.

Baxter, D. M., and Warrington, E. K. (1986). Ideational agraphia: A single case study. *Journal of Neurology, Neurosurgery and Psychiatry, 49,* 369–374.

Beattie, G., and Butterworth, B. (1979). Contextual probability and word frequency as determinants of pauses in spontaneous speech. *Language and Speech, 22,* 201–211.

Beauvois, M.-F. (1982). Optic aphasia: A process of interaction between vision and language. *Philosophical Transactions of the Royal Society of London B, 298,* 35–47.

Beauvois, M. F., and Derouesné, J. (1979). Phonological alexia: three dissociations. *Journal of Neurology, Neurosurgery, and Psychiatry, 42,* 1115–1124.

Beauvois, M.-F., and Derouesné, J. (1981). Lexical or orthographic agraphia. *Brain, 104*, 21–49.

Beauvois, M.-F., Saillant, B., Meininger, V., and Lhermitte, F. (1978). Bilateral tactile aphasia: A tactoverbal dysfunction. *Brain, 101*, 381–401.

Beland, R., Caplan, D., and Nespoulous, J.-L. (1990). The role of abstract phonological representations in word production: Evidence from phonemic paraphasias. *Journal of Neurolinguistics, 5*, 125–164.

Benson, D. F. (1979). *Aphasia, alexia and agraphia*. London: Churchill Livingstone.

Benson, D. F., and Geschwind, N. (1971). Aphasia and related cortical disturbances. In A. B. Baker, and L. H. Baker (Eds.), *Clinical Neurology* New York: Harper and Row.

Berko-Gleason, J., Goodglass, H., Obler, L., Green, E., Hyde, M. R., and Weintraub, S. (1980). Narrative strategies of aphasic and normal-speaking subjects. *Journal of Speech and Hearing Research, 23*, 370–382.

Berndt, R. S. (1987). Symptom co-occurence and dissociation in the interpretation of agrammatism. In M. Coltheart, G. Sartori, and R. Job (Eds.), *The cognitive neuropsychology of language* (pp. 221–232). London: Lawrence Erlbaum.

Berndt, R., and Caramazza, A. (1980). A redefinition of the syndrome of Broca's aphasia. *Applied Psycholinguistics, 1*, 225–278.

Berndt, R. S., and Mitchum, C. C. (1990). Auditory and lexical information sources in immediate recall: Evidence from a patient with a deficit to the phonological short-term store. In G. Vallar, and T. Shallice (Eds.), *Neuropsychological impairments of short-term memory* (pp. 115–144). Cambridge: Cambridge University Press.

Berwick, R. C., and Weinberg, A. (1984). *The grammatical basis of linguistic performance: Language use and acquisition*. Cambridge, Mass.: MIT Press.

Besner, D., Twilley, L., McCann, R. S., and Seergobin, K. (1990). On the association between connectionism and data: Are few words necessary? *Psychological Review, 97*, 432–446.

Bever, T. G. (1970). The cognitive basis for linguistic structures. In J. R. Hayes (Ed.), *Cognition and the development of language* New York: Wiley.

Bihrle, A. M., Brownell, H. H., Powelson, J. A., and Gardner, H. (1986). Comprehension of humourous and non-humourous materials by left and right brain-damaged patients. *Brain and Cognition, 5*, 399–411.

Blumstein, S. (1973a). *A phonological investigation of aphasic speech*. The Hague: Mouton.

Blumstein, S. (1973b). Some phonological implications of aphasic speech. In H. Goodglass, and S. Blumstein (Eds.), *Psycholinguistics and aphasia* (pp. 123–137). Baltimore: Johns Hopkins University Press.

Blumstein, S. E. (1988). Approaches to speech production deficits in aphasia. In F. Boller, and J. Grafman (Ed.), *Handbook of neuropsychology. Vol. 1* (pp. 349–365). Amsterdam: Elsevier.

Blumstein, S. E. (1990). Phonological deficits in aphasia: Theoretical perspectives. In A. Caramazza (Ed.), *Cognitive neuropsychology and neurolinguistics: Advances in models of cognitive function and impairment* (pp. 33–54). Hillsdale, N.J.: Lawrence Erlbaum.

Blumstein, S. E., Baker, E., and Goodglass, H. (1977a). Phonological factors in auditory comprehension in aphasia. *Neuropsychologia, 15,* 19–30.

Blumstein, S., Cooper, W. E., Zurif, E. B., and Caramazza, A. (1977b). The perception and production of voice-onset time in aphasia. *Neuropsychologia, 15,* 371–383.

Blumstein, S. E., Cooper, W. E., Goodglass, H., Statlander, S., and Gottlieb, J. (1980). Production deficits in aphasia: A voice-onset time analysis. *Brain and Language, 9,* 153–170.

Blumstein, S. E., Milberg, W., and Schrier, R. (1982). Semantic processing in aphasia: Evidence from an auditory lexical decision task. *Brain and Language, 17,* 301–315.

Blumstein, S., Katz, B., Goodglass, H., Shrier, R., and Dworetsky, B. (1985). The effects of slowed speech on auditory comprehension in aphasia. *Brain and Language, 24,* 246–265.

Bock, J. K. (1985). Discourse Structure and Mental Models. In T. Carr (Ed.), *The development of reading skills: New directions for child development* (pp. 55–75). San Francisco: Jossey-Bass.

Bock, J. K. (1986). Meaning, sound, and syntax: Lexical priming in sentence production. *Journal of Experimental Psychology: Learning, Memory, and Cognition, 12,* 575–587.

Bock, J. K., and Irwin, D. E. (1980). Syntactic effects of information availability in sentence production. *Journal of Verbal Learning and Verbal Behavior, 19,* 467–484.

Bock, J. K., and Warren, R. K. (1985). Conceptual accessibility and syntactic structure in sentence formulation. *Cognition, 21,* 47–67.

Bradley, D. C. (1979). Lexical representation of derivational relation. In M. Aronoff, and M.-L. Kean (Ed.), *Juncture* Cambridge, Mass.: MIT Press.

Bradley, D. C., Garrett, M. F., and Zurif, E. B. (1980). Syntactic deficits in Broca's aphasia. In D. Caplan (Ed.), *Biological studies of mental processes* (pp. 269–286). Cambridge, Mass.: MIT Press.

Bransford, J. D., and McCarrell, N. S. (1977). A sketch of a cognitive approach to comprehension: Some thoughts about understanding what it means to comprehend. In P. N. Johnson-Laird, and P. C. Wason (Ed.), *Thinking: Reading in cognitive science* (pp. 377–399). Cambridge: U.K.: Cambridge University Press.

Bresnan, J. (1982). *The mental representation of grammatical relations.* Cambridge, Mass.: MIT Press.

Brookshire, R. H., and Nicholas, L. E. (1984). Comprehension of directly and indirectly stated main ideas and details in discourse by brain-damaged and non-brain–damaged listeners. *Brain and Language, 21*, 21–36.

Brown, R., and McNeill, D. (1966). The "tip of the tongue" phenomenon. *Journal of Verbal Learning and Verbal Behavior, 5*, 325–337.

Brownell, H. H., and Gardner, H. (1988). Neuropsychological insights into humour. In J. Durant, and J. Miller (Eds.), *Laughing matters* (pp. 17–34). Essex, U.K.: Longman Scientific.

Brownell, H. H., Michel, D., Powelson, J. A., and Gardner, H. (1983). Surprise but not coherence: Sensitivity to verbal humor in right hemisphere patients. *Brain and Language, 18*, 20–27.

Brownell, H. H., Potter, H. H., Bihrle, A. M., and Gardner, H. (1986). Inference deficits in right brain-damaged patients. *Brain and Language, 27*, 310–321.

Bub, D., and Kertesz, A. (1982a). Evidence for lexicographic processing in a patient with preserved written over oral single word naming. *Brain, 105*, 697–717.

Bub, D., and Kertesz, A. (1982b). Deep agraphia. *Brain and Language, 17*, 146–165.

Bub, D., and Lewine, J. (1988a). The nature of half-field processing for words as a function of hemispheric specialization. *Brain and Language, 14*, 16–53.

Bub, D. N., and Lewine, J. (1988b). Different modes of word recognition in the left and right visual fields. *Brain and Language, 33*, 161–188.

Bub, D., Cancelliere, A., and Kertesz, A. (1985). Whole-word and analytic translation of spelling-to-sound in a non-semantic reader. In K. E. Patterson, M. Coltheart, and J. C. Marshall (Ed.), *Surface dyslexia* (pp. 15–34). London: Lawrence Erlbaum.

Bub, D., Black, S., and Behrmann, M. (1986). *Are there two orthographic lexicons? Evidence from a case of surface dyslexia.* Nashville, Tenn.: Academy of Aphasia.

Bub, D., Black, S., Howell, J., and Kertesz, A. (1987). Damage to input and output buffers—What's a lexicality effect doing in a place like that? In E. Keller, and M. Gopnick (Ed.), *Motor and Sensory Processes of Language* (pp. 83–110). Hillsdale, N.J.: Lawrence Erlbaum.

Bub, D. N., Black, S., Hampson, E., and Kertesz, A. (1988). Semantic encoding of pictures and words: Some neuropsychological observations. *Cognitive Neuropsychology, 5*, 27–66.

Bub, D., Black, S., and Howell, J. (1989). Word recognition and orthographic context effects in a letter-by-letter reader. *Brain and Language, 36*, 357–376.

Buckingham, H. (1980). On correlating aphasic errors with slips of the tongue. *Applied Psycholinguistics, 1*, 199–220.

Burani, C., and Caramazza, A. (1987). *Representation and processing of derived words*. Manuscripts of the Cognitive Science Center; Baltimore: Johns Hopkins University.

Butler-Hinz, S., Caplan, D., and Waters, G. S. (1990). Characteristics of syntactic comprehension deficits following closed head injury versus left cerebrovascular accident. *Journal of Speech and Hearing Research, 33,* 269–280.

Butterworth, B. (1979). Hesitation and the production of verbal paraphasias and neologisms in jargon aphasia. *Brain and Language, 8,* 133–161.

Butterworth, B. (1982). Speech errors: Old data in search of new theories. In A. Cutler (Ed.), *Slips of the tongue in language production* (pp. 73–108). The Hague: Mouton.

Butterworth, B. L. (1985). Jargon aphasia: Processes and strategies. In S. Newman, and R. Epstein (Eds.), *Current perspectives in dysphasia* Edinburgh: Churchill Livingstone.

Butterworth, B., and Howard, D. (1987). Paragrammatisms. *Cognition, 26,* 1–38.

Butterworth, B., Howard, D., and McLoughlin, P. (1984). The semantic deficit in aphasia: The relationship between semantic errors in auditory comprehension and picture naming. *Neuropsychologia, 22,* 409–426.

Butterworth, B., Campbell, R., and Howard, D. (1986). The uses of short-term memory: A case study. *Quarterly Journal of Experimental Psychology, 38,* 705–737.

Byng, S. (1988). Sentence comprehension deficit: Theoretical analysis and remediation. *Cognitive Neuropsychology, 5,* 629–676.

Campbell, R. (1983). Writing non-words to dictation. *Brain and Language, 19,* 153–178.

Cantor, G. J., Trost, J. E., and Burns, M. S. (1985). Contrasting speech patterns in apraxia of speech and phonemic paraphasia. *Brain and Language, 24,* 204–222.

Caplan, D. (1983). A note on the "word order problem" in agrammatism. *Brain and Language, 20,* 155–165.

Caplan, D. (1985). Syntactic and semantic structures in agrammatism. In M.-L. Kean (Ed.), *Agrammatism* (pp. 125–152). New York: Academic Press.

Caplan, D. (1986). In defense of agrammatism. *Cognition, 24,* 263–276.

Caplan, D. (1987a). Agrammatism and the co-indexation of traces: Comments on Grodzinsky's reply. *Brain and Language, 30,* 191–193.

Caplan, D. (1987b). Discrimination of normal and aphasic subjects on a test of syntactic comprehension. *Neuropsychologia, 25,* 173–184.

Caplan, D. (1987c). *Neurolinguistics and Linguistic Aphasiology.* Cambridge: Cambridge University Press.

Caplan, D. (1988). The biological basis for language. In F. J. Newmeyer (Ed.), *Linguistics: The Cambridge survey III. Language: Psychological and biological aspects* (pp. 237–255). Cambridge: Cambridge University Press.

Caplan, D. (1991a). Language processing and language disorders as revealed through studies of syntactic comprehension. In F. Boller, and J. Grafman (Eds.), *Handbook of neuropsychology* (pp. 311–341). Amsterdam: Elsevier.

Caplan, D. (1991b). Agrammatism is a theoretically coherent aphasic category. *Brain and Language, 110,* 274–281.

Caplan, D. (in press). Review of Grodzinksy: Theoretical perspectives on language deficits. *Applied Psycholinguistics.*

Caplan, D., and Bub, D. (1990). *Psycholinguistic assessment of aphasia.* Presented at American Speech and Hearing Association Conference, Seattle, Wash.

Caplan, D., and Evans, K. L. (1990). The effects of syntactic structure on discourse comprehension in patients with parsing impairments. *Brain and Language, 39,* 206–234.

Caplan, D., and Futter, C. (1986). Assignment of thematic roles to nouns in sentence comprehension by an agrammatic patient. *Brain and Language, 27,* 117–134.

Caplan, D., and Hildebrandt, N. (1986). Language deficits and the theory of syntax. A reply to Grodzinsky. *Brain and Language, 27,* 168–177.

Caplan, D., and Hildebrandt, N. (1988a). *Disorders of syntactic comprehension.* Cambridge, Mass.: MIT Press.

Caplan, D., and Hildebrandt, N. (1988b). Specific deficits in syntactic comprehension. *Aphasiology, 2,* 255–258.

Caplan, D., and Hildebrandt, N. (1989). Disorders affecting comprehension of syntactic form: Preliminary results and their implications for theories of syntax and parsing. *Canadian Journal of Linguistics, 33,* 477–505.

Caplan, D., and Waters, G. (in press). Issues arising regarding the nature and consequences of reproduction conduction aphasia. In S. E. Kohn (Ed.), *Conduction aphasia.* Hillsdale: Lawrence Erlbaum.

Caplan, D., Kellar, L., and Locke, S. (1972). Inflection of neologisms in aphasia. *Brain, 95,* 169–172.

Caplan, D., Baker, C., and Dehaut, F. (1985). Syntactic determinants of sentence comprehension in aphasia. *Cognition, 21,* 117–175.

Caplan, D., Vanier, M., and Baker, C. (1986a). A case study of reproduction conduction aphasia: I. Word production. *Cognitive Neuropsychology, 3,* 99–128.

Caplan, D., Vanier, M., and Baker, C. (1986b). A case study of reproduction conduction aphasia: II. Sentence comprehension. *Cognitive Neuropsychology, 3,* 129–146.

Caramazza, A. (1988). Some aspects of language processing revealed through the analysis of acquired aphasia: The lexical system. *11*, 395–421.

Caramazza, A. (1989). When is enough enough? A Comment on Grodzinsky and Marek. *Brain and Language, 33*, 390–399.

Caramazza, A., and Berndt, R. S. (1985). A multicomponent view of agrammatic Broca's aphasia. In M. L. Kean (Ed.), *Agrammatism* (pp. 27–64). New York: Academic Press.

Caramazza, A., and Hillis, A. (1989). The disruption of sentence production: A case of selected deficit to positional level processing. *Brain and Language, 35*, 625–650.

Caramazza, A., and Hillis, A. E. (1990). Where do semantic errors come from? *Cortex, 26*, 95–122.

Caramazza, A., and Zurif, E. (1976). Dissociation of algorithmic and heuristic processes in language comprehension: Evidence from aphasia. *Brain and Language, 3*, 572–582.

Caramazza, A., Hersch, H., and Torgerson, W. S. (1976). Subjective structures and operations in semantic memory. *Journal of Verbal Learning and Verbal Behavior, 15*, 103–118.

Caramazza, A., Berndt, R. S., and Basili, A. G. (1983). The Selective Impairment of Phonological Processing: A Case Study. *Brain and Language, 18*, 128–174.

Caramazza, A., Miceli, G., and Villa, G. (1986). The role of the (output) phonological buffer in reading, writing and repetition. *Cognitive Neuropsychology, 3*, 37–76.

Caramazza, A., Miceli, G., Villa, G., and Romani, C. (1987). The role of the grapheme buffer in spelling: Evidence from a case of acquired dysgraphia. *Cognition, 26*, 59–85.

Caramazza, A., Laudanna, A., and Romani, C. (1988). Lexical access and inflectional morphology. *Cognition, 28*, 297–332.

Caramazza, A., Hillis, A. E., Rapp, B. C., and Romani, C. (1990). The multiple semantics hypothesis: Multiple confusions? *Cognitive Neuropsychology, 7*, 161–189.

Carpenter, R., and Rutherford, D. (1973). Acoustic cue discrimination in adult aphasia. *Journal of Speech and Hearing Research, 16*, 534–544.

Carr, T. H., McCauley, C., Sperber, R. D., and Parmalee, C. M. (1982). Words, pictures and priming: On semantic activation, conscious identification and the automaticity of information processing. *Journal of Experimental Psychology: Human Perception and Performance, 8*, 757–777.

Cattell, J. M. (1886). The time taken up by cerebral operations. *Mind, 11*, 220–242.

Charcot, J. M. (1883). Les varietes de l'aphasie. *Progres Medical, 23, 24, 25, 27*, 44.

Charolles, M. (1978). Introduction aux problèmes de la cohérence des textes. *Langue française, 38,* 7–41.

Chertkow, H., and Bub, D. (1990). Semantic memory loss in Alzheimer's Disease: What do indirect measures measure? *Brain, 113,* 397–417.

Chertkow, H., and Bub, D. (1991). Semantic memory in dementia. In M. Schwartz (Ed.), *Modular approaches to dementia* (pp. 207–244). Cambridge, Mass.: MIT Press.

Chertkow, H., Bub, D., and Caplan, D. (in press). Stages of semantic memory: Evidence from dementia. *Cognitive Neuropsychology.*

Chertkow, H., Bub, D., and Seidenberg, M. S. (1989). Priming and semantic memory loss in Alzheimer's Disease. *Brain and Language, 36,* 420–446.

Chocolle, R., Chedru, F., Botte, M. C., Chain, F., and Lhermitte, F. (1975). Etude psychoacoustique d'un cas de 'surdité corticale'. *Neuropsychologia, 13,* 163–172.

Chomsky, N. (1955). *The logical structure of linguistic theory.* New York: Plenum.

Chomsky, N. (1957). *Syntactic structures.* The Hague: Mouton.

Chomsky, N. (1965). *Aspects of the theory of syntax.* Cambridge, Mass.: MIT Press.

Chomsky, N. (1970). Remarks on nominalizations. In R. A. Jacobs, and P. S. Rosenbaum (Eds.), *Readings in English transformation grammar* Boston: Ginn.

Chomsky, N. (1981). *Lectures on government and binding.* Dordrecht: Foris.

Chomsky, N. (1985). *Knowledge of language: Its nature, origin, and use.* New York: Praeger.

Chomsky, N., and Halle, M. (1968). *The Sound Pattern of English.* New York: Harper and Row.

Church, K. W. (1987). Phonological parsing and lexical retrieval. *Cognition, 25,* 53–70.

Clark, H., and Clark, E. (1977). *Psychology and language.* New York: Harcourt Brace Jovanovich.

Clarke, R. G. B., and Morton, J. (1983). The effects of priming in visual word recognition. *Quarterly Journal of Experimental Psychology, 35,* 79–96.

Clements, G. N., and Keyser, S. J. (1983). *CV phonology. A generative theory of the syllable.* Cambridge, Mass.: MIT Press.

Clifton, C., and Ferreira, F. (1987). Modularity in sentence comprehension. In J. L. Garfield (Ed.), *Modularity in Knowledge Representation and Natural-Language Understanding* (pp. 277–290). Cambridge, Mass: MIT Press.

Cohen, R., Kelter, S., and Woll, G. (1980). Analytical competence and language impairment in aphasia. *Brain and Language, 10,* 331–347.

Collins, A. M., and Loftus, E. F. (1975). A spreading-activation theory of semantic processing. *Psychological Review, 82*, 407–428.

Colsher, P. L., Cooper, W. E., and Graff-Radford, N. (1987). Intonational variability in the speech of right-hemisphere damaged patients. *Brain and Language, 32*, 379–383.

Coltheart, M. (1978). Lexical access in simple reading tasks. In B. Underwood (Ed.), *Strategies of Information Processing* (pp. 151–215). London: Academic Press.

Coltheart, M. (1980). Deep dyslexia: A right-hemisphere hypothesis. In M. Coltheart, K. E. Patterson, and J. C. Marshall (Eds.), *Deep dyslexia* (pp. 326–380). London: Routledge.

Coltheart, M. (1982). The psycholinguistic analysis of acquired dyslexias: Some illustrations. *Philosophical Transactions of the Royal Society of London B, 298*, 151–163.

Coltheart, M., and Byng, S. (1983). *Phonological spelling (surface dysgraphia) and its relationship to phonological reading (surface dyslexia): A developmental case study.* Paper presented at Conference on Cognitive Neuropsychology of Language, Venice.

Coltheart, M., Besner, D., Jonasson, J. T., and Davelaar, E. (1979). Phonological Encoding in the Lexical Decision Task. *Quarterly Journal of Experimental Psychology, 31*, 489–507.

Coltheart, M., Patterson, J., Byng, S., Prior, M., and Riddoch, J. (1983). Surface dyslexia. *Quarterly Journal of Experimental Psychology, 35A*, 469–495.

Coltheart, M., Patterson, J., and Marshall, J. C. (1980). *Deep dyslexia.* London: Routledge.

Coltheart, M., Patterson, K. E., and Marshall, J. C. (1987). Deep dyslexia since 1980. In M. Coltheart, K. E. Patterson, and J. C. Marshall (Ed.), *Deep dyslexia (2nd edition)* (pp. 407–451). London: Routledge and Kegan Paul.

Cooper, F. S., Delattre, P. C., Liberman, A. M., Borst, J. M., and Gerstman, L. J. (1952). Some experimental on the perception of synthetic speech sounds. *Journal of the Acoustic Society of America, 24*, 597–608.

Cooper, W. E., and Sorensen, J. M. (1981). *Fundamental frequency in sentence production.* New York: Springer-Verlag.

Coslett, H. B., Rothi, L. J., Valenstein, E., and Heilman, K. (1986). Dissociations of writing and praxis: Two cases in point. *Brain and Language, 28*, 357–369.

Coslett, H. B., and Saffran, E. M. (1988). Evidence for preserved reading in "pure alexia." *Brain, 112*, 327–359.

Coughlan, A. K., and Warrington, E. K. (1981). The impairment of verbal semantic memory: A single case study. *Journal of Neurology, Neurosurgery and Psychiatry, 44*, 1079–1083.

Crain, S., and Fodor, J. D. (1985). How can grammars help parsers? In D. Dowty, L. Kartunnen, and A. Zwicky (Eds.), *Natural language parsing* (pp. 94–128). Cambridge: Cambridge University Press.

Crain, S., and Steedman, M. (1985). On not being led up the garden path: The use of context by the psychological syntax parser. In D. Dowty, L. Kartunnen, and A. M. Zwicky (Eds.), *Natural language parsing: psycholinguistic, computational and theoretical perspectives* (pp. 320–358). Cambridge: Cambridge University Press.

Cutting, J. E. (1972). Plucks and bows are categorically perceived, sometimes. *Perception and Psychophysics, 31*, 462–476.

Damasio, H., and Damasio, A. R. (1980). The anatomical basis of conduction aphasia. *Brain, 103*, 337–350.

Danly, M., Cooper, W., and Shapiro, B. (1983). Fundamental frequency, language processing, and linguistic structure in Wernicke's aphasia. *Brain and Language, 19*, 1–24.

Danly, M., and Shapiro, B. (1982). Speech prosody in Broca's aphasia. *Brain and Language, 16*, 171–190.

Darley, F. L., Aronson, A. E., and Brown, J. R. (1975). *Motor Speech Disorders.* Toronto: W.B. Saunders.

De Bleser, R. (1987). From Agrammatism to paragrammatism: German Aphasiological Traditions and Grammatical Disturbances. *Cognitive Neuropsychology, 4*, 187–256.

Dejerine, J. (1891). Sur un cas de cecité verbale avec agraphie, suivi d'autopsie. *Compte rendu des séances de la société de biologie, 3*, 197–201.

Dejerine, J. (1892). Contribution à l'étude anatomoclinique et clinique des differentes variétés de cecité verbale. *Memories de la Société de Biologie, 4*, 61–90.

Dejerine, J., and Pellisier, A. (1914). Contribution a l'étude de le cecité verbale pure. *l'Encephale, 7*, 1–34.

Delis, D. C., Wapner, W., Gardner, H., and Moses, J. A., Jr. (1983). The contribution of the right hemisphere to the organization of paragraphs. *Cortex, 19*, 43–50.

Dell, G. S. (1984). Representation of serial order in speech: Evidence from the repeated phoneme effect in speech errors. *Journal of Experimental Psychology: Learning, Memory, and Cognition, 10*, 222–233.

Dell, G. S. (1986). A spreading activation theory of retrieval in sentence production. *Psychological Review, 93*(3), 283–321.

Dell, G. S. (1988). The retrieval of phonological forms in production: Tests of predictions from a connectionist model. *Journal of Memory and Language, 27*, 124–142.

Dell, G. S., and Reich, P. A. (1981). Stages in sentence production: An analysis of speech error data. *Journal of Verbal Learning and Verbal Behavior, 20*, 611–629.

Dell, G. S., McKoon, G., and Ratcliff, R. (1983). The activation of antecedent information during the processing of anaphoric reference in reading. *Journal of Verbal Learning and Verbal Behavior, 22,* 121–132.

Denes, G., and Semenza, C. (1975). Auditory modality-specific anomia: evidence from a case of pure word deafness. *Cortex, 11,* 401–411.

DeRenzi, E., and Fagiolini, P. (1978). Normative data and screening power of shortened version of the Token Test. *Cortex, 14,* 41–49.

DeRenzi, E., and Vignolo, L. A. (1962). The Token Test: A sensitive test to detect receptive disturbances in aphasics. *Brain, 85,* 665–678.

de Villiers, J. G. (1974). Quantitative aspects of agrammatism in aphasia. *Cortex, 10,* 36–54.

Divenyi, P. L., and Robinson, A. J. (1989). Non-linguistic auditory capabilities in aphasia. *Brain and Language, 37,* 290–326.

Drewnowski, A., and Healy, A. F. (1977). Detection errors on *the* and *and*: Evidence for reading units larger than the word. *Memory and Cognition, 5,* 636–647.

Drewnowski, A., and Healy, A. F. (1980). Missing -ing in reading: Letter detection errors on word endings. *Journal of Verbal Learning and Verbal Behavior, 19,* 247–262.

Dunn, L. M. (1965). *Expanded manual for the Peabody Picture Vocabulary Test.* Circle Pines, Minn.: American Guidance Service.

Eggert, G. H. (1977). *Wernicke's works on aphasia.* The Hague: Mouton.

Eimas, P. D., Siqueland, E. R., Jusczyk, P., and Vigorito, J. (1971). Speech perception in infants. *Science, 171,* 303–306.

Ellis, A. W. (1979b). Slips of the pen. *Visible Language, 13,* 265–282.

Ellis, A. W. (1982). Spelling and writing (and reading and speaking). In A. W. Ellis (Ed.), *Normality and pathology in cognitive function.* London: Academic Press.

Elman, J. L. (1989). Connectionist approaches to acoustic/phonetic processing. In W. Marslen-Wilson (Ed.), *Lexical representation and process* (pp. 227–260). Cambridge, Mass.: MIT Press.

Elman, J. L., and McClelland, J. L. (1984). Speech perception as a cognitive process: The interactive activation model. In N. Lass (Ed.), *Speech and language: Vol. 10.* New York: Academic Press.

Ellman, J. L., and McClelland, J. L. (1986). Exploiting the lawful variability in the speech wave. In J. Perkell, and D. Klatt (Ed.), *Invariance and variability in speech processes.* Hillsdale, N.J.: Lawrence Erlbaum.

Emmorey, K. D. (1987). The neurological substrates for prosody aspects of speech. *Brain and Language, 30,* 305–320.

Engdahl, E. (1983). Parasitic gaps. *Linguistics and Philosophy, 6,* 5–34.

Eriksen, C. W., Pollock, M. D., and Montague, W. E. (1970). Implicit speech: Mechanisms in perceptual encoding? *Journal of Experimental Psychology, 84,* 502–507.

Farah, M. J. (1990). *Visual agnosia*. Cambridge, Mass.: MIT Press.

Fay, D., and Cutler, A. (1977). Malapropisms and the structure of the mental lexicon. *Linguistic Inquiry, 8*, 505–520.

Ferreira, F., and Clifton, C. (1986). The independence of syntactic processing. *Journal of Memory and Language, 25*, 348–368.

Fletcher, C. R. (1981). Short-term memory processes in text comprehension. *Journal of Verbal Learning and Verbal Behavior, 20*, 564–574.

Flores d'Arcais, G. B. (1975). Some perceptual determinants of sentence construction. In G. B. Flores d'Arcais (Ed.), *Studies in perception* Milan: Martello.

Fodor, J. A. (1983). *The modularity of mind*. Cambridge, Mass.: MIT Press.

Fodor, J. A. (1990). *Modularity in sentence processing*. Paper presented at the City University of New York Conference on Sentence Processing.

Fodor, J. A., Bever, T. G., and Garrett, M. F. (1974). *The psychology of language*. New York: McGraw-Hill.

Fodor, J. D. (1978). Parsing strategies and constraints on transformations. *Linguistic Inquiry, 9*, 427–473.

Ford, M., Bresnan, J., and Kaplan, R. (1982). A competence-based theory of syntactic closure. In J. Bresnan, and R. Kaplan (Ed.), *The mental representation of grammatical relations* (pp. 727–796). Cambridge, Mass.: MIT Press.

Forster, K. I. (1979). Levels of Processing and the Structure of the Language Processor. In W. E. Cooper, and E. C. T. Walker (Ed.), *Sentence processing* (pp. 27–85). Hillsdale, N. J.: Erlbaum.

Fowler, C. A., Napps, S., and Feldman, L. B. (1985). Relations among regular and irregular morphologically related words in the lexicon as revealed by repetition priming. *Memory and Cognition, 13*, 241–255.

Frauenfelder, U. H., and Tyler L. K. (1987). The process of spoken word recognition: An introduction. *Cognition, 25*, 1–20.

Frazier, L., Clifton, C., and Randall, J. (1983). Filling gaps: Decision principles and structure in sentence comprehension. *Cognition, 13*, 187–222.

Frazier, L. (1987a). Sentence processing: A tutorial review. In M. Coltheart (Ed.), *Attention and performance XII: The psychology of reading* (pp. 559–586). London: Lawrence Erlbaum.

Frazier, L. (1987b). Theories of sentence processing. In J. Garfield (Ed.), *Modularity in knowledge representation and natural-language processing* (pp. 291–307). Cambridge, Mass.: MIT Press.

Frazier, L. (1989). Against lexical generation of syntax. In W. Marslen-Wilson (Ed.), *Lexical representation and process* (pp. 505–528). Cambridge, Mass.: MIT Press.

Frazier, L., and Clifton, C. (1989). Successive cyclicity in the grammar and the parser. *Language and Cognitive Processes, 4*, 93–126.

Frazier, L., and Fodor, J. D. (1978). The sausage machine: A new two-stage parsing model. *Cognition, 6*, 291–325.

Frederiksen, C. H., Bracewell, R. J., Breuleux, A., and Renaud, A. (1990). The cognitive representation and processing of discourse: Function and dysfunction. In Y. Joanette, and H. H. Brownell (Eds.), *Discourse Ability and Brain Damage: Theoretical and Empirical Perspectives* New York: Springer-Verlag.

Freedman-Stern, R., Ulatowska, H. K., Baker, T., and Delacoste, C. (1984). Disruption of written language in aphasia: A case study. *Brain and Language, 22*, 181–205.

Friederici, A. D. (1981). Production and comprehension of prepositions in aphasia. *Neuropsychologia, 19*, 191–199.

Friederici, A. D. (1982). Syntactic and semantic processes in aphasic deficits: The availability of prepositions. *Brain and Language, 15*, 249–258.

Friedman, A., and Bourne, L. E. (1976). Encoding the levels of information in pictures and words. *Journal of Experimental Psychology: General, 105*(2), 169–190.

Friedman, R. B. (1982). Mechanisms of reading and spelling in a case of alexia without agraphia. *Neuropsychologia, 20*, 533–545.

Friedrich, F. J., Glenn, C. G., and Marin, O. S. M. (1984). Interruption of phonological coding in conduction aphasia. *Brain and Language, 22*, 266–291.

Fromkin, V. A. (1971). The non-anomalous nature of anomalous utterances. *Language, 47*, 27–52.

Fromkin, V. A. (1973). *Speech errors as linguistic evidence.* The Hague: Mouton.

Funnell, E. (1983). Phonological processing in reading: New evidence from acquired dyslexia. *British Journal of Psychology, 74*, 159–180.

Funnell, E., and Allport, D. A. (1987). Non-linguistic cognition and word meanings. Neuropsychological exploration of common mechanisms. In D. A. Allport, D. Mackay, W. Prinz, and E. Scheerer (Ed.), *Language perception and production* (pp. 367–400). London: Academic Press.

Gandour, J., and Dardarananda, R. (1982). Voice onset time in aphasia: Thai I: Perception. *Brain and Language, 17*, 24–34.

Gandour, J., and Dardarananda, R. (1984). Voice onset time in aphasia: Thai II: Production. *Brain and Language, 23*, 177–205.

Gardner, H., Albert, M., and Weintraub, S. (1975). Comprehending a word: The influence of speed and redundancy on auditory comprehension in aphasia. *Cortex, 11*, 155–162.

Garnsey, S., Tanenhaus, M. K., and Chapman, R. (1987). *Evoked potential measures of sentence comprehension.* Proceedings of the Ninth Annual Meeting of the Cognitive Science Society, Portland.

Garrett, M. F. (1975). The analysis of sentence production. In G. Bower (Ed.), *Psychology of learning and motivation: Vol. 9.* (pp. 137–177). New York: Academic Press.

Garrett, M. F. (1976). Syntactic processes in sentence production. In R. J. Wales, and E. Walker (Eds.), *New approaches to language mechanisms* (pp. 231–255). Amsterdam: North-Holland.

Garrett, M. F. (1978). Word and sentence perception. In R. Held, H. W. Liebowitz, and H.-L. Teuber (Eds.), *Handbook of sensory physiology: Vol. 8: Perception* (pp. 611–623). Berlin: Springer-Verlag.

Garrett, M. F. (1980). Levels of processing in sentence production. In B. Butterworth (Ed.), *Language production: Vol 1: Speech and Talk* (pp. 177–220). London: Academic Press.

Garrett, M. F. (1982). Production of speech: Observations from normal and pathological language use. In A. W. Ellis (Ed.), *Normality and pathology in cognitive functions* (pp. 19–75). London: Academic Press.

Garrett, M. F. (1984). The organization of processing structure for language production: Applicaations to aphasic speech. In D. Caplan, A. R. Lecours, and A. Smith (Ed.), *Biological perspectives of language* (pp. 172–193). Cambridge, Mass.: MIT Press.

Gazdar, G., Klein, E., Pullum, J., and Sag, I. (1985). *Generalized phrase structure grammar.* Cambridge, Mass.: Harvard University Press.

Gazzaniga, M. S. (1983). Right hemisphere language following brain bisection: A 20-year perspective. *American Psychologist, 38,* 525–549.

Gee, J. P., and Grosjean, F. (1983). Performance structures: A psycholinguistic and linguistic appraisal. *Cognitive Psychology, 15,* 411–458.

Geschwind, N. (1965). Disconnection syndromes in animals and man. *Brain, 88,* 237–294, 585–644.

Geschwind, N., and Fusillo, M. (1966). Color naming defects in association with alexia. *Archives of Neurology, 15,* 137–146.

Gibson, E. J., and Guinet, L. (1971). Perception of inflections in brief visual presentations of words. *Journal of Verbal Learning and Verbal Behavior, 10,* 182–189.

Glanzer, M., and Cunitz, A. R. (1966). Two storage mechanisms in free recall. *Journal of Verbal Learning and Verbal Behavior, 5,* 351–360.

Glanzer, M., Dorfman, D., and Kaplan, B. (1981). Short-term storage in the processing of text. *Journal of Verbal Learning and Verbal Behavior, 20,* 656–670.

Glushko, R. J. (1979). The organization and activation of orthographic knowledge in reading aloud. *Journal of Experimental Psychology: Human Perception and Performance, 5*(4), 674–691.

Goldblum, M,-C. (1985). Word comprehension in surface dyslexia. In K. E. Patterson, J. C. Marshall, and M. Coltheart (Ed.), *Surface dyslexia:*

Neuropsychological and cognitive studies of phonological reading (pp. 175–206). London: Erlbaum.

Goldman, N. (1975). Conceptual generation. In R. Schank (Ed.), *Conceptual information processing* Amsterdam: North-Holland.

Goldsmith, J. (1976). *Autosegmental phonology.* Ph.D. dissertation, Department of Linguistics, MIT, Cambridge, Mass.

Goodglass, H. (1973). Studies on the grammar of aphasics. In H. Goodglass, and S. Blumstein (Ed.), *Psycholinguistics and aphasia* Baltimore: John Hopkins University Press.

Goodglass, H. (1976). Agrammatism. In H. Whitaker, and H. A. Whitaker (Eds.), *Studies in neurolinguistics* (pp. 237–260). New York: Academic Press.

Goodglass, H. (1990). Inferences from cross-modal comparisons of agrammatisim. In L. Menn, and L. K. Obler (Ed.), *Agrammatic Aphasia: A cross-language narrative sourcebook* (pp. 1365–1368). Philadelphia: John Benjamins.

Goodglass, H., and Baker, E. (1976). Semantic field, naming, and auditory comprehension in aphasia. *Brain and Language, 3,* 359–374.

Goodglass, H., and Berko, J. (1960). Agrammatism and inflectional morphology in English. *Journal of Speech and Hearing Research, 3,* 257–267.

Goodglass, H., and Geschwind, N. (1976). Language disorders (aphasia). In E. C. Carterette, and Friedman (Eds.), *Handbook of Perception* New York: Academic Press.

Goodglass, H., Gleason, J. B., Bernholtz, N., and Hyde, M. R. (1972). Some linguistic structures in the speech of a Broca's aphasic. *Cortex, 8,* 191–212.

Goodglass, H., and Kaplan, E. (1972). *The assessment of aphasia and related disorders, 1st edition.* Philadelphia: Lea & Febiger.

Goodglass, H., and Kaplan, E. (1982). *The assessment of aphasia and related disorders, 2nd edition.* Philadelphia: Lea & Febiger.

Goodglass, H., Kaplan, E., Weintraub, S., and Ackerman, N. (1976). The "tip of the tongue" phenomenon in aphasia. *Cortex, 12,* 145–153.

Goodman, R. A., and Caramazza, A. (1986). Aspects of the spelling process: Evidence from a case of acquired dysgraphia. *Language and Cognitive Processes, 1,* 263–296.

Gordon, B., and Caramazza, A. (1982). Lexical decision for open- and closed-class words: Failure to replicate differential frequency sensitivity. *Brain and Language, 15,* 143–160.

Gough, P. B., and Cosky, M. J. (1977). One second of reading again. In N. J. Castellan, D. B. Pisoni, and G. R. Potts (Ed.), *Cognitive Theory* (pp. 271–288). Hillsdale, N.J.: Erlbaum.

Greene, R. L., and Crowder, R. G. (1984). Modality and suffix effects in the absence of auditory stimulation. *Journal of Verbal Learning and Verbal Behavior, 23,* 371–382.

Grice, H. P. (1975). Logic and conversation. In P. Cole, and J. L. Morgan (Eds.), *Syntax and Semantics: Vol 3: Speech Acts* (pp. 41–58). New York: Academic Press.

Grodzinsky, Y. (1984). The syntactic characterization of agrammatism. *Cognition, 16,* 99–120.

Grodzinsky, Y. (1986). Language deficits and the theory of syntax. *Brain and Language, 27,* 135–159.

Grodzinsky, Y. (1988). Syntactic representations in agrammatic aphasia: The case of prepositions. *Language and Speech, 31*(2), 115–134.

Grodzinksy, Y. (1990). *Theoretical perspectives on language deficits.* Cambridge, Mass.: MIT Press.

Grodzinsky, Y., and Marek, A. (1988). Algorithmic and heuristic processes revisited. *Brain and Language, 33,* 316–325.

Grodzinsky, Y., and Pierce, A. (1987). *Neurolinguistic evidence for syntactic passive.* Amherst: University of Massachusetts.

Grosjean, F., and Gee, J. P. (1987). Prosodic structure and spoken word recognition. *Cognition, 25,* 135–156.

Grosz, B. J., Pollack, M. E., and Sidner, C. L. (1989). Discourse. In M. Posner (Ed.), *Foundations of cognitive science* (pp. 437–468). Cambridge, Mass.: MIT Press.

Grosz, B.J., and Sidner, C.L. (1986). Attention, intentions, and the structure of discourse. *Computational Linguistics, 12,* 175–204.

Hagiwara, H., and Caplan, D. (1990). Syntactic comprehension in Japanese aphasics: Effects of category and thematic role order. *Brain and Language, 38,* 159–170.

Halle, M., and Monahan, K. P. (1985). Segmental phonology in modern English. *Linguistic inquiry, 16,* 57–116.

Halle, M., and Stevens, K. N. (1964). Speech recognition: A model and a program for research. In J. A. Fodor and J. J. Katz (Ed.), *The structure of language: Reading in the philosophy of language* (pp. 604–612). Englewood Cliffs, N.J.: Prentice Hall.

Halle, M., and Vergnaud, J.-R. (1980). Three-dimensional phonology. *Journal of Linguistic Research, 1,* 83–105.

Halliday, M. A. K., and Hasan, R. (1976). *Cohesion in English.* London: Longman.

Hampton, J. A. (1979). Polymorphous concepts in semantic memory. *Journal of Verbal Learning and Verbal Behavior, 18,* 441–461.

Hanna, P. R., Hanna, J. S., Hodges, R. E., and Rudorf, E. H. (1966). *Phoneme-grapheme correspondences as cues to spelling improvement*. Washington, D.C.: U.S. Dept. of Health, Education and Welfare.

Hansen, D., and Rodgers, T. (1968). An exploration of psycholinguistic units in initial reading. In K. S. Goodman (Ed.), *The psycholinguistic nature of the reading process* (pp. 56–68). Detroit: Wayne State University Press.

Hart, J., Berndt, R. S., and Caramazza, A. (1985). Category-specific naming deficit following cerebral infarction. *Nature, 316,* 439–440.

Hatfield, F. M. (1985). Visual and phonological factors in acquired agraphia. *Neuropsychologia, 23,* 13–29.

Hatfield, F. M., and Patterson, K. E. (1983). Phonological spelling. *Quarterly Journal of Experimental Psychology, 35A,* 451–468.

Hatfield, F. M., Howard, D., Barber, J., Jones, C., and Morton, J. (1977). Object naming in aphasics: The lack of the effect of context or realism. *Neuropsychologia, 15,* 717–727.

Heeschen, C. (1985). Agrammatism vs. paragrammatism: A fictitious opposition. In M.-L. Kean (Ed.), *Agrammatism* (pp. 207–248). London: Academic Press.

Heilman, K. M., and Scholes, R. J. (1976). The nature of comprehension errors in Broca's, conduction, and Wernicke's aphasics. *Cortex, 12,* 258–265.

Henderson, L. (1982). *Orthography and word recognition in reading*. London: Academic Press.

Henderson, L. (1985a). Issues in the modelling of pronunciation assembly in normal reading. In J. C. Marshall, M. Coltheart, and K. Patterson (Eds.), *Surface dyslexia* (pp. 459–508). London: Erlbaum.

Henderson, L. (1985b). Toward a psychology of morphemes. In A. W. Ellis (Ed.), *Progress in the psychology of language* (pp. 15–68). London: LEA Ltd.

Henderson, V. W., Friedman, R. B., Teng, E. L., and Weiner, J. M. (1984). Left hemisphere pathways in reading: Inferences from pure alexia without hemianopia. *Neurology, 35,* 962.

Hildebrandt, N. (1987). *A linguistically based parsing analysis of aphasics' comprehension of referential dependencies*. Ph.D. dissertation, Linguistics, McGill University, Montreal.

Hildebrandt, N., Caplan, D., and Evans, K. (1987). The man$_i$ left t$_i$ without a trace: A case study of aphasic processing of empty categories. *Cognitive Neuropsychology, 4,* 257–302.

Hildyard, A., and Olsen, D. R. (1978). Memory in infants and the comprehension of oral and written discourse. *Discourse Processes, 1,* 91–117.

Hillis, A., and Caramazza, A. (1989). The graphemic buffer and attentional mechanisms. *Brain and Language, 36,* 208–235.

Hillis, A., Rapp, B., Romani, C., and Caramazza, A. (1990). Selective impairment of semantics in lexical processing. *Cognitive Neuropsychology, 7,* 191–243.

Holland, A. L., Fromm, D., and Swindell, C. S. (1986). The labeling problem in aphasia: An illustrative case. *Journal of Speech and Hearing Disorders, 51,* 176–180.

Holmes, V. M. (1987). Syntactic parsing: In search of the garden path. In M. Coltheart (Ed.), *Attention and performance XII: The psychology of reading* (pp. 587–600). London: Lawrence Erlbaum.

Horn, L. R. (1988). Pragmatic theory. In F. J. Newmeyer (Ed.), *Linguistics: The Cambridge Survey: Vol. 1: Linguistic theory: Foundations* (pp. 113–145). Cambridge: Cambridge University Press.

Hotopf, W. H. N. (1980). Slips of the pen. In U. Frith (Ed.), *Cognitive processes in spelling* (pp. 287–309). London: Academic Press.

Hotopf, W. H. N. (1983). Lexical slips of the pen the tongue: What they tell us about language production. In B. Butterworth (Ed.), *Language production, Volume 2* (pp. 147–199). London: Academic Press.

Howard, D. (1985). *The semantic organization of the lexicon: Evidence from aphasia.* Ph.D. dissertation, Psychology, University College, London.

Howard, D., and Franklin, S. (1987). Three ways for understanding written words and their use in two contrasting cases of surface dyslexia. In D. A. Allport, D. Mackay, W. Prinz, and E. Scheerer (Eds.), *Language perception and production: Common processes in listening, speaking, reading and writing* (pp. 340–366). London: Academic Press.

Howard, D., and Orchard-Lisle, V. (1984). On the origin of semantic errors in naming: Evidence from the case of a global aphasic. *Cognitive Neuropsychology, 1,* 163–190.

Huber, W., and Gleber, J. (1982). Linguistic and nonlinguistic processing of narratives in aphasia. *Brain and Language, 16,* 1–18.

Huff, F. J., Corkin, S., and Growdon, J. H. (1986). Semantic impairment and anomia in Alzheimer's Disease. *Brain and Language, 28,* 235–249.

Humphreys, G. W., and Evett, L. J. (1985). Are there independent lexical and nonlexical routes in word processing? An evaluation of the dual-route theory of reading. *The Behavioral and Brain Sciences, 8,* 689–740.

Humphreys, G. W., and Riddoch, M. J. (1984). Routes to object constancy: Implications from neurological impairments of object constancy. *Quarterly Journal of Experimental Psychology, 36A,* 385–415.

Humphreys, G. W., Riddoch, M. J., and Quinlan, P. T. (1985). Interactive processes in perceptual organisation: Evidence from visual agnosia. In M. I. Posner, and O. S. M. Marin (Eds.), *Attention and performance XI.* Hillsdale, N.J.: Lawrence Erlbaum.

Humphreys, G. W., Riddoch, M. J., and Quinlan, P. T. (1988). Cascade processes in picture identification. *Cognitive Neuropsychology, 5,* 67–104.

Itoh, M., Sasanuma, S., Tatsumi, I. F., Murakami, S., Fukusako, Y., and Suzuki, T. (1982). Voice onset time characteristics in apraxia of speech. *Brain and Language, 17,* 193–210.

Itoh, M., Sasanuma, S., and Ushijima, T. (1979). Velar movements during speech in a patient with apraxia of speech. *Brain and Language, 7,* 227–239.

Itoh, S., Sasanuma, S., and Hirose, H. (1980). Abnormal articulatory dynamics in a patient with apraxia of speech: X-ray microbeam observation. *Brain and Language, 11,* 66–75.

Jackendoff, R. (1975). Morphological and semantic regularities in the lexicon. *Language, 51,* 639–671.

Jakobson, R. (1941). *Kindersprache, Aphasie und allgemeine Lautgesetze.* Uppsala, Sweden: Universitets Arsskrift.

Jakobson, R., Fant, G. M., and Halle, M. (1963). *Preliminaries to speech analysis.* Cambridge, Mass.: MIT Press.

Jarvella, R. V. (1970). Effects of syntax on running memory span for connected discourse. *Psychonomic Science, 19,* 235–236.

Jarvella, R. V. (1971). Syntactic processing of connected speech. *Journal of Verbal Learning and Verbal Behavior, 10,* 409–416.

Jassem, W., Hill, D. R., and Witten, I. H. (1984). Isochrony in English speech: Its statistical validity and linguistic relevance. In D. Gibbon, and H. Richter (Eds.), *Intonation, accent and rhythm* Berlin: De Gruyter.

Jauhianen, T., and Nuutila, A. (1977). Auditory perception of speech and speech sounds in recent and recovered cases of aphasia. *Brain and Language, 6,* 47–51.

Jerger, J., Weikers, N. J., Sharbrough, F. J., and Jerger, S. (1969). Bilateral lesions of the temporal lobe: A case study. *Acta Oto-Laryngologica, 258,* 1–51.

Joanette, Y., Keller, E., and Lecours, A.-R. (1980). Sequence of phonemic approximations in aphasia. *Brain and Language, 11,* 30–44.

Joanette, Y., Goulet, P., Ska, B., and Nespoulous, J.-L. (1986). Informative content of narrative discourse in right-brain-damaged right-handers. *Brain and Language, 29,* 81–105.

Job, R., and Sartori, G. (1984). Morphological decomposition: Evidence from crossed phonological dyslexia. *Quarterly Journal of Experimental Psychology, 36A,* 435–458.

Johnson-Laird, P. N. (1983). *Mental models: Towards a cognitive science of language inference and consciousness.* Cambridge: Cambridge University Press.

Johnston, J. C. (1978). A test of the sophisticated guessing theory of word perception. *Cognitive Psychology, 10,* 123–153.

Kail, M. (1989). Cue validity, cue cost and processing types in sentence comprehension in French and Spanish. In B. MacWhinney and E. Bates (Eds.), *A cross-linguisitic study of sentence processing* (pp. 77–117). Cambridge: Cambridge University Press.

Kanshepolsky, J., Kelley, J. J., and Wagner, J. D. (1973). A cortical auditory disorder: Clinical audiologic and pathologic aspects. *Neurology, 23,* 699–705.

Kaplan, E., Goodglass, H., and Weintraub, S. (1976). *The Boston Naming Test.* Boston: Veterans Administration.

Kay, J., and Marcel, A. J. (1981). One process not two in reading aloud: Lexical analogies do the work of non-lexical rules. *Quarterly Journal of Experimental Psychology, 33A,* 397–413.

Kay, J., and Patterson, K. E. (1985). Routes to meaning in surface dyslexia. In K. E. Patterson, J. C. Marshall, and M. Coltheart (Ed.), *Surface dyslexia: Neuropsychological and cognitive studies of phonological reading* (pp. 79–104). London: Erlbaum.

Kean, M.-L. (1977). The linguistic interpretation of aphasic syndromes: Agrammatism in Broca's aphasia, an example. *Cognition, 5,* 9–46.

Kean, M.-L. (1982). Three perspectives for the analysis of aphasic syndromes. In M. A. Arbib, D. Caplan, and J. C. Marshall (Ed.), *Neural models of language processes* (pp. 173–201). New York: Academic Press.

Kean, M.-L. (Ed.) (1985). *Agrammatism.* New York: Academic Press,

Keenan, J. M. (1978). *Inferring causal connections in prose comprehension.* In Proceedings of the Annual Meeting of the American Psychological Association, Toronto, Canada.

Keenan, J. M., and Kintsch, W. (1974). The identification of explicitly and implicitly presented information. In W. Kintsch (Ed.), *The representation of meaning in memory* (pp. 153–165). Hillsdale, N.J.: Erlbaum.

Kelly, M. H., and Bock, J. K. (1988). Stress in time. *Journal of Experimental Psychology: Human Perception and Performance, 14,* 389–403.

Kelso, J. A. S., Tuller, B., and Harris, K. S. (1986). A theoretical note on speech timing. In J. S. Perkell, and D. Klatt (Ed.), *Invariance and variability in speech processes* Hillsdale, N.J.: Lawrence Erlbaum.

Kempen, G. (1988). Language generation systems. In I. Batori, W. Lenders, and W. Putschke (Ed.), *Computational linguistics: An international handbook on computer oriented language research and applications* (pp. 471–480). Berlin: de Gruyter.

Kempen, G., and Huijbers, P. (1983). The lexicalization process in sentence production and naming: Indirect election of words. *Cognition, 14,* 185–209.

Kempen, G., and Hoenkamp, E. (1987). An incremental procedural grammar for sentence formulation. *Cognitive Science, 11,* 201–258.

Kempley, S. T., and Morton, J. (1982). The effects of priming with regularly and irregularly related words in auditory word recognition. *British Journal of Psychology, 73,* 441–454.

Kent, R. D. (1986). Is a paradigm change needed? *Journal of Phonetics, 14,* 111–115.

Kent, R. D., and Rosenbek, J. C. (1983). Acoustic patterns of apraxia of speech. *Journal of Speech and Hearing Research, 26,* 231–249.

Kertesz, A. (1979a). *Aphasia and associated disorders: Taxonomy, localization and recovery.* New York: Grune & Stratton.

Kertesz, A. (1979b). Visual agnosia: The dual deficit of perception and recognition. *Cortex, 15,* 403–419.

Kertesz, A., and Poole, E. (1974). The aphasia quotient: The taxonomic approach to measurement of aphasic disability. *Canadian Journal of Neurological Sciences, 1,* 7–16.

Kertesz, A., Harlock, W., and Coates, R. (1979). Computer tomographic localization, lesion size, and prognesis in aphasia and nonverbal impairment. *Brain and Language, 8,* 34–50.

Kertesz, A., Sheppard, A., and MacKenzie, R. (1982). Localization in transcortical sensory aphasia. *Archives of Neurology, 39,* 475–478.

Kimball, J. (1973). Seven principles of surface structure parsing in natural language. *Cognition, 2,* 15–47.

Kinsbourne, M., and Rosenfield, D. B. (1974). Agraphia selective for written spelling: An experimental case study. *Brain and Language, 1,* 215–225.

Kinsbourne, M., and Warrington, E. K. (1962a). A variety of reading disability associated with right hemisphere lesions. *Journal of Neurology, Neurosurgery and Psychiatry, 25,* 339–344.

Kinsbourne, M., and Warrington, E. K. (1962b). A disorder of simultaneous form perception. *Brain, 85,* 461–486.

Kintsch, W., and Keenan, J. (1973). Reading rate and retention as a function of the number of propositions in the base structure of sentences. *Cognitive Psychology, 6,* 257–274.

Kintsch, W., and van Dijk, T. A. (1978). Toward a model of text comprehension and production. *Psychological Review, 85,* 363–394.

Kintsch, W., Kozminsky, E., Streby, W. J., McKoon, G., and Keenan, J. M. (1975). Comprehension and recall of text as a function of content variables. *Journal of Verbal Learning and Verbal Behavior, 14,* 196–214.

Kiparsky, P. (1982). From cyclic phonology to lexical phonology. In H. van der Hulst, and N. Smith (Ed.), *The structure of phonological representations: Vol. 1.* Dordrecht, Netherlands, Foris.

Klapp, S. T., Anderson, W. G., and Berrian, R. W. (1973). Implicit speech in reading, reconsidered. *Journal of Experimental Psychology, 100,* 368–374.

Klatt, D. H. (1979). Speech perception: A model of acoustic-phonetic analysis and lexical access. In R. A. Cole (Ed.), *Perception and production of fluent speech* Hillsdale, N.J.: Lawrence Erlbaum.

Klatt, D. H. (1986). The problem of variability in speech recognition and in models of speech perception. In J. Perkell, and D. Klatt (Eds.), *Invariance and variability in speech processes.* Hillsdale, N.J.: Lawrence Erlbaum.

Klatt, D. H. (1989). Review of selected models of speech perception. In W. Marslen-Wilson (Ed.), *Lexical representation and process* (pp. 169–226). Cambridge, Mass.: MIT Press.

Kleiman, G. (1975). Speech recording in reading. *Journal of Verbal Learning and Verbal Behavior., 14,* 323–329.

Kohn, S. E. (1984). The nature of the phonological disorder in conduction aphasia. *Brain and Language, 23,* 97–115.

Kohn, S. E., and Smith, K. L. (1990). Between-word speech errors in conduction aphasia. *Cognitive Neuropsychology, 7,* 133–156.

Kohn, S. E., Smith, K. L., and Arsenault, J. K. (1990). The remediation of conduction aphasia via sentence repetition: A case study. *British Journal of Disorders of Communication, 25,* 45–60.

Kolers, P. A. (1966). Talking and reading bilingually. *American Journal of Psychology, 79,* 357–376.

Kolk, H. H., and van Grunsven, J. J. F. (1985). Agrammatism as a variable phenomenon. *Cognitive Neuropsychology, 2,* 347–384.

Kosslyn, S. M., Flynn, R. A., Amsterdam, J. B., and Wang, G. (1990). Components of high level vision: A cognitive neuroscience analysis and accounts of neurological syndromes. *Cognition, 34,* 203–278.

Kremin, H. (1985). Routes and strategies in surface dyslexia and dysgraphia. In K. E. Patterson J. C. Marshall, and M. Coltheart (Ed.), *Surface dyslexia: Neuropsychological and cognitive studies of phonological reading* (pp. 105–138). London: Erlbaum.

Kuhl, P. K., and Miller, J. D. (1974). Discrimination of speech sounds by the chinchilla: /t/ vs /d/ in CV syllables. *Journal of the Acoustical Society of America, 56, suppl. 2,* S217.

Kuhl, P. K., and Miller, J. D. (1975). Speech perception by the chinchilla: Voiced-voiceless distinction in alveolar plosive consonants. *Science, 190,* 69–72.

Labov, W. (1973). The boundaries of words and their meanings. In C.-J. N. Bailey, and R. W. Shuy (Ed.), *New ways of analyzing variation in English* (pp. 340–373). Washington, D.C.: Georgetown University Press.

Lachter, J., and Bever, T. G. (1988). The relation between linguistic structure and associative theories of language learning: A constructive critique of some connectionist learning models. *Cognition, 28,* 195–247.

Lahiri, A., and Marslen-Wilson, W. (1991). The mental representation of lexical form: A phonological approach to the recognition lexicon. *Cognition, 38*, 245–294.

Lapointe, S. (1983). Some issues in the linguistic description of agrammatism. *Cognition, 14*, 1–39.

Lashley, K. S. (1929). *Brain mechanisms and intelligence.* Chicago: University of Chicago Press.

Lashley, K. S. (1950). In search of the engram. *Symposium of the Society for Experimental Biology, 4*, 454–482.

Lasnik, H., and Uriagereka, J. (1988). *A course in GB syntax: Lectures on binding and empty categories.* Cambridge, Mass.: MIT Press.

Laudanna, A., Badecker, W., and Caramazza, A. (1989). Priming homographic stems. *Journal of Memory and Language, 28*, 531–546.

Lecours, A. R., and Lhermitte, F. (1969). Phonemic paraphasias: Linguistic structures and tentative hypotheses. *Cortex, 5*, 193–228.

Lecours, A. R., Lhermitte, F., and Bryans, B. (1983). *Aphasiology.* London: Balliere Tindall.

Lesser, R. (1986). *Comprehension of Linguistic Cohesion After Right Brain Damage.* Presented at INS, Veldhoven, Netherlands.

Levelt, W. J. M. (1983). Monitoring and self-repair in speech. *Cognition, 14*, 41–104.

Levelt, W. J. M. (1989). *Speaking: From intention to articulation.* Cambridge, Mass.: MIT Press.

Levelt, W. J. M., Schriefers, H., Vorberg, D., Meyer, A. S., Pechmann, T., and Havinga, J. (1991). The time course of lexical access in speech production: A study of picture naming. *Psychological Review, 98*, 122–142.

Levine, D. N., Calvanio, R., and Popovics, A. (1982). Language in the absence of inner speech. *Neuropsychologia, 20*(4), 391–401.

Levy, B. A. (1975). Vocalization and suppression effects in sentence memory. *Journal of Experimental Child Psychology, 14*, 304–316.

Levy, B. A. (1977). Reading: Speech and meaning processes. *Journal of Verbal Learning and Verbal Behavior, 16*, 623–638.

Lhermitte, F., and Beauvois, M.-F. (1973). A visual-speech disconnexion syndrome: Report of a case with optic-aphasia, agnosic alexia and colour agnosia. *Brain, 96*, 695–714.

Liberman, A. M. (1970). Some characteristics of perception in the speech mode. *Perception and Its Disorders, 48*, 238–254.

Liberman, A. M., and Mattingly, I. G. (1985). The motor theory of speech perception revised. *Cognition, 21*, 1–36.

Liberman, A. M., and Studdert-Kennedy, M. (1978). Phonetic perception. In R. Held, H. Leibowitz, and H.-L. Teuber (Eds.), *The handbook of sensory physiology: Vol. 8: Perception* (pp. 143–178). Heidelberg: Springer-Verlag.

Liberman, A. M., Cooper, F. S., Shankweiler, D. P., and Studdert-Kennedy, M. (1967). Perception of the speech code. *Psychological Review, 74*, 431–461.

Liberman, A. M., Isenberg, D., and Rakerd, B. (1981). Duplex perception of cues for stop consonants: Evidence for a phonetic mode. *Perception and Psychophysics, 30*, 133–143.

Liberman, M., and Prince, A. (1977). On stress and linguistic rhythm. *Linguistic Inquiry, 8*, 249–336.

Lichtheim, L. (1885). On aphasia. *Brain, 7*, 433–484.

Lieberman, P., and Blumstein, S. E. (1990). *Speech physiology, speech perception, and acoustic phonetics.* Cambridge, U.K.: Cambridge University Press.

Lichtheim, L. (1885). On aphasia. *Brain, 7*, 433–484.

Lindsley, J. R. (1975). Producing simple utterances: How far do we plan? *Cognitive Psychology, 7*, 1–19.

Lindsley, J. R. (1976). Producing simple utterances: Details of the planning process. *Journal of Psycholinguistic Research, 5*, 331–351.

Linebarger, M. C. (1990). Neuropsychology of sentence parsing. In A. Caramazza (Ed.), *Cognitive neuropsychology and neurolinguistics: Advances in models of cognitive function and impairment* (pp. 55–122). Hillsdale, N.J.: Lawrence Erlbaum.

Linebarger, M. C., Schwartz, M. F., and Saffran, E. M. (1983a). Sensitivity to grammatical structure in so-called agrammatic aphasics. *Cognition, 13*, 361–392.

Linebarger, M. C., Schwartz, M. F., and Saffran, E. M. (1983b). Syntactic processing in agrammatism: A reply to Zurif and Grodzinsky. *Cognition, 15*, 207–214.

Lukatela, K., Crain, S., and Shankweller, D. (1988). Sensitivity to inflectional morphology in agrammatism: Investigation of a highly inflected language. *Brain and Language, 33*, 1–15.

Luria, A. R. (1947). *Traumatic Aphasia.* Reprinted in translation (1971). The Hague: Mouton.

Luria, A. R. (1973). *The working brain.* New York: Basic Books.

Mack, M., and Blumstein, S. E. (1983). Further evidence of acoustic invariance in speech production: The stop-glide contrast. *Journal of the Acoustical Society of America, 73*, 1739–1750.

MacKay, D. (1970). Spoonerisms: The structure of errors in the serial order of speech. *Neuropsychologia, 8*, 323–350.

MacKay, D. (1972). The structure of words and syllables: Evidence from errors in speech. *Cognitive Psychology, 3*, 210–227.

MacKay, D. G. (1978). Derivational rules and the internal lexicon. *Journal of Verbal Learning and Verbal Behavior, 17*, 61–71.

MacNeilage, P. (1982). Speech production mechanisms in aphasia. In S. Griller, B. Lindblum, J. Lubker, and A. Person (Eds.), *Speech Motor Control* (pp. 43–60). Oxford: Pergamon.

MacWhinney, B. (1989). Competition and connectionism. In B. MacWhinney, and E. Bates (Eds.), *A cross-linguistic study of sentence processing* (pp. 422–457). Cambridge: Cambridge University Press.

Mandler, J. M., and Johnson, N. S. (1977). Remembrance of things parsed: Story structure and recall. *Cognitive Psychology, 9,* 111–151.

Manelis, L. (1974). The effect of meaningfulness in tachistoscopic word perception. *Perception and Psychophysics, 16,* 182–192.

Manelis, L., and Tharp, D. A. (1977). The processing of affixed words. *Memory and Cognition, 4,* 53–61.

Marcel, A. J. (1980). Surface dyslexia and beginning reading: A revised hypothesis of the pronunciation of print and its impairments. In M. Coltheart, K. E. Patterson, and J. C. Marshall (Ed.), *Deep dyslexia* (pp. 227–258). London: Routledge.

Marcel, A. J. (1983a). Conscious and unconscious perception: Experiments on visual masking and word recognition. *Cognitive Psychology, 15,* 197–237.

Marcel, A. J. (1983b). Conscious and unconscious perception: An approach to the relations between phenomenal experience and perceptual processes. *Cognitive Psychology, 15,* 238–300.

Marcus, M. P. (1980). *A theory of syntactic recognition for natural language.* Cambridge, Mass.: MIT Press.

Margolin, D. I. (1984). The neuropsychology of writing and spelling: Semantic, phonological, motor and perceptual processes. *Quarterly Journal of Experimental Psychology, 36A,* 459–489.

Margolin, D. I., and Binder, L. (1984). Multiple component agraphia in a patient with atypical cerebral dominance: An error analysis. *Brain and Language, 22,* 26–40.

Margolin, D. I., Marcel, A. J., and Carlson, N. R. (1985). Common mechanisms in dysnomia and post-semantic surface dyslexia: Processing deficits and selective attention. In K. E. Patterson, J. C. Marshall, and M. Coltheart (Ed.), *Surface dyslexia: Neuropsychological and cognitive studies of phonological reading* (pp. 139–174). London: Erlbaum.

Marr, D. (1982). *Vision.* San Francisco: W. H. Freeman.

Marshall, J. C., and Newcombe, F. (1973). Patterns of paralexia: A psycholinguistic approach. *Journal of Psycholinguistic Research, 2*(3), 175–199.

Marslen-Wilson, W. D. (1973). Linguistic structure and speech shadowing at very short latencies. *Nature, 244,* 522–523.

Marslen-Wilson, W. D. (1987). Functional parallelism in spoken word-recognition. *Cognition, 25,* 71–102.

Marslen-Wilson, W. D. (1989). Access and integration: Projecting sounds onto meaning. In W. Marslen-Wilson (Ed.), *Lexical representation and process* (pp. 2–24). Cambridge, Mass.: MIT Press.

Marslen-Wilson, W. D., and Tyler, L. K. (1976). Memory and levels of processing in a psycholinguistic context. *Journal of Experimental Psychology: Human Learning and Memory, 2*, 112–119.

Marslen-Wilson, W. D., and Tyler, L. K. (1980). The temporal structure of spoken language understanding. *Cognition, 8*, 1–71.

Marslen-Wilson, W., and Tyler, L. K. (1987). Against modularity. In J. L. Garfield (Ed.), *Modularity in knowledge representation and natural-language understanding* (pp. 37–62). Cambridge, Mass.: MIT Press.

Marslen-Wilson, W. D., and Welsh, A. (1978). Processing interactions and lexical access during word recognition in continuous speech. *Cognitive Psychology, 10*, 29–63.

Martin, R. C. (1987). Articulatory and phonological deficits in short-term memory and their relation to syntactic processing. *Brain and Language, 32*, 159–192.

Martin, R. C., and Caramazza, A. (1979). Classification in well-defined and ill-defined categories: Evidence for common processing strategies. *Journal of Experimental Psychology: General, 109*, 320–353.

Martin, R. C., Wetzel, W. F., Blossom-Stach, C., and Feher, E. (1989). Syntactic loss versus processing deficit: An assessment of two theories of agrammatism and syntactic comprehension deficits. *Cognition, 32*, 157–191.

McCarthy, J. (1979). *Formal problems in Semitic phonology and morphology.* Ph.D. dissertation, Department of Linguistics, MIT, Cambridge, Mass.

McCarthy, R. A., and Warrington, E. K. (1984). A two-route model of speech production: Evidence from aphasia. *Brain, 107*, 463–485.

McCarthy, R. A., and Warrington, E. K. (1985). Category specificity in an agrammatic patient: The relative impairment of verb retrieval and comprehension. *Neuropsychologia, 23*, 709–727.

McCarthy, R. A., and Warrington, E. K. (1987a). Understanding: A function of short-term memory? *Brain, 110*, 1565–1578.

McCarthy, R. A., and Warrington, E. K. (1987b). The double-dissociation of short-term memory for lists and sentences: Evidence from aphasia. *Brain, 110*, 1545–1563.

McCarthy, R. A., and Warrington, E. K. (1988). *Evidence for modality-specific* meaning systems in the brain. *Nature, 334.*

McCarthy, R. A., and Warrington, E. K. (1990). Neuropsychological studies of short-term memory. In G. Vallar, and T. Shallice (Ed.), *Neuropsychological Impairments of Short-Term Memory* Cambridge: Cambridge University Press.

McClelland, J. L. (1976). Preliminary letter identification in the perception of words and non-words. *Journal of Experimental Psychology: Human Perception and Performance, 2*, 80–91.

McClelland, J., and Kawamoto, A. (1986). Mechanisms of sentence processing: Assigning role to constituents. In J. McClelland, and D. Rumelhart (Eds.), *Parallel distributed processing*. Cambridge, Mass.: MIT Press.

McClelland, J. L., and Johnston, J. C. (1977). The role of familiar units in perception of words and non-words *Perception and Psychophysics, 22*, 249–261.

McClelland, J. L., and Rumelhart, D. E. (1981). An interaction model of context effects in letter perception: Part I. An account of basic findings. *Psychology Review, 88*, 375–407.

McClelland, J. L., St. John, M., and Taraban, R. (1989). Sentence comprehension: A parallel distributed processing approach. *Language and Cognitive Processes, 4*, 287–336.

McDonald, J., and MacWhinney, B. (1989). Maximum likelihood models for sentence processing. In B. MacWhinney, and E. Bates (Eds.), *A cross-linguistic study of sentence processing* (pp. 397–422). Cambridge: Cambridge University Press.

McKoon, G., and Ratcliff, R. (1980). The comprehension processes and memory structures involved in anaphoric reference. *Journal of Verbal Learning and Verbal Behavior, 19*, 668–682.

KcKoon, G., Keenan, J., and Kintsch, W. (1974). Response latencies to explicit and implicit statements as a function of the delay between reading and test. In W. Kintsch (Ed.), *The Representation of meaning in memory* (pp. 166–176). Hillsdale, N.J.: Erlbaum.

Menn, L. (1990). Agrammatism in English: Two case studies. In L. Menn, and L. K. Obler (Ed.), *Agrammatic aphasia: A cross-language narrative sourcebook* (pp. 117–178). Philadelphia: John Benjamins.

Menn, L., and Obler, L. (Eds.) (1990a). *Agrammatic aphasia: A cross-language narrative sourcebook*. New York: John Benjamins.

Menn, L., and Obler, L. K. (1990b). Cross-language data and theories of agrammatism. In L. Menn, and L. K. Obler (Ed.), *Agrammatic aphasia: A cross-language narrative sourcebook* (pp. 369–390). Philadelphia: John Benjamins.

Metz-Lutz, M.-N., and Dahl, E. (1983). Analysis of word comprehension in a case of pure word deafness. *Brain and Language, 23*, 13–25.

Meyer, D. E., and Schvaneveldt, R. W. (1971). Facilitation in recognizing pairs of words: Evidence for a dependence between retrieval operations. *Journal of Experimental Psychology, 90*, 227–234.

Meyer, D. E., Schvaneveldt, R. W., and Ruddy, M. G. (1974). Functions of graphemic and phonemic codes in visual word recognition. *Memory and Cognition, 2*, 309–321.

Miceli, G., and Caramazza, A. (1988). Dissociation of inflectional and derivational morphology. *Brain and Language, 35,* 24–65.

Miceli, G., Gainotti, G., Caltagirone, C., and Masullo, C. (1980). Some aspects of phonological impairment in aphasia. *Brain and Language, 11,* 159–169.

Miceli, G., Mazzucchi, A., Menn, L., and Goodglass, H. (1983). Contrasting cases of Italian agrammatic aphasia without comprehension disorder. *Brain and Language, 19,* 65–97.

Miceli, G., Silveri, M., Villa, G., and Caramazza, A. (1984). On the basis for the agrammatic's difficulty in producing main verbs. *Cortex, 20,* 207–220.

Miceli, G., Silveri, M. C., Romani, C., and Caramazza, A. (1989). Variation in the pattern of omissions and substitutions of grammatical morphemes in the spontaneous speech of so-called agrammatic patients. *Brain and Language, 36,* 447–492.

Miceli, G., Giustolisi, L., and Caramazza, A. (1990). *The interaction of lexical and non-lexical processing mechanisms: Evidence from anomia.* Baltimore: The Cognitive Neuropsychology Laboratory, The Johns Hopkins University.

Michel, F., and Andreewsky, E. (1983). Deep dysphasia: An auditory analog of deep dyslexia in the auditory modality. *Brain and Language, 18,* 212–223.

Milberg, W., and Blumstein, S. E. (1981). Lexical decision and aphasia: Evidence for semantic processing. *Brain and Language, 14,* 371–385.

Miller, D., and Ellis, A. W. (1987). Speech and writing errors in "neologistic jargonaphasia": A lexical activation hypothesis. In M. Coltheart, G. Sartori, and J. R. (Ed.), *The Cognitive Neuropsychology of Language* London: Lawrence Erlbaum.

Miller, G. A., and Johnson-Laird, P. N. (1976). *Language and perception.* Cambridge, Mass.: Harvard University Press.

Miller, G. A., and Nicely, P. E. (1955). An analysis of perceptual confusions among some English consonants. *Journal of the Acoustical Society of America, 27,* 338–352.

Milner, B. (1966). Amnesia following operation on the temporal lobes. In C. W. M. Whitty, and O. L. Zangwill (Eds.), *Amnesia* (pp. 109–133). London: Butterworths.

Monrad-Krohn, G. H. (1974). Dysprosody of altered "melody of language". *Brain, 70,* 405–423.

Monsell, S. (1985). Repetition and the lexicon. In A. W. Ellis (Ed.), *Progress in the psychology of language* Hillsdale, N.J.: Lawrence Erlbaum.

Monsell, S. (1987). On the relation between lexical input and output pathways for speech. In A. Allport, D. MacKay, W. Prinz, and E. Sheerer (Eds.), *Language perception and production* London: Academic Press.

Morris, W. (1969). *The American heritage dictionary of the English language.* Boston: Houghton Mifflin.

Morton, J. (1964). A preliminary functional model for language behavior. *Audiology, 3,* 216–225.

Morton, J. (1969). The interaction of information in word recognition. *Psychological Review, 76,* 165–178.

Morton, J. (1970). A functional model of memory. In D. A. Norman (Ed.), *Models of human memory* New York: Academic Press.

Morton, J. (1979a). Facilitation in word-recognition experiments causing changes in the logogen model. In P. A. Kolers, M. E. Wrolstad, and H. Bouma (Eds.), *Processing of visible language* New York: Plenum.

Morton, J. (1979b). Word recognition. In J. Morton, and J. C. Marshall (Eds.), *Psycholinguistics (Series 2)* (pp. 109–156). London: Elek.

Morton, J. (1980). Two auditory parallels to deep dyslexia. In M. Coltheart, K. Patterson, and J. C. Marshall (Eds.), *Deep dyslexia* (pp. 189–197). London: Routledge.

Morton, J., and Patterson, K. E. (1980). A new attempt at an interpretation, or, an attempt at a new interpretation. In M. Coltheart, K. E. Patterson, and J. C. Marshall (Eds.), *Deep dyslexia* (pp. 91–118). London: Routledge.

Murphy, G. L. (1985a). Processes of understanding anaphora. *Journal of Memory and Language, 24,* 290–303.

Murphy, G. L. (1985b). Psychological explanations of deep and surface anaphora. *Journal of Pragmatics, 9,* 785–813.

Murphy, G. L. (1990). The psycholinguistics of discourse comprehension. In Y. Joanette, and H. H. Browneli (Ed.), *Discourse Ability and brain damage: Theoretical and empirical perspectives* (pp. 28–49). New York: Springer-Verlag.

Murphy, G. L., and Brownell, H. H. (1985). Category differentiation in object recognition: Typicality constraints on the basic category advantage. *Journal of Experimental Psychology: Learning, Memory and Cognition, 11,* 70–84.

Murrell, G. A., and Morton, J. (1974). Word recognition and morphemic structure. *Journal of Experimental Psychology, 102,* 963–968.

Naeser, M. A., and Hayward, R. W. (1978). Lesion localization in aphasia with cranial computed tomography and the Boston diagnostic aphasia examination. *Neurology, 28,* 545–551.

Nespoulous, J.-L., Dordain, M., Perron, C., Ska, B., Bub, D., Caplan, D., Mehler, J., and Lecours, A.-R. (1988). Agrammatism in sentence production without comprehension deficits: Reduced availability of syntactic structures and/or of grammatical morphemes? A case study. *Brain and Language, 33,* 273–295.

Nespoulous, J. L., Joanette, Y., Beland, R., Caplan, D., and Lecours, A. R. (1984). Phonological disturbances in aphasia: Is there a "markedness" effect in aphasic phonemic errors? In F. C. Rose (Ed.), *Progress in aphasiology: Advances in neurology.* New York: Raven Press.

Newcombe, F., and Marshall, J. C. (1985). Reading and writing by letter sounds. In K. E. Patterson, J. C. Marshall, and M. Coltheart (Ed.), *Surface dyslexia: Cognitive and neuropsychological studies of phonological reading* (pp. 35–52). Hillsdale: Lawrence Erlbaum.

Newell, A., and Simon, H. A. (1972). *Human problem solving.* Englewood Cliffs, N.J.: Prentice-Hall.

Nooteboom, S. (1972). *Production and perception of vowel duration.* Unpublished doctoral dissertation, Utrecht University.

Nooteboom, S. (1973). The tongue slips into patterns. In V. Fromkin (Ed.), *Speech errors as linguistic evidence.* The Hague: Mouton.

Obler, L. K., and Albert, M. L. (1979). *Action naming test.* Unpublished, Boston.

O'Connor, R. E. (1975). *An investigation into the word frequency effect.* Unpublished honors thesis, Psychology, Monash University.

Ohala, J. J. (1978). Production of tone. In V. Fromkin (Ed.), *Tone: A linguistic survey.* New York: Academic Press.

Ojemann, G. (1983). Brain organization for language from the perspective of electrical stimulation mapping. *Behavioural and Brain Sciences, 6,* 189–230.

Ostrin, R. (1982). *Framing the production problem in agrammatism.* Unpublished paper, Psychology, University of Pennsylvania.

Ostrin, R., and Schwartz, M. F. (1986). Reconstructing from a degraded trace: A study of sentence repetition in agrammatism. *Brain and Language, 28,* 328–345.

Ostrin, R. K., Schwartz, M. F., and Saffrin, E. M. (1983). *The influence of syntactic complexity in the elicited production of agrammatic aphasics.* Paper Presented at the Annual Meeting of the Academy of Aphasia, Minneapolis, MN.

Paivio, A. (1971). *Imagery and verbal processes.* London: Holt, Rinehart & Winston.

Paivio, A. (1975). Perceptual comparisons through the mind's eye. *Memory and Cognition, 3,* 635–647.

Paivio, A. (1978). Dual coding: Theoretical issues and empirical evidence. In J. M. Scandura, and C. J. Brainerd (Eds.), *Structure/process models of complex human behavior* Leiden, Netherlands: Nordhoff.

Parisi, D. (1987). Grammatical disturbances of speech production. In M. Coltheart, G. Sartori, and R. Job (Eds.), *The cognitive neuropsychology of language* (pp. 201–220). London: Lawrence Erlbaum.

Pate, D. S., Saffran, E., M., and Martin, N. (1987). Specifying the nature of the production impairment in a conduction aphasic: A case study. *Language and Cognitive Processes, 2,* 43–84.

Patterson, K. E. (1980). Derivational errors. In M. Coltheart, K. E. Patterson, and J. C. Marshall (Eds.), *Deep dyslexia* (pp. 286–306). London: Routledge.

Patterson, K. E. (1982). The relation between reading and phonological coding: Further neuropsychological observations. In A. W. Ellis (Ed.), *Normality and pathology in cognitive functions* (pp. 77–111). London: Academic Press.

Patterson, K. E. (1986). Lexical but nonsemantic spelling? *Cognitive Neuropsychology, 3,* 341–367.

Patterson, K. E., and Besner, D. (1984). Is the right hemisphere literate? *Cognitive Neuropsychology, 1,* 315–342.

Patterson, K. E., and Kay, J. (1982). Letter-by-letter reading: Psychological descriptions of a neurological syndrome. *Quarterly Journal of Experimental Psychology, 34A,* 411–441.

Patterson, K. E., and Morton, J. (1985). From orthography to phonology: An attempt at an old interpretation. In K. E. Patterson, M. Coltheart, and J. C. Marshall (Ed.), *Surface dyslexia* (pp. 335–359). London: Erlbaum.

Patterson, K., Seidenberg, M. S., and McClelland, J. L. (1989). Connections and disconnections: Acquired dyslexia in a computational model of reading processes. In R. Morris (Ed.), *Parallel distributed processing: Implications for psychology and neurobiology* (pp. 131–181). New York: Oxford University Press.

Perecman, E., and Kellar, L. (1981). The effect of voice and place among aphasic, nonaphasic right-damaged, and normal subjects on a metalinguistic task. *Brain and Language, 12,* 213–223.

Perfetti, C. A., and Goldman, S. R. (1974). Thematization and sentence retrieval. *Journal of Verbal Learning and Verbal Behavior, 13,* 70–79.

Perfetti, C. A., and Goldman, S. R. (1975). Discourse functions of thematization and topicalization. *Journal of Psycholinguistic Research, 4,* 257–271.

Pesetsky, D. (1979). *Russian morphology and texical theory.* Unpublished manuscript, Department of Linguistics, Massachusetts Institute of Technology.

Peterson, S. E., Fox, P. T., Posner, M. I., Mintun, M., and Raichle, M. E. (1988). Positron emission tomographic studies of the cortical anatomy of single-word processing. *Nature, 331,* 585–589.

Pike, K. (1945). *The intonation of American English.* Ann Arbor: University of Michigan Press.

Pinker, S., and Prince, A. (1988). On language and connectionism: Analysis of a parallel distributed processing model of language acquisition. *Cognition, 28,* 73–194.

Pisoni, D. B., and Luce, P. A. (1987). Acoustic-phonetic representations in word recognition. *Cognition, 25,* 21–52.

Porch, B. E. (1971). *The Porch Index of Communicative Ability: Administration, scoring and interpretation.* Palo Alto, Calif.: Consulting Psychologists.

Posner, M. I., and Snyder, C. R. (1975). Attention and cognitive control. In R. L. Solso (Ed.), *Information processing and cognition* (pp. 55–85). New York: Erlbaum.

Posner, M. I., Peterson, S. E., Fox, P. T., and Raichle, M. E. (1988). Localization of cognitive operations in the human brain. *Science, 240,* 1627–1632.

Postman, L., and Phillips, L. W. (1965). Short-term temporal changes in free recall. *Quarterly Journal of Experimental Psychology, 17,* 132–138.

Potter, M. C. (1979). Mundane symbolism: The relations among names, objects and ideas. In N. Smith, and M. B. Franklin (Eds.), *Symbolic functioning in childhood* Hillsdale, N.J.: Lawrence Erlbaum.

Potter, M. C., and Faulconer, B. A. (1975). Time to understand pictures and words. *Nature, 253,* 437–438.

Prentice, J. L. (1967). Effects of cuing actor vs. cuing object on word order in sentence production. *Psychonomic Science, 8,* 163–164.

Pulleyblank, D. (1986). *Tone lexical phonology.* Dordrecht: Reidel.

Radford, A. (1988). *Transformational grammar: A first course.* Cambridge: Cambridge University Press.

Rapp, B., and Caramazza, A. (1990). *Lexical deficits.* Baltimore: The Cognitive Neuropsychology Laboratory, Johns Hopkins University.

Ratcliff, G., and Newcombe, F. (1982). Object recognition: Some deductions from the clinical evidence. In A. W. Ellis (Ed.), *Normally and pathology in cognitive function* (pp. 147–171). London: Academic Press.

Reicher, G. M. (1969). Perceptual recognition as a function of meaningfulness of stimulus material. *Journal of Experimental Psychology, 81(2),* 274–280.

Reinhart, T. (1983). *Anaphora and semantic interpretation.* London: Croom Helm.

Reisner, P. (1972). *Storage and retrieval of polymorphemic words in the internal lexicon.* Unpublished Ph.D. thesis, Psychology, Lehigh University, Bethlehem, Pa.

Riedel, K., and Studdert-Kennedy, M. (1985). Extending formant transitions may not improve aphasics' perception of stop consonant place of articulation. *Brain and Language, 24,* 223–232.

Riddoch, M. J., and Humphreys, G. W. (1987). Visual object processing in optic aphasia: A case of semantic access agnosia. *Cognitive Neuropsychology, 4,* 131–185.

Riddoch, M. J., Humphreys, G. W., Coltheart, M., and Funnell, E. (1988). Semantic systems or system? Neuropsychological evidence re-examined. *Cognitive Neuropsychology, 5,* 3–25.

Ripich, D. N., and Terrell, B. Y. (1988). Patterns of discourse cohesion and coherence in Alzheimer's disease. *Journal of Speech and Hearing Disorders, 53,* 8–15.

Rips, L. J., Shoben, E. J., and Smith, E. E. (1973). Semantic distance and the verification of semantic relations. *Journal of Verbal Learning and Verbal Behavior, 12*, 1–20.

Rizzi, L. (1985). Two notes on the linguistic interpretation of Broca's Aphasia. In M.-L. Kean (Ed.), *Agrammatism* (pp. 153–164). London: Academic Press.

Roeltgen, D. P., and Heilman, K. M. (1984). Lexical agraphia: Further support for the two system hypothesis of linguistic agraphia. *Brain, 107*, 811–827.

Roman, M., Brownell, H. H., Potter, H. H., Seibold, M. S., and Gardner, H. (1987). Script knowledge in right hemisphere-damaged and in normal elderly adults. *Brain and Language, 31*, 151–170.

Rosati, G., and De Bastiani, P. (1979). Pure agraphia: A discrete form of aphasia. *Journal of Neurology, Neurosurgery and Psychiatry, 42*, 266–269.

Rosch, E. (1973). On the internal structure of perceptual and semantic categories. In T. E. Moore (Ed.), *Cognitive Development and the Acquisition of Language.* New York: Academic Press.

Rosch, E. (1975). Cognitive representations of semantic categories. *Journal of Experimental Psychology: General, 104*, 192–233.

Rosch, E., and Mervis, C. B. (1975). Family resemblance: Studies in the internal structure of categories. *Cognitive Psychology, 7*, 573–605.

Rosch, E. H. (1973). Natural categories. *Cognitive Psychology, 4*, 328–350.

Rosenberg, B., Zurif, E., Brownell, H., Garrett, M., and Bradley, D. (1985). Grammatical class effects in relation to normal and aphasic sentence processing. *Brain and Language, 26*, 287–303.

Ross, E., and Mesulam, M. (1979). Dominant language functions of the right hemisphere? Prosody and emotional gesturing. *Archives of Neurology, 36*, 144–148.

Roth, E. H., and Shoben, E. J. (1980). Unpublished data, University of Illinois, Champaign, Ill., cited in E. E. Smith and D. L. Medin (1991).

Rothi, L. J., and Heilman, K. M. (1981). Alexia and agraphia with spared spelling and letter recognition abilities. *Brain and Language, 12*, 1–13.

Rubenstein, H., Lewis, S. S., and Rubenstein, M. A. (1971). Evidence for phonemic recoding in visual word recognition. *Journal of Verbal Learning and Verbal Behavior, 19*, 645–657.

Rubin, G. S., Becker, C. A., and Freeman, R. H. (1979). Morphological structure and its effect on visual word recognition. *Journal of Verbal Learning and Verbal Behavior, 18*, 757–767.

Rumelhart, D. E., and McClelland, J. L. (1982). An interactive activation model of context effects in letter perception, Part 2: The contextual enhancement effect and some tests and extensions of the model. *Psychological Review, 89*, 60–94.

Rumelhart, D. E., Lindsay, P. J., and Norman, D. A. (1972). A process model for long-term memory. In E. Tulving, and W. Donaldson (Eds.), *Organization and memory*. New York: Academic Press.

Ryalls, J. (1986). What constitutes a primary disturbance of speech prosidy?: A reply to Shapiro and Danly. *Brain and Language, 29*, 183–187.

Ryalls, J. H. (1986). An acoustic study of vowel production in aphasia. *Brain and Language, 29*, 48–67.

Saffran, E. M., and Marin, O. S. M. (1975). Immediate memory for word lists and sentences in a patient with deficient auditory short-term memory. *Brain and Language, 2*, 420–433.

Saffran, E. M., Marin, O., and Yeni-Komshian, G. (1976). An analysis of speech perception and word deafness. *Brain and Language, 3*, 209–228.

Saffran, E. M., Bogyo, L. C., Schwartz, M. F., and Marin, O. S. M. (1980a). Does deep dyslexia reflect right-hemisphere reading? In M. Coltheart, K. E. Patterson, and J. C. Marshall (Eds.), *Deep dyslexia* (pp. 381–406). London: Routledge.

Saffran, E. M., Schwartz, M. F., and Marin, O. (1980b). The word order problem in agrammatism II: Production. *Brain and Language, 10*, 263–280.

Salame, P., and Baddeley, A. (1982). Disruption of short-term memory by unattended speech: Implications for the structure of short-term memory. *Journal of Verbal Learning and Verbal Behavior, 21*, 150–164.

Samuel, A. G. (1981). Phonemic restoration: Insights from a new methodology. *Journal of Experimental Psychology: General, 110*, 474–494.

Sartori, G., and Job, R. (1988). The oyster with four legs: A neuropsychological study on the interaction of visual and semantic information. *Cognitive Neuropsychology, 5*, 105–132.

Schnitzer, M. L. (1972). *Generative phonology: Evidence from aphasia*. University Park, Pa.: Pennsylvania State University.

Schonle, T. W., Grabe, K., and Winig, P., et al. (1987). Electromagnetic articulography: Use of alternating magnetic fields for tracking movements of multiple points inside and outside the vocal tract. *Brain and Language, 31*, 26–35.

Schuell, H., Jenkins, J. J., and Jimenez-Pabon, E. (1964). *Aphasia in adults: Diagnosis, prognosis and treatment*. New York: Harper & Row.

Schwartz, M. (1984). What the classical aphasia categories can't do for us, and why. *Brain and Language, 21*, 1–8.

Schwartz, M. F. (1987). Patterns of speech production deficits within and across aphasic syndromes: Application of a psycholinguistic model. In M. Coltheart, G. Sartori, and R. Job (Ed.), *The Cognitive Neuropsychology of Language* (pp. 163–199). London: Lawrence Erlbaum.

Schwartz, M. F., Saffran, E. M., and Marin, O. S. M. (1980a). Fractionating the reading process in dementia: Evidence for word-specific print-to-sound associations. In M. Coltheart, K. E. Patterson, and J. C. Marshall (Eds.), *Deep dyslexia* (pp. 259–269). London: Routledge.

Schwartz, M., F. Saffran, E., and Marin, O. (1980b). The word order problem in agrammatism I: Comprehension. *Brain and Language, 10,* 249–262.

Schwartz, M. F., Linebarger, M. C., and Saffran, E. M. (1985). The status of the syntactic deficit theory of agrammatism. In M.-L. Kean (Ed.), *Agrammatism* (pp. 83–124). New York: Academic Press.

Schwartz, M. F., Linebarger, M. C., Saffran, E. M., and Pate, D. S. (1987). Syntactic transparency and sentence interpretation in aphasia. *Language and Cognitive Processes, 2,* 85–113.

Searle, J. R. (1969). *Speech acts: An essay in the philosophy of language.* Cambridge: Cambridge University Press.

Seidenberg, M. S. (1989). Reading complex words. In G. N. Carlson, and M. K. Tanenhaus (Ed.), *Linguistic Structure in Language Processing* (pp. 53–106). Dordrecht: Kluwer.

Seidenberg, M. S., and McClelland, J. L. (1989). A distributed, developmental model of word recognition and naming. *Psychological Review, 96,* 523–568.

Seidenberg, M. S., and McClelland, J. L. (1990). More words but still no lexicon: Reply to Besner et al. *Psychological Review, 97,* 447–452.

Seidenberg, M. S., and Tanenhaus, M. K. (1979). Orthographic effects on rhyme monitoring. *Journal of Experimental Psychology: Human Learning and Memory, 5(6),* 546–554.

Seidenberg, M. S., Tanenhaus, M. K., Leiman, J. M., and Bienkowski, M. A. (1982). Automatic access of the meanings of ambiguous words in context: Some limitations of knowledge-based processing. *Cognitive Psychology, 14,* 489–537.

Seidenberg, M. S., Waters, G. S., Barnes, M. A., and Tanenhuas, M. K. (1984). When does irregular spelling or pronunciation influence word recognition? *Journal of Verbal Learning and Verbal Behavior, 23,* 383–404.

Selkirk, E. (1984). *Phonology and syntax: The relation between sound and structure.* Cambridge, Mass.: MIT Press.

Sells, P. (1985). *Lectures on contemporary syntactic theories.* Chicago: University of Chicago Press.

Shallice, T. (1981). Phonological agraphia and the lexical route in writing. *Brain, 104,* 412–429.

Shallice, T. (1987). Impairments of semantic processing: Multiple dissociations. In M. Coltheart, G. Sartori, and R. Job (Eds.), *The cognitive neuropsychology of language* (pp. 111–127). London: Lawrence Erlbaum.

Shallice, T. (1988a). *From neuropsychology to mental structure.* Cambridge: Cambridge University Press.

Shallice, T. (1988b). Specialisation within the semantic system. *Cognitive Neuropsychology, 5,* 133–142.

Shallice, T., and Butterworth, B. (1977). Short-term memory impairment and spontaneous speech. *Neuropsychologia, 15,* 729–735.

Shallice, T., and McCarthy, R. (1985). Phonological reading: From patterns of impairment to possible procedures. In K. E. Patterson, J. C. Marshall, and M. Coltheart, (Ed.), *Surface Dyslexia: Neuropsychological and Cognitive Studies of Phonological Reading* (pp. 361–398). London: Erlbaum.

Shallice, T., and Saffran, E. M. (1986). Lexical processing in the absence of explicit word identification; Evidence from a letter-by-letter reader. *Cognitive Neuropsychology, 3,* 429–458.

Shallice, T., and Warrington, E. K. (1970). Independent functioning of verbal memory stores: A neuropsychological study. *Quarterly Journal of Experimental Psychology, 22,* 261–273.

Shallice, T., and Warrington, E. K. (1977). Auditory-verbal short-term memory impairment and conduction aphasia. *Brain and Language, 4,* 479–491.

Shallice, T., and Warrington, E. K. (1980). Single and multiple component central dyslexic syndromes. In M. Coltheart, K. E. Patterson, and J. C. Marshall (Ed.), *Deep dyslexia* (pp. 119–145). London: Routledge & Kegan Paul.

Shallice, T., Warrington, E. K., and McCarthy, R. (1983). Reading without semantics. *Quarterly Journal of Experimental Psychology, 35A,* 111–138.

Shallice, T., McLeod, P., and Lewis, K. (1985). Isolating cognitive modules with the dual-task paradigm: Are speech perception and production separate processes? *Quarterly Journal of Experimental Psychology, 37A,* 507–532.

Shankweiler, D., and Studdert-Kennedy, M. (1967). Identification of consonants and vowels presented to left and right ears. *Quarterly Journal of Experimental Psychology, 19,* 59–63.

Shapiro, B., and Danly, M. (1985). The role of the right hemisphere in the control of speech prosody in propositional and effective context. *Brain and Language, 25,* 19–36.

Stattuck-Hufnagel, S. (1979). Speech errors as evidence for a serial order mechanism in sentence production. In W. E. Cooper, and E. C. T. Walker (Ed.), *Sentence processing: Psycholinguistic studies presented to Merrill Gerrett* (pp. 295–342). Hillsdale, N.J: Lawrence Erlbaum.

Shattuck-Hufnagel, S. (1986). The role of word onset consonants in speech production planning: New evidence from speech error patterns. In E. Keller, and M. Gopnik (Eds.), *Motor and sensory processes in language* (pp. 17–51). Hillsdale, N.J.: Lawrence Erlbaum.

Stattuck-Hufnagel, S., and Klatt, D. (1979). The limited use of distinctive features and markedness in speech production: Evidence from speech error data. *Journal of Verbal Learning and Verbal Behavior, 18,* 44–55.

Shewan, C. M., Leeper, H. A., and Booth, J. C. (1984). An analysis of voice onset time (VOT) in aphasic and normal subjects. In J. Rosenbek, M. McNeil, and A. Aronson (Eds.), *Apraxia of speech: Physiology, acoustics, linguistics, management* San Diego: College-Hill Press.

Shieber, S. (1985). *An introduction to unification-based approaches to grammar.* Chicago: University of Chicago Press.

Shiffrin, R. M., and Schneider, W. (1977). Controlled and automatic human information processing: II. Perceptual learning, automatic attending, and a general theory. *Psychological Review, 84,* 127–190.

Shinn, P., and Blumstein, S. E. (1983). Phonetic disintegration in aphasia: Acoustic analysis of spectral characteristics for place of articulation. *Brain and Language, 20,* 90–114.

Silveri, M. C., and Gainotti, G. B. (1987). *Interaction between vision and language in category specific semantic impairment for living things.* Unpublished manuscript.

Slobin, D. I. (1966). Grammatical transformations and sentence comprehension in childhood and adulthood. *Journal of Verbal Learning and Verbal Behavior, 2,* 219–227.

Slowiaczek, M. L., and Clifton, C. J. (1980). Subvocalization and Reading for Meaning. *Journal of Verbal Learning and Verbal Behavior, 19,* 573–582.

Smith, E. E., and Medin, D. L. (1981). *Categories and Concepts.* Cambridge, Mass.: Harvard University Press.

Smith, E. E., Shoben, E. J., and Rips, L. J. (1974). Structure and process in semantic memory: A featural model for semantic decisions. *Psychological Review, 81,* 214–241.

Smith, P. T., and Sterling, C. M. (1982). Factors affecting the perceived morphemic structure of written words. *Journal of Verbal Learning and Verbal Behavior, 21,* 704–721.

Smith, S., and Bates, E. (1987). Accessibility of case and gender contrasts for assignment of agent-object relations in Broca's aphasics and fluent anomics. *Brain and Language, 30,* 8–32.

Smith, S., and Mimica, I. (1984). Agrammatism in a case-inflected language: Comprehension of agent-object relations. *Brain and Language, 13,* 274–290.

Snodgrass, J. G. (1984). Concepts and their surface representations. *Journal of Verbal Learning and Verbal Behavior, 23,* 3–22.

Snodgrass, J. G., and Jarvella, R. J. (1972). Some linguistic determinants of word classification times. *Psychonomic Science, 27,* 220–222.

Sokal, R. R. (1977). Classification: Purposes, principles, progress, prospects. In P. N. Johnson-Laird, and P. C. Wason (Ed.), *Thinking: Readings in cognitive science* (pp. 185–198). Cambridge, U.K.: Cambridge University Press.

Sperber, D., and Wilson, D. (1986). *Relevance: Communication and cognition.* Cambridge, Mass.: Harvard University Press.

Sridhar, S. N. (1988). *Cognition and sentence production: A cross-linguistic study.* New York: Springer.

Stachowiak, F.-J., Huber, W., Poeck, K., and Kerschensteiner, M. (1977). Text comprehension in aphasia. *Brain and Language, 4,* 177–195.

Stanners, R. F., Neiser, J. J., Hernon, W. P., and Hall, R. (1979). Memory representation for morphologically related words. *Journal of Verbal Learning and Verbal Behavior, 18,* 399–412.

Steedman, M. J., and Johnson-Laird, P. N. (1980). The production of sentences, utterances and speech acts: Have computers anything to say? In B. Butterworth (Ed.), *Language production: Vol 1. Speech and talk.* London: Academic Press.

Steinberg, D., and Krohn, R. (1975). The psychological validity of Chomsky and Halle's Vowel Shift Rule. In E. Koerner, J. Odmark, and J. Shaw (Ed.), *The transformational-generative paradigm and modern linguistic theory* (pp. 233–259). Amsterdam: John Benjamins.

Stemberger, J., and MacWhinney, B. (1986). Frequency and the lexical storage of regularly inflected forms. *Memory and Cognition, 14,* 17–26.

Stemberger, J. P. (1982). The nature of segments in the lexicon: Evidence from speech errors. *Lingua, 56,* 235–259.

Stemberger, J. P. (1983a). The nature of /r/ and /l/ in English: Evidence from speech errors. *11, Journal of Phonetics* 139–147.

Stemberger, J. P. (1983b). *Speech errors and theoretical phonology: A review.* Bloomington: Indiana Linguistics Club.

Stemberger, J. P. (1985). An interactive action model of language production. In A. W. Ellis (Ed.), *Progress in the psychology of language: Vol. 1* (pp. 143–186). Hillsdale, N.J.: Lawrence Erlbaum.

Sternberg, S., Monsell, S., Knoll, R. L., and Wright, C. E. (1978). The latency and duration of rapid movement sequences: Comparisons of speech and typewriting. In G. E. Stelmach (Ed.), *Information processing in motor control and learning* (pp. 118–152). New York: Academic Press.

Stevens, K. N. (1983). Design features of speech sound systems. In P. F. MacNeilage (Ed.), *The Production of Speech* (pp. 247–261). New York: Springer-Verlag,

Stevens, K. N. (1986). *Models of phonetic recognition II: A feature-based model of speech recognition.* Proceedings of the Montreal Satellite Symposium on Speech Recognition (Twelfth International Congress on Acoustics). McGill University, Montreal.

Stevens, K. N., and Blumstein, S. E. (1981). The search for invariant acoustic correlates of phonetic features. In P. D. Elmas, and J. L. Miller (Ed.), *Perspectives on the study of speech* (pp. 1–38). New Jersey: Erlbaum.

Stevens, K. N., Fant, G., and Hawkins, S. (1987). Some acoustical and perceptual correlates of nasal vowels. In R. Channon, and L. Shockey (Eds.), *In Honor of Ilse Lehiste Puhendusteos* (pp. 241–254). The Netherlands: Foris.

Stowe, L. A. (1986). Parsing WH-constructions: Evidence for on-line gap location. *Language and Cognitive Processes, 1,* 227–245.

Stowe, L. A. (1989). Thematic structures and sentence comprehension. In G. Carlson, and M. Tanenhaus (Eds.), *Linguistic structure in language processing* (pp. 319–357). Dordrecht, Netherlands, Kluwer.

Strub, R. L., and Gardner, H. (1974). The repetition defect in conduction aphasia: Mnestic or linguistic? *Brain and Language, 1,* 241–255.

Studdert Kennedy, M. (1982). On the dissociation of auditory and phonetic perception. In R. Carison and B. Cranstrom (Ed.), *Representation of speech in the peripheral auditory system* (pp. 9–25).

Swinney, D. A. (1979). Lexical access during sentence comprehension: (Re)consideration of context effects. *Journal of Verbal Learning and Verbal Behavior, 18,* 645–659.

Swinney, D., Zurif, E., and Nicol, J. (1988). The effects of focal brain damage on sentence processing: An examination of the neurological organization of a mental module. *The Journal of Cognitive Neuroscience, 1,* 25–37.

Taft, M. (1976). *Morphological and syllabic analysis in word recognition.* Unpublished Ph.D. thesis, Psychology, Monash University, Australia.

Taft, M. (1979). Recognition of affixed words and the word frequency effect. *Memory and Cognition, 7,* 263–272.

Taft, M. (1981). Prefix stripping revisited. *Journal of Verbal Learning and Verbal Behavior, 20,* 289–297.

Taft, M. (1985). The decoding of words in lexical access: A review of the morphographic approach. In D. Besner, T. Waller, and G. MacKinnon (Eds.), *Reading research: Advances in theory and practice* (pp. 83–123). New York: Academic Press.

Taft, M., and Forster, K. (1975). Lexical storage and retrieval of prefixed words. *Journal of Verbal Learning and Verbal Behavior, 14,* 638–647.

Taft, M., and Forster, K. I. (1976). Lexical storage and retrieval of polymorphemic and polysyllabic words. *Journal of Verbal Learning and Verbal Behavior, 15,* 607–620.

Taft, M., and Hambly, G. (1985). The influence of orthography on phonological representations in the lexicon. *Journal of Memory and Language, 24,* 320–335.

Tallal, P., and Newcombe, F. (1978). Impairment of auditory perception and language comprehension in dysphasia. *Brain and Language, 5,* 13–24.

Tanenhaus, M. K., and Carlson, G. N. (1989). Lexical structure and language comprehension. In W. Marslen-Wilson (Ed.), *Lexical Representation and Process* (pp. 529.–561). Cambridge, Mass.: MIT Press.

Tanenhaus, M. K., and Lucas, M. M. (1987). Context effects in lexical processing. *Cognition, 25,* 213–234.

Tanenhaus, M. K., Stowe, L., and Carlson, G. (1985a). *The interaction of lexical expectation and pragmatics in parsing filler-gap constructions.* Proceedings of the Seventh Annual Cognitive Science Society Meeting, Irrine, CA.

Tanenhaus, M. K., Carlson, G. N., and Seidenberg, M. S. (1985b). Do listeners compute linguistic representations? In L. K. Dowty and A. Z. D. Dowty (Eds.), *Natural language parsing* (pp. 359–408). Cambridge: Cambridge University Press.

Taraban, R., and McClelland, J. (in press). The role of semantic constraints in interpreting prepositional phrases. *Journal of Memory and Language,*

Thorndyke, P. W. (1977). Cognitive structures in comprehension and memory of narrative discourse. *Cognitive Psychology, 9,* 77–110.

Tissot, R. J., Mounin, G., and Lhermitte, F. (1973). *L'agrammatisme.* Brussels: Dessart.

Townsend, D. J. (1983). Thematic processing in sentences and texts. *Cognition, 13,* 223–261.

Treiman, R. (1983). The structure of spoken syllables: Evidence from novel word games. *Cognition, 15,* 49–74.

Treiman, R. (1984). On the status of final consonant clusters in English syllables. *Journal of Verbal Learning and Verbal Behavior, 23,* 343–356.

Trost, J. E., and Canter, G. J. (1974). Apraxia of speech in patients with Broca's aphasia: A study of phoneme production accuracy and error patterns. *Brain and Language, 1,* 63–79.

Trubetzkoy, N. S. (1939). *Grundzuge der Phonologie.* Prague: Travaux du Cercle Linguistique de Prague.

Tulving, E. (1972). Episodic and semantic memory. In E. Tulving, and W. Donaldson (Eds.), *Organization of Memory* (pp. 381–403). New York: Academic Press.

Tulving, E. (1983). *Elements of Episodic Memory.* Oxford: Oxford University Press.

Turner, E., and Rommetveit, R. (1968). Focus of attention in recall of active and passive sentences. *Journal of Verbal Learning and Verbal Behavior, 7,* 543–548.

Tversky, A. (1977). Features of similarity. *Psychological Review, 84,* 327–352.

Tyler, L. (1985). Real-time comprehension processes in agrammatism: A case study. *Brain and Language, 26*, 259–275.

Tyler, L., and Wessels, J. (1983). Quantifying contextual contributions to word-recognition processes. *Perception and Psychophysics, 34*, 409–420.

Tyler, L. K. (1989). The role of lexical representations in language comprehension. In W. Marslen-Wilson (Ed.), *Lexical representation and process* (pp. 439–462). Cambridge, Mass.: MIT Press.

Tyler, L. K. (in press). *Spoken Language Comprehension: An Experimental Approach to Disordered and Normal Processing.* Cambridge, Mass.: MIT Press.

Tyler, L. K., and Cobb, H. (1987). Processing bound grammatical morphemes in context: The case of an aphasic patient. *Language and Cognitive Processes, 2*, 245–262.

Tyler, L. K., and Marslen-Wilson, W. D. (1977). The on-line effects of semantic context on syntactic processing. *Journal of Verbal Learning and Verbal Behavior, 16*, 683–692.

Tyler, L. K., Behrens, S., Cobb, H., and Marslen-Wilson, W. (1990). Processing distinctions between stems and affixes: Evidence from a non-fluent aphasic patient. *Cognition, 36*, 129–153.

Ulatowska, H. K., North, A. J., and Macaluso-Haynes, S. (1981). Production of narrative and procedural discourse in aphasia. *Brain and Language, 13*, 345–371.

Ulatowska, H. K., Freedman-Stern, R., Weiss-Doyel, A., and Macaluso-Haynes, S. (1983a). Production of narrative discourse in aphasia. *Brain and Language, 19*, 317–334.

Ulatowska, H. K., Doyel, A. W., Stern, R. F., Haynes, S. M., and North, A. J. (1983b). Production of procedural discourse in aphasia. *Brain and Language, 18*, 315–341.

Ulatowska, H. K., Allard, L., and Chapman, S. B. (1991). Narrative and procedural discourse in aphasia. In Y. Joanette, and H. H. Brownell (Ed.), *Discourse Ability in Brain Damage: Theoretical and Empirical Perspectives* New York: Springer-Verlag.

Vallar, G., and Baddeley, A. D. (1984a). Fractionation of working memory: Neuropsychological evidence for a phonological short-term store. *Journal of Verbal Learning and Verbal Behavior, 23*, 151–161.

Vallar, G., and Baddeley, A. D. (1984b). Phonological short-term store, phonological processing and sentence comprehension: A neuropsychological case study. *Cognitive Neuropsychology, 1*, 121–142.

Vallar, G., and Baddeley, A. D. (1987). Phonological short-term store and sentence processing. *Cognitive Neuropsychology, 4*, 417–438.

Vanderwart, M. (1984). Priming by pictures in lexical decision. *Journal of Verbal Learning and Verbal Behavior, 23*, 67–83.

van Dijk, T. A. (1977). Semantic macro structures and knowledge frames in discourse comprehension. In M. A. Just, and P. A. Carpenter (Eds.), *Cognitive processes in comprehension* (pp. 3–32). Hillsdale, N.J.: Lawrence Erlbaum.

van Dijk, T. A., and Kintsch, W. (1983). *Strategies of Discourse Comprehension.* New York: Academic Press.

van Galen, G. P., and Teulings, H. L. (1983). The independent monitoring of form and scale factors in handwriting. *Acta Psychologia, 54,* 9–22.

van Orden, G. C. (1987). A ROWS is a ROSE: Spelling, sound, and reading. *Memory and Cognition, 15*(3), 181–198.

van Orden, G. C., Johnston, J. C. and Hale, B. L. (1988). Word identification in reading proceeds from spelling to sound to meaning. *Journal of Experimental Psychology Learning, Memory, and Cognition, 14*(3), 371–384.

Varney, N. L. (1984). Phonemic imperception in aphasia. *Brain and Language, 21,* 85–94.

van Wijk, C. (1987). The PSY behind PHI: A psycholinguistic model for performance structures. *Journal of Psycholinguistic Research, 60,* 185–199.

von Stockert, T. R. (1972). Recognition of syntactic structure in aphasic patients. *Cortex, 8,* 322–334.

von Stockert, T. R., and Bader, L. (1976). Some relations of grammar and lexicon in aphasia. *Cortex, 12,* 49–60.

Waller, M., and L. Darley, F. L. (1978). The influence of context on the auditory comprehension of paragraphs by aphasic subjects. *Journal of Speech and Hearing Research, 21,* 732–745.

Wanner, E., and Maratsos, M. (1978). An ATN approach to comprehension. In M. M. Halle, G. Miller, and J. Bresnan (Eds.), *Linguistic theory and psychological reality* (pp. 119–161). Cambridge, Mass.: MIT Press.

Warrington, E. K. (1975). The selective impairment of semantic memory. *Quarterly Journal of Experimental Psychology, 27,* 635–657.

Warrington, E. K. (1981a). Concrete word dyslexia. *British Journal of Psychology, 72,* 175–196.

Warrington, E. K. (1981b). Neuropsychological studies of verbal semantic systems. *Philosophical Transactions of the Royal Society of London, B295,* 411–423.

Warrington, E. K. (1982). Neuropsychological studies of object recognition. *Philosophical Transactions of the Royal Society of London, B298,* 15–33.

Warrington, E. K., and McCarthy, R. (1983). Category specific access dysphasia. *Brain, 106,* 859–878.

Warrington, E. K., and McCarthy, R. (1987). Categories of knowledge: Further fractionation and an attempted integration. *Brain, 110,* 1273–1296.

Warrington, E. K., and Rabin, P. (1971). Visual span of apprehension in patients with unilateral cerebral lesions. *Quarterly Journal of Experimental Psychology, 23,* 423–431.

Warrington, E. K., and Shallice, T. (1969). The selective impairment of auditory verbal short-term memory. *Brain, 92,* 885–896.

Warrington, E. K., and Shallice, T. (1979). Semantic access dyslexia. *Brain, 102,* 43–63.

Warrington, E. K., and Shallice, T. (1980). Word-form dyslexia. *Brain, 103,* 99–112.

Warrington, E. K., and Shallice, T. (1984). Category specific semantic impairments. *Brain, 107,* 829–853.

Waters, G., Caplan, D., and Hildebrandt, N. (1987). Working memory and written sentence comprehension. In M. Coltheart (Ed.), *Attention and performance XII: The psychology of reading* (pp. 531–555). London: Lawrence Erlbaum.

Waters, G. S., and Seidenberg, M. S. (1985). Spelling-sound effects in reading: Time-course and decision criteria. *Memory and Cognition, 13*(6), 557–572.

Waters, G. S., Caplan, D., and Hildebrandt, N. (1991). On the structure and function role of auditory-verbal short-term memory in sentence comprehension: A case study. *Cognitive Neuropsychology, 8,* 81–126.

Waugh, N. C., and Norman, D. A. (1965). Primary memory. *Psychological Review, 72,* 89–104.

Wegner, M. L., Brookshire, R. H., and Nicholas, L. E. (1984). Comprehension of main ideas and details in coherent and noncoherent discourse by aphasic and non-aphasic listeners. *Brain and Language, 21,* 37–51.

Weinberg, A. (1987). Language Processing and Linguistic Explanation. In M. Coltheart (Ed.), *Attention and performance XII: The psychology of reading* (pp. 673–688). London: Lawrence Erlbaum.

Wepman, J. M. (1958). *Auditory discrimination test.* Chicago.: Language Research Associates.

Wernicke, C. (1874). *Der aphasische Symptomenkomplex.* Breslau: Cohn & Weigart, Reprinted in translation in *Boston Studies in Philosophy of Science, 4,* 34–97.

Wernicke, C. (1908). The aphasia symptom complex. In A. Church (Ed.), *Diseases of the nervous system* (pp. 265–324). New York: Appleton.

Wheeler, D. D. (1970). Processes in word recognition. *Cognitive Psychology, 1,* 59–85.

Wickelgren, W. A. (1969). Context-sensitive coding, associated memory, and serial order in (speech) behavior. *Psychological Review, 76,* 1–15.

Wickelgren, W. A. (1976). Network strength theory of storage and retrieval dynamics. *Psychological Review, 83,* 466–478.

Wickelgren, W. A. (1976). Phonetic code and serial order. In E. C. Carterette, and M. P. Friedman (Eds.), *Handbook of Perception: Vol. 7.* New York: Academic Press.

Wiegel-Crump, C., and Koenigsknecht, R. A. (1973). Tapping the lexical store of the adult aphasic: Analysis of the improvement made in word retrieval skills. *Cortex, 9,* 411–418.

Williams, E. (1981). X features. In S. Tavakolian (Ed.), *Language acquisition and linguistic theory.* Cambridge, Mass.: MIT Press.

Wing, A. M., and Baddeley, A. D. (1980). Spelling errors in handwriting: A corpus and a distributional analysis. In U. Frith (Ed.), *Cognitive processes in spelling* (pp. 251–285). London: Academic Press.

Wittgenstein, L. (1953). *Philosophical Investigations.* Oxford: Blackwell.

Wolpert, I. (1924). Die Simultanagnosie—Storung der Gesamtauffassung. *Zeitschrift fur die gesamte Neurologie und Psychiatrie, 93,* 397–415.

Young, A. W., and Ellis, A. W. (1985). Different methods of lexical access for words presented in the left and right visual hemifields. *Brain and Language, 24,* 326–358.

Zue, V. W. (1986). *Models of speech recognition III: The role of analysis by synthesis in phonetic recognition.* Proceedings of the Montreal Satellite Symposium on Speech Recognition (Twelfth International Congress on Acoustics), McGill University, Montreal.

Zurif, E., and Caramazza, A. (1976). Psycholinguistic structures in aphasia: Studies in syntax and semantics. In H. Whitaker, and H. Whitaker (Ed.), *Studies in neurolinguistics: Vol. 1* (pp. 261–292). New York: Academic Press.

Zurif, E., and Grodzinsky, Y. (1983). Sensitivity to grammatical structure in agrammatic aphasics: A reply to Linebarger, Schwartz, and Saffran. *Cognition, 15,* 207–214.

Zurif, E. B. (1984). Psycholinguistic interpretation of the aphasis. In D. Caplan, A. R. Lecours, and A. Smith (Eds.), *Biological perspectives on language* (pp. 158–171). Cambridge, Mass.: MIT Press.

Zwitserlood, P. (1985). *Activation of word candidates during spoken word recognition.* Manuscript presented at the Psychonomic Society Meeting, Boston.

Patient Index

Author Index

Subject Index

197–204, 207, 214, 229, 415. *See also* Grapheme; Graphemic representation

PAL. *See* Psycholinguistic Assessment of Language

Paragrammatism, 237, 245, 331, 341–342, 344, 347–350, 357. *See also* Aphasia; Language disorders

Paralexia. *See also* Error
morphological, 237, 241–242, 247–248, 416
semantic, 182–186, 416

Parallel distributed processing models (PDP). *See* Reading; Writing

Paraphasia. *See also* Error
morphological, 246
phonemic, 120, 131, 134, 137–146, 155, 157n7, 246, 329, 412, 430, 436
semantic, 121, 132, 329, 412
syntactic, 355

Parser, 271–277, 278–280, 283–286, 293, 295–297, 299–300, 304, 309–310, 312n5, 313n6, 375, 411. *See also* Late closure; Minimal attachment; Syntactic structures
sausage-machine, 310

Pattern-action rule, 272, 313n6. *See also* Syntactic structures

PDP. *See* Parallel distributed processing models

Peabody Picture Vocabulary Test, 92, 406. *See also* Aphasia battery

PET. *See* Positron emission tomography

Phoneme, 6, 20–24, 26, 60n1–2, 109, 111–116, 131–133, 137, 142, 159–161, 199, 246–247, 324, 328, 408. *See also* Acoustic-phonetic processing; Articulation; Co-articulation; Distinctive features; Grapheme-to-phoneme translation; Phonological processing
identification from acoustic correlates, 27–32, 36
role in auditory word recognition, 36–37, 39

Phoneme-grapheme translation. *See* Grapheme-to-phoneme translation

Phoneme restoration effect, 45–46. *See also* Phonological processing; Word recognition

Phonetics. *See* Acoustic-phonetic processing

Phonetic spellout, 117. *See also* Acoustic-phonetic processing

Phonological agraphia, 171, 192–194, 203. *See also* Agraphia
category-specific, 194–196
visual aspects, 196–197

Phonological alexia, 241. *See also* Error

Phonological buffer, 118–119, 150–153, 412

Phonological clitic, 123, 324, 334

Phonological cueing. *See* Cueing

Phonological dyslexia, 176–178, 183, 204, 239–341, 247. *See also* Dyslexia

Phonological features. *See* Distinctive features

Phonological lexicon, 109–110, 120–121, 132–135, 150, 152–153, 156n2, 179, 412, 426, 431, 433. *See also* Lexicon

Phonological phrase, 124

Phonological processing, 26–27, 36–41, 45, 115–120, 131–146, 320. *See also* Language-related tasks; Phonology
lexical vs. nonlexical routes, 149–154, 157n9–10

Phonological processing disorders, 47–48, 50–52, 54–59, 77, 203, 404. *See also* Error; Language disorders
access vs. storage disorder, 157n6
of representation access, 131–136